Advance praise for
The Vagina Bible

"Gunter approachably, respectfully, and even playfully presents a huge amount of reproductive and sexual health education information to women with the assurance that they can use it."
—*Publishers Weekly* (starred review)

"Dr. Jen Gunter is a fountain of critically important information, and she's funny as hell. Buy this book if you have a vagina or if you spend any time at all in reasonably close proximity to one."
—Ayelet Waldman, *New York Times* bestselling author of
A Really Good Day

"This book is basically everything you've ever wanted to know about the vagina but were afraid to ask."
—Imani Gandy, @angryblacklady, Senior Legal Analyst, Rewire News

"*The Vagina Bible*—Dr. Jen Gunter's savvy, detailed, funny, and wise guide to female health—should be required reading for every woman seeking smart information about her body. I don't say this often, but it's a don't-miss book."
—Deborah Blum, *New York Times* bestselling author of *The Poison Squad*

"Men who want to understand the experiences of their partners or provide sound guidance to their daughters should turn to *The Vagina Bible*. Jen Gunter offers authoritative information with her trademark clarity and good humor."
—Carl Zimmer, author of *She Has Her Mother's Laugh: The Powers, Perversions, and Potential of Heredity*

"Reading *The Vagina Bible* is like having the realest, most honest talk ever with your best friend—if your best friend happened to be a leading expert in women's health. I want to give this book to everyone I know."
—Rachel Hawkins, *New York Times* bestselling author

"In a time where pseudoscience has a large foothold, it is vital that physicians and scientists meet readers where they live. With *The Vagina Bible*, Dr. Gunter has done exactly that! A vital book that will undoubtedly have a profound impact."
—Mark Shapiro, MD, founder and host, Explore the Space podcast

"Whether she is debunking Freud or providing the lowdown on the science of sex, Dr. Jen Gunter provides a frank, funny, and thoroughly science-informed perspective. Gunter pulls no punches and provides a clear and concise summation of the facts on every vagina-related topic you can think of. Seriously. Everything. The world needs more Jen!"

> —Professor Timothy Caulfield, author of *Is Gwyneth Paltrow Wrong About Everything?*

"Dr. Jen Gunter is the vagina's most passionate defender and publicist. *The Vagina Bible* is a practical, informative, and hilarious guide to women's health, but it's also a biography of the most misunderstood and mysterious part of the human body. The vagina gets the star treatment—and it's about time!"

> —Elaine Lui, @laineygossip, author of *Listen to the Squawking Chicken* and co-host of *The Social*

"*The Vagina Bible* is a marvel of medical writing: precise, funny, passionate, and furious. In her engaged and amusing writing voice, Dr. Gunter's expertise becomes accessible instead of distancing; this book will become a model for how to write about health and science, more generally."

> —Kevin Patterson, MD, author of *News from the Red Desert*

"Full of accurate information that separates myth from medicine, *The Vagina Bible* should be on every nightstand and in every hotel room."

> —Dr. Judy Melinek, co-author with T. J. Mitchell of the *New York Times* bestseller *Working Stiff*

"Dr. Gunter shines a much needed light on this very private subject, aiming to bring facts, confidence, and joy into the personal lives of readers."

> —Miranda Esmonde-White, author of *Aging Backwards*

"Dr. Jen Gunter's *The Vagina Bible* brilliantly dispels myths and imparts knowledge with large doses of wit, wisdom, and invaluable advice. This empowering and engaging resource belongs on every woman's bookshelf."

> —Ami McKay, author of *The Birth House*

"*The Vagina Bible* is written for all women but should also be read by men, and it has special relevance for health care providers, the media, and celebrities promoting 'wellness products.' It is truly a one-stop shop for the latest science and facts about the vagina and vulva."

> —Lori A. Brotto, PhD, Canada Research Chair in Women's Sexual Health, executive director of the Women's Health Research Institute, and author of *Better Sex Through Mindfulness*

THE VAGINA BIBLE

The Vulva and the Vagina—
Separating the Myth
from the Medicine

JEN GUNTER, MD

CITADEL PRESS
Kensington Publishing Corp.
www.kensingtonbooks.com

CITADEL PRESS BOOKS are published by

Kensington Publishing Corp.
119 West 40th Street
New York, NY 10018

PUBLISHER'S NOTE
The reader is advised that this book is not intended to be a substitute for an assessment by, and advice from, an appropriate medical professional(s).

All Kensington titles, imprints, and distributed lines are available at special quantity discounts for bulk purchases for sales promotions, premiums, fund-raising, educational, or institutional use. Special book excerpts or customized printings can also be created to fit specific needs. For details, write or phone the office of the Kensington sales manager: Kensington Publishing Corp., 119 West 40th Street, New York, NY 10018, attn: Sales Department; phone 1-800-221-2647.

CITADEL PRESS and the Citadel logo are Reg. U.S. Pat. & TM Off.

ISBN-13: 978-0-8065-3931-7
ISBN-10: 0-8065-3931-3

First trade paperback printing: September 2019

10 9 8 7

Printed in the United States of America

Library of Congress CIP data is available.

First electronic edition: September 2019

ISBN-13: 978-0-8065-3935-5
ISBN-10: 0-8065-3935-6

For every woman
who has ever been told—usually by some dude—
that she is too wet, too dry, too gross, too loose,
too tight, too bloody, or too smelly.
This book is for you.

Contents

SYMPTOMS   325

PUTTING IT ALL TOGETHER   371

Introduction

I HAVE A VAGENDA: for *every woman* to be empowered with *accurate information* about the vagina and vulva.

One of the core tenets of medicine is informed consent. We doctors provide information about risks and benefits and then, armed with that information, our patients make choices that work for their bodies. This only works when the information is accurate and unbiased. Finding this kind of data can be challenging, as we have quickly passed through the age of information and seem to be stalled in the age of misinformation.

Snake oil and the lure of a quick fix have been around for a long time, and so false, fantastical medical claims are nothing new. However, sorting myth from medicine is getting harder and harder.

In addition to social media feeds that constantly display medical messaging of variable quality, there are the demands of a headline-driven news cycle that constantly requires new content—even when it doesn't exist. With women's bodies, there are even more forces of misdirection at work. Pseudoscience and those who peddle it are invested in misinformation, but so is the patriarchy.

Obsessions with reproductive tract purity and cleansing date back to a time when a woman's worth was measured by her virginity and how many children she might bear. A vagina and uterus were currency. Playing on these fears awakens something visceral. It's no wonder the words "pure," "natural," and "clean" are used so often to market products to women.

Members of the media and celebrity influencers tap into these fears with articles about and products to prevent vaginal mayhem, as if the vagina (which evolved to stretch and tear to deliver a baby long before suture material was invented) is somehow so fragile that it is constantly in a state of near catastrophe.

Why *The Vagina Bible* instead of *The Vagina and Vulva Bible*? Because that is how we collectively talk about the lower reproductive tract (the vagina and vulva). Medically, the vagina is only the inside, but language evolves and words take on new meaning. For example, "catfish" and "text" both have additional meanings that I could never have imagined when I was growing up. "Gut" is from the Old English for the intestinal tract, usually meaning the lower part (from the stomach on down) but not always. It's actually a very imprecise term; yet it has been embraced by the medical community and is even the name of a leading journal dedicated to the study of the alimentary (digestive) tract, the liver, biliary tree, and pancreas.

I have been in medicine for thirty-three years, and I've been a gynecologist for twenty-four of them. I've listened to a lot of women, and I know the questions they ask as well as the ones they want to ask but don't quite know how.

The Vagina Bible is everything I want women to know about their vulvas and vaginas. It is my answer to every woman who has listened to me pass on information in the office or online and then wondered, "How did I not know this?"

You can read the book in order from front to back or visit specific chapters or even sections as they speak to you. It's all good! I hope over the years many pages will become worn as you go back to double-check what a doctor told you in the office, to research a product that makes wild claims about improving vaginas and vulvas, or help a friend or sexual partner out with an anatomy lesson.

Misinforming women about their bodies serves no one. And I'm here to help end it.

—*Jen Gunter, MD*

Getting Started

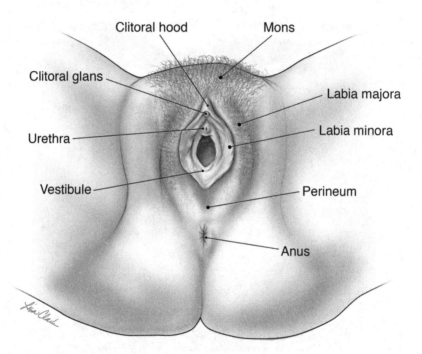

Clitoral hood

Mons

Clitoral glans

Labia majora

Labia minora

Urethra

Vestibule

Perineum

Anus

Image 1: The vulva. ILLUSTRATION BY LISA A. CLARK, MA, CMI.

CHAPTER 1

The Vulva

No woman has ever benefited by learning less about her body.

The vulva is the ultimate multitasker—it is the most important organ for sexual pleasure, it protects the tissues at the vaginal opening, it is built to handle the irritation of urine and feces, and it can deliver a baby and heal as if nothing happened. And do it all again.

Oh, yeah—and multiple orgasms.

The penis and scrotum have nothing on the vulva.

The problem? The vulva is often neglected. A lot of this vulvar neglect is a result of patriarchal society's lack of investment in and fear of female sexual pleasure. When we exclude the vulva from conversations about women's bodies and sexuality, we erase the organ responsible for female orgasm. We also make it harder for women to communicate with their health care providers.

The most important basic anatomic point of the lower genital tract: the vulva is the outside (where your clothes touch your skin) and the vagina is the inside. The transition zone between the vulva and vagina is called the vestibule.

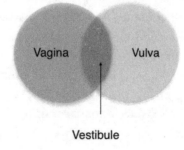

The main structures of the vulva are as follows (refer to Image 1 on page 2):

- Mons
- Labia majora (outer lips)
- Labia minora (inner lips)
- The glans clitoris (the part of the clitoris that is visible)
- The clitoral hood
- The vestibule
- The opening of the urethra (the tube that drains the bladder)
- The perineum (the area between the vestibule and the anus)

We are also going to invite the anus to the vulva's party, even though technically it is part of the gastrointestinal tract and not the reproductive tract. Many vulvar conditions affect the anus, and women often have a hard time getting help for anal concerns—doctors often hear "woman" and "down there" and deflect to the gynecologist. Some women are also interested in information about anal sex, and fecal incontinence can be a consequence of vaginal delivery.

The History of Clitoral Neglect

Going way back, medically speaking—as in Hippocrates (although there is a belief among many academics that Hippocrates wasn't even a real person)—male physicians rarely performed pelvic exams on women or even dissected female cadavers, as it was considered inappropriate or insensitive for a man to touch a woman outside of a marital relationship. As there were no female physicians, everything first written about women's bodies in ancient medical textbooks and taught to the first physicians was what women and midwives passed along to men, who in turn interpreted the information as they saw fit. So medicine has been steeped in mansplaining from the start.

Most ancient physicians, probably like many other males of the time, were unsure of the role of the clitoris and likely thought it unimportant. This stands in sharp contrast to the anatomic glory of the penis. In medicine, all body surfaces are assigned a front or back, which we call ventral (front) or dorsal (back). If you look at a person standing straight in a neutral position (arms at the side and palms facing forward), the face, chest, and palms of the hands are on the ventral side, and the back and the back of the hands are dorsal. This convention is applied differently to the penis, because of course it is. The neutral stance for a man, according to the anatomists of old, was a massive, skyward-pointing erection. Except, of course, men don't walk around with constant erections, and so when you look at a man in what most people would consider the resting state—meaning a flaccid penis—the part that faces you is not the "front" of the penis but actually the dorsal or back surface, and the undersurface is the ventral.

It's not really a small point; it is a wonderful (in a tragicomic kind of way) encapsulation of how society, including medicine, is obsessed with erections, while the clitoris barely registers as a footnote. The clitoris, when it was considered by ancient physicians at all, was believed to be the female version of the penis. But lesser. (I'm sorry, but the organ, capable of multiple orgasms, that only exists for pleasure is not lesser. It is the gold standard.) Clitoral neglect wasn't confined to medicine. Think about all those ancient Greek statues with defined scrotum and penises (although the penises are on the small side because sexuality was apparently at odds with intellectual pursuits and so a big brain, not a big penis, was the ideal). The vulvas of the time were but mysterious mounds concealed by crossed legs.

Around 1000 A.D., Persian and Arab physicians began to take more interest in the clitoris, but given the constraints imposed on male physicians touching a naked woman or even a female cadaver, work was slow. By the end of the 17th century, descriptions of female anatomy, including the clitoris, were quite accurate, anatomically speaking. Some anatomists who made these advancements are memorialized in the names of the structures they accurately described—Gabriele Fallopio (fallopian tubes; also invented the first condom and studied it in a clinical trial!) and Caspar Bartholin (Bartholin's glands).

By 1844, the anatomist Georg Ludwig Kobelt published such detailed work that his anatomic descriptions of the clitoris rival those we have today. However, his work was essentially ignored (as was almost everything that had led up to it), likely due to a combination of the expansion of Victorian beliefs (essentially the dangers of female sexuality) and Freud popularizing the false belief that the clitoris produced an "immature" orgasm.

For many years, discussing female sexuality in the doctor's office was taboo, but that oppression is not a failing unique to medicine. In 1938, a Los Angeles teacher, Helen Hulick, was held in contempt of court for daring to show up in pants to testify as a witness and for refusing to change into a dress when the male judge insisted. She was given a five-day jail sentence. Much of women's health, especially sexual health, was deemed unimportant or irrelevant because that is how women were viewed.

Physicians in the '20s and '30s truly believed the vagina was filled with dangerous bacteria. Of course, that idea is absurd, and you don't need a medical degree to reach that conclusion. If the vagina were perpetually in such a state of infectious near-catastrophe, women would never have survived, evolutionarily speaking. The narrative of a dirty vagina did, however, fit the societal goal of female oppression.

A male-dominated profession, a male-dominated society with little interest in women's experiences and opinions about their own bodies, a penis-centric view of female sexuality, and the belief propagated by Freud's work that the clitoris was unimportant are a lot of obstacles to overcome. The clitoris, being largely internal, is practically also harder to study than the penis. Eventually, anatomic studies using female cadavers to dissect the clitoris were allowed, but it is important to note the limitations of the work. Most cadaveric studies involve a few bodies; seven is considered a lot. Cadavers are expensive and not readily available. Many cadavers are also older subjects, and clitoral volume reduces after menopause; in one cadaveric study, all subjects were between seventy and eighty years old. The preservation process also distorts the clitoris. Before the advent of MRI (magnetic resonance imaging), it wasn't really possible to know exactly how the clitoris in a living woman was positioned or how it engorges with blood in response to sexual stimulation.

Anatomic knowledge has come a long way. While I don't remember each anatomy lecture from medical school and residency, I still have my textbooks. Two were printed in 1984 and another in 1988. The two that are specific for OB/GYN are anatomically correct clitoris-wise, but the general anatomy book (1984) devoted three pages of illustrations (two in color) to the penis, with the clitoris relegated to an inset image in an upper outer corner—*and* the entire structure is the worst shade of puce. It's also called a "miniature penis."

As if.

The Clitoris

The clitoris has one purpose: sexual pleasure. It is the only structure in the human body solely designed for pleasure.

Structurally, think of the clitoris as an inverted Y, but each side has two sets of arms. The very tip of the Y is folded and is the only visible part. This is known as the glans, which is partially covered by the prepuce (clitoral hood). The inverted Y sits on top of the urethra, with the two arms draped over either side.

Beneath the surface, you find the following:

- **THE BODY:** The part of the inverted Y that folds on itself. It is 2–4 cm in length. Connected to the pubic bone with a ligament.
- **THE ROOT:** Connects the clitoral body with the crura. The erectile parts of the clitoris converge here. It is very important for sensation because it's very superficial (beneath the skin right above the urethra).

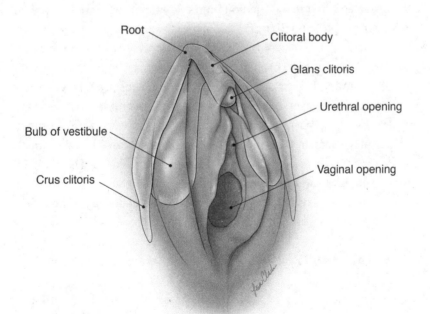

Image 2: Clitoral anatomy. ILLUSTRATION BY LISA A. CLARK, MA, CMI.

- **THE CRURA ("CRUS" IS THE SINGULAR):** The outside arms of the inverted Y (some people also describe them as looking like the arms of a wishbone). They are 5–9 cm in length, and there is one on each side, approximately beneath the labia majora.
- **THE CLITORAL (ALSO CALLED VESTIBULAR) BULBS:** The inside arms of the inverted Y. They are 3–7 cm in length and are in contact with the outside of the urethra and vagina.

Because the clitoris is so intimate with the urethra and the lower walls of the vagina, many experts feel a better terminology is the *clitorourethrovaginal complex.*

All parts of the clitoris are involved in sexual sensation and all parts are erectile, meaning they can engorge with blood, becoming firmer. The glans has the highest concentration of nerves and the least amount of erectile tissue. The body and the crura have the most erectile tissue. The presence of sexually responsive nerves and erectile tissue in all parts of the clitoris likely explains why there are reports of women who were born without a clitoral glans, women who have had surgery that removed the urethra (and likely parts of the clitoris that were connected), and women who have endured female genital mutilation (FGM) who are still able to achieve orgasm. This tells us that all of the clitorourethrovaginal complex is capable of sexual sensation. It means there are a lot of sexually responsive areas to explore. This can be for fun, discovering the results from sexually stimulating various areas (sexploration at its best). This can also be in search of orgasm. For some women the glans clitoris may not be the best pathway to orgasm, so moving sexual stimulation to other areas may help achieve orgasm. This information about the clitoris being so much more than the glans may also give hope to women who have endured injury to their clitoral glans—for example as a consequence of cancer surgery or FGM—although obviously, it does not make up for the loss.

The Labia and Mons

The mons and the two sets of labia, the labia majora and labia minora, exist to enhance sexual pleasure and to protect the vestibule (vaginal opening).

The mons is the area of skin and fatty tissue from just above the pubic bone down to the clitoral hood—the fat pad raises the tissue a little, and this may offer a mechanical barrier of sorts. The labia majora are folds of hair-bearing skin and fatty tissue that extend from the mons to just below the vestibule. They are filled with different kinds of glands. They are generally 7–12 cm in length, but if yours are larger or smaller, that is just fine.

The labia minora do not have fat, but they have erectile tissue, so they engorge or swell with sexual stimulation. At the level of the glans, they divide into two folds; the top forms the clitoral hood (prepuce) while the bottom is called the frenulum and sits under the glans. The glans of the clitoris is nestled between these folds, so traction on the labia minora enhances sexual pleasure. The labia minora are filled with specialized nerve endings important for sexual response, especially along their edge. They are capable of distinguishing touch on a very fine scale.

The labia minora may or may not protrude beyond the labia majora, and there is no "normal" size or shape. They can range from < 1 cm in width to 5 cm, but wider would not be considered medically abnormal. They may be asymmetric—think of them as sisters, not twins.

The Skin of the Vulva

Under the microscope, all skin looks like a brick wall—cells are stacked on top of each other in layers upon multiple layers. The very bottom layer has specialized cells called basal cells. Basal cells produce new skin cells that are pushed up towards the top, like a conveyor belt. The cells develop as they move upwards, producing a protein called keratin that serves as waterproofing and makes the cells tougher so they can resist injury. At the surface, the skin cells release fatty substances that provide protection against trauma and infection, as well as trapping moisture. The cells in the top layer are dead, and they are brushed off with everyday wear and tear, or with trauma. A new layer is replaced approximately every thirty days.

The mons and labia majora have sweat glands (eccrine glands) that secrete perspiration through pores directly onto the skin. They also have vellus hair (fine, peach fuzz–like hair) and pubic hair; both provide a mechanically protective barrier and trap moisture. As each pubic hair is attached to a nerve ending, tugging or friction on the hair may have a role in sexual stimulation.

Inside the hair follicle of each pubic and vellus hair is a sebaceous gland that produces sebum, an oily substance that keeps the skin soft and pliable and contributes to the waterproofing. Pubic hair follicles also have specialized sweat glands called apocrine glands (also found in the armpit) that become active during puberty. They empty a specialized oily sweat with trace amounts of hormones and pheromones onto the hair shaft. Skin bacteria convert the secretions from apocrine sweat glands into odorous compounds, which are responsible for the typical, intense apocrine sweat smell. The true function of the apocrine sweat glands is not known, but as they develop and become functional around puberty and secrete pheromones, it is likely they had or still have some role in sexual attraction.

The skin of the labia minora has fewer layers and less keratin. These skin changes become more pronounced as you move towards the vaginal opening (vestibule). The labia minora has no hair, but it does have sebaceous glands. Less keratin, thinner skin, and no hair makes the labia minora more vulnerable to trauma and irritants.

Secretions from the sebaceous and apocrine glands mix with fatty substances produced by the skin cells and form a layer called the acid mantle—a film on the surface of the skin that helps protect against bacteria, viruses, and other contaminants. The pH of the vulvar skin is around 5.3–5.6, so just slightly acidic (water has a pH of 7.0, which is considered neutral).

Melanin

Skin, hair, and the irises of your eyes all get their color from the pigment melanin, which is produced by specialized skin cells called melanocytes in the basal layer. Interestingly, the vulva has more melanocytes than many other body parts, yet it is the same skin tone as almost everywhere else (with the exception of palms and soles, which can be lighter). Medicine still can't explain how your back has fewer melanocytes than your vulva but they end up the same or a very similar tone.

While melanin absorbs and reflects ultraviolet light and provides protection from the sun, melanocytes also respond to biological, physical, and chemical stimuli and are part of the immune system.

The Vestibule

The junction between the vagina and the vulva is the vestibule, and the urethra is located in the vestibule. Technically the vestibule is external, but the skin is similar to what you would find in the vagina: it's mucosal skin, meaning there is very little keratin and the cells are filled with *glycogen*, a storage sugar. There is also no hair or sebum, so the tissue is primarily protected physically by the labia minora.

There are also two sets of specialized glands—the top pair are Skene's glands, which are similar to the prostate in men (studies show that they secrete tiny amounts of prostate-specific antigen, or PSA). The Bartholin's glands sit at the bottom on either side of the vestibule. They both may contribute a small amount of lubrication.

Anal Sphincters

The anus has two muscular rings called the internal and the external sphincter. The mucosa of the anus is highly innervated (full of nerves) because the tissue has to distinguish between solid and liquid stool as well as gas, in addition to coordinating the socially appropriate time for emptying. This rich network of nerves is why some people find anal sex very stimulating. It is also why hemorrhoids or fissures (small breaks in the skin) hurt so very much.

The internal sphincter is the most important in terms of stool continence. It is responsible for about 80 percent of fecal continence.

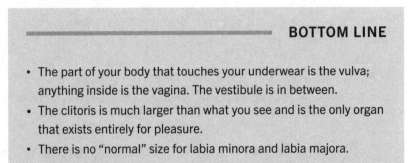

BOTTOM LINE

- The part of your body that touches your underwear is the vulva; anything inside is the vagina. The vestibule is in between.
- The clitoris is much larger than what you see and is the only organ that exists entirely for pleasure.
- There is no "normal" size for labia minora and labia majora.

- Labia minora, labia majora, and the mons contribute to both sexual pleasure and protection of the vagina opening.
- The pH of the vulvar skin is acidic, between 5.3 and 5.6.

CHAPTER 2

The Vagina

THE VAGINA IS A FIBROMUSCULAR TUBE that connects the vulva with the cervix. I realize this is the least sexy way to describe something that brings so much pleasure. Personally, I'd love to use a different term, as vagina means "sheath" in Latin, and I hate having female anatomy defined in terms of how it fits with a penis. Medically, the vagina starts at the hymen, so just inside the vestibule.

Why Do We Even Have a Hymen?

Evolutionary biologists have not been able to answer this question.

Some experts have postulated that a hymen may once have served to prove to a male mate that he wouldn't be raising another man's child, but there are several reasons why that seems improbable and ridiculously patriarchal. The hymen can tear from physical activity, and approximately 50 percent of teens who report sexual activity still have an intact hymen, meaning it is a highly unreliable "virginity indicator." This "preserving purity" theory also implies that, evolutionarily speaking, only the first child has value, but for most of human history 30–50 percent of newborns did not survive their first year. It makes no sense to invest a supposedly precious biological resource for a sexual encounter that may not provide a child who lives—or even produce a child at all.

Another proposed theory is that the hymen evolved to make first sex painful so women would only have sex with a "bonded" male partner. However, it's pretty clear that for the majority of women, their sexual debut is not painful enough that they are going to hold out for some hypothetical Mr. Right. If it hurt that much, we wouldn't have so many teen pregnancies. Also, if the evolutionary goal was to keep the first sex disappointing enough that women wouldn't bother to look elsewhere and hence stay with their "first man," it seems counterproductive to have such an amazing organ as the clitoris be fully functional early in the reproductive years.

My theory is the hymen was at one point in human history a physical barrier for protection. Before puberty, the mucosa (skin) of the vagina is very sensitive to irritants. If a prepubertal girl gets even a small amount of dirt in her vagina, the dirt can cause a profuse inflammatory reaction. Estrogen, fat pads in the mons and labia majora, pubic hair, and labia minora—essentially all of the protective mechanisms for the lower vagina—don't develop until puberty. So I believe the hymen was a pre-puberty physical barrier against dirt and debris. As we evolved and began to walk upright, physically taking the vaginal opening farther away from dirt, the need for a physical barrier for the lower vagina lessened, and evolution became less invested in a rigid, physically protective hymen. This would explain why we now have so many variations in hymen shape: it is simply no longer biologically important.

In a fetus, the vagina starts as a solid tube. The cells from the inside gradually disappear—this proceeds from top (the cervix) to bottom. Any remnants that remain at the lower part of the vagina are the hymen, which can be a ring, crescent shaped, have holes, or even be absent altogether. Sometimes larger portions of cells are left behind, which can lead to a band of vaginal tissue that runs horizontally or vertically. This band is called a septum. A septum can be flimsy and break easily with a tampon or penetration during sex, but it can also be very thick; rarely, it can even obstruct the vagina. The presence of a septum should be considered for any teen who has not had a period by the age of sixteen, any women who is unable to insert a tampon, fingers, a penis, or have a speculum exam due to pain, and any woman who has a feeling of an obstruction with vaginal penetration.

Vagina: The Basics

The vagina is lined with specialized skin called mucosa. The mucosa is arranged in accordion-like folds or ridges called rugae—some women may perceive these as "bumps" or a roughness. The best visual for rugae is a king-sized fitted sheet on a queen-sized bed.

The mucosa sits atop a layer of smooth muscle, which is technically the outer wall of the vagina. Smooth muscle is a type of muscle not under voluntary control (your gut is also made of smooth muscle). While not all the functions of the vaginal smooth muscle are well known, it is believed it moves blood and vaginal discharge towards the vaginal opening. If the muscle contractions become uncoordinated or spasm excessively, this can cause pain. There is data that suggests that some women who have painful periods have more spasms or uncoordinated activity of their vaginal smooth muscle.

The rugae and smooth muscle allow the vagina to be collapsed at rest with the walls touching, keeping air out, and then to stretch for penetration or for a vaginal delivery. Everyone (okay, the patriarchy) seems very impressed with the ability of a penis to grow, but the few centimeters of change that a penis can muster up pales in comparison with the vagina's ability to stretch.

The vaginal smooth muscle is surrounded by a network of blood vessels. The rich blood flow is one of the reasons the vagina typically heals well after injury.

Vaginal length can vary significantly. The back wall (closer to the rectum) is longer and can range from 5.1 to 14.4 cm, and the front wall ranges from 4.4 to 8.4 cm. Your body size and shape are not predictive of your vaginal length. The vagina gets wider as you move from the vaginal opening towards the cervix.

The pelvic floor

The pelvic floor muscles (PFM) are two layers of muscles that wrap around the vagina and the vaginal opening. These muscles provide structural support for organs, assist with continence (bladder and bowel), contract during orgasm, and also help with stability of your core and posture. On average, the pelvic floor muscles contract 3–15 times during an

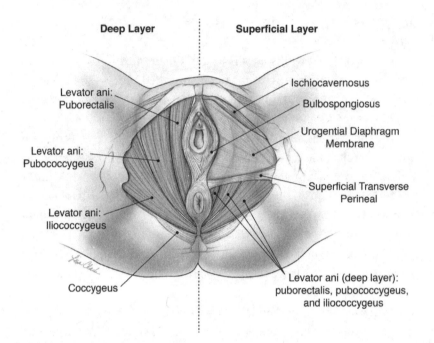

Image 3: Pelvic floor muscles. ILLUSTRATION BY LISA A. CLARK, MA, CMI.

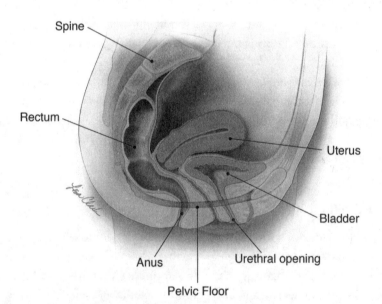

Image 4: Female pelvic floor (sagittal view). ILLUSTRATION BY LISA A. CLARK, MA, CMI.

orgasm. We know this because there have been studies where women have stimulated themselves to orgasm in a highly monitored setting. (I always wonder how people get funding for these kinds of studies!)

The superficial layer is directly beneath the skin of the vulva and is made of three muscles: ischiocavernosus, bulbospongiosus, and superficial transverse perineal. The point where the superficial transverse perineal, bulbospongiosus, and the anal sphincter come together is called the perineal body.

The deeper layer of muscles extends from the pubic bone from front to back, out to the hips, and back to the coccyx (tailbone), like a hammock. There are openings for the urethra, vagina, and rectum. This deeper layer, called the levator ani, is a made up of three muscles: the puborectalis, pubococcygeus, and the iliococcygeus.

The muscles in your pelvic floor are not typically in your conscious control—you don't think about emptying your bladder or bowel or about having an orgasm, you just do. Once we get enough motor and sensory control, we train the bladder and bowel to work relatively independently, like a computer program that runs in the background. Evolutionarily speaking, these activities were likely off-loaded from the consciousness because if we had to be constantly aware of regulating bladder and bowel function, we would never have crawled out of the swamp!

Weakness or tearing of the pelvic floor, most commonly caused by childbirth, can contribute to incontinence (both bladder and bowel) and pelvic organ prolapse (descending of the pelvic organs and structures). If the pelvic floor becomes too tight, the resulting muscle spasm can lead to pain with sex and pelvic pain.

The vaginal mucosa

The mucosa (skin) of the vagina is about twenty-eight cell layers thick. Like the vulva, there is a layer of basal cells constantly producing new cells. Unlike in the vulva, the cells of the vagina are filled with glycogen, a storage sugar. They also have much less keratin than the vulva cells, making the surface of the vagina slightly less waterproof than the vulva. This allows a small amount of fluid to leave the bloodstream and leak between the cells of the vagina to become part of the vaginal discharge. This fluid is called transudate. The reduced waterproofing also means some substances can be absorbed from the vagina into the bloodstream.

The vaginal mucosa turns over much faster than the vulvar skin—a new layer is produced every ninety-six hours. There are several biological reasons:

- **FRICTION:** No matter how gentle you are with a finger, toy, tongue, or penis, friction will rub off the top layer of cells, and this needs to be repaired quickly. If heterosexual sex led to prolonged internal injury, that would dramatically affect our ability to procreate.
- **NUTRITION FOR THE ECOSYSTEM:** The surface layer of cells sheds approximately every four hours for a woman of reproductive age. These dead cells are filled with the storage sugar glycogen (made of thousands of glucose molecules), which feeds the bacteria that keeps the vagina healthy. Up to 3 percent of vaginal secretions are glycogen.
- **CONFUSING THE BAD BACTERIA:** The dead cells floating in the vagina work like a decoy. They are the first cells encountered by pathogenic (potentially harmful) bacteria. If this bacteria attaches to these free-floating cells, it gets flushed out as part of the vaginal discharge.

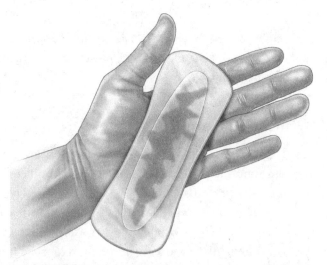

Image 5: Hand holding pad with discharge. ILLUSTRATION BY LISA A. CLARK, MA, CMI.

Vaginal ecosystem

The vagina typically produces 1–3 ml of discharge in twenty-four hours, but up to 4 ml has been reported as normal. For perspective, 4 ml is a completely soaked mini pad, and the image below contains a very normal amount—2 ml.

Based on my anecdotal experience, and from what I hear from colleagues around the country, more and more women erroneously believe that any vaginal discharge is abnormal. I don't know if this is because mainstream porn frequently looks dry, women don't talk much about their discharge, more women are removing all their pubic hair and so discharge that would normally be trapped now appears on underwear, or the fact that there are shelves of products in drugstores designed to "tame" a healthy, wet vagina.

Vaginal discharge is made of secretions from the cervix, the glands at the vaginal opening (Bartholin's and Skene's), various substances made by the healthy bacteria, cells that have been shed from the vaginal surface, and a small amount of transudate (fluid that leaks across from the bloodstream).

One of the most well-known bacteria in the vagina is the *Lactobacillus* species (spp.), often referred to as *lactobacilli*. These are healthy bacteria that protect the vagina. The lactobacilli produce lactic acid, which keeps the vaginal pH between 3.5 and 4.5 (acidic), making it harder for many bacteria and viruses to thrive. Lactobacilli also make proteins called bacteriocins that kill or inhibit the growth of pathogenic (harmful) bacteria—think of bacteriocins like homemade antibiotics. Lactobacilli bind to the mucosal (skin) cells in the vagina, preventing other bacteria from binding. Lactobacilli also produce hydrogen peroxide, which we used to believe had a role in vaginal defense mechanisms (that theory has fallen out of favor).

There are many different species of lactobacilli. The four main ones in terms of the vagina are *L. crispatus*, *L. jensenii*, *L. iners*, and *L. gasseri*. We are now only beginning to understand the full role of the different lactobacilli species, and so what today we think we know could change. For example, when I was in training everyone thought *L. acidophilus* was most common, but that was because it was one of the only types of lactobacilli that could be grown easily in a lab. With the advent of DNA technology, we have been able to get a better evaluation of the vaginal microbiome because we don't have to coax bacteria to grow. We currently believe *L. iners* is the most prevalent species; 84 percent of women have this bacteria, and it dominates the vaginal microbiome for 34 percent of women. Comparatively, *L. acidophilus* likely has a minor role, if it even has any at all.

Each woman has one of five community states of vaginal bacteria. Four are dominated by *Lactobacillus* spp. (73 percent of women); the remaining 27 percent have few lactobacilli and instead have a diverse collection of other bacteria. There are many factors that go into the vaginal bacteria communities, and it is likely a complex combination of genetics and environment. White and Asian women are more likely to have lactobacilli-dominant vaginal communities, whereas approximately 40 percent of African American and Hispanic women have other, non-lactobacilli bacterial communities. The more lactobacilli, the more acidic the vaginal pH, so women who have non-lactobacilli-dominant communities may have a slightly elevated vaginal pH (in the 4.7–5.0 range).

This does not mean that those 40 percent of African American and Hispanic women have unhealthy vaginal bacteria; rather, this is a normal variant. We are only beginning to understand the vaginal microbiome, and many factors besides lactobacilli go into vaginal health.

Vaginal pH increases during menses due to the blood itself, which has a pH of 7.35. Blood also binds lactobacilli, so lactobacilli levels are reduced with bleeding. This is one explanation for why women are most susceptible to infections at the end of their menstrual periods, as they have the lowest counts of good bacteria as well as a higher pH. In addition, blood is also a good medium for bacterial growth.

SHOULD I GET MY VAGINAL MICROBIOME TESTED? There is at least one test on the market that allows you to assess some of the bacteria in your microbiome and, given the expansion of the at-home medical-testing market, we can likely expect more. Given what we currently know about the vaginal microbiome, there are a few issues with this testing. The first is that your microbiome can fluctuate from day to day for a variety of reasons—it can even be different in the morning and the evening of one day. A single snapshot, or even three snapshots on different days, is not very helpful. If I took a picture of your hair at 4 P.M. one day, that would not be representative of how your hair looks day to day, nor would it tell me how to wash your hair or what hair-care products to choose.

Another issue with home testing is worry. We know that some women normally have a healthy microbiome with low levels of lactobacilli. A home test evaluating lactobacilli might erroneously identify these women as having an abnormal microbiome and cause worry.

Finally, we have no idea how to use information from home microbiome testing and no way to replace or augment the microbiome. One day these tests may be useful, but as of today, in 2019, they are not.

BOTTOM LINE

- The folds in the vagina are called rugae.
- The length of the vagina is not related to overall size and body shape.
- Vaginal discharge is typically 1–3 ml a day.
- The vagina has a lot of sugar in the form of glycogen to feed the good bacteria (see chapter 7 for more on food and your vagina).
- There are five different communities of vaginal bacteria.

CHAPTER 3

Vaginas and Vulvas in Transition

SEX IS THE DESIGNATION OF A PERSON as male or female based on biological characteristics, such as anatomy and/or hormones. Sex can be assigned at birth or changed. Gender is your sense of who you are—male, female, both, or neither. A transgender individual is a person whose gender identity differs from their assigned sex at birth.

There are approximately 1 to 1.4 million transgender women and men in the United States. In addition to medical concerns, many face health care providers unfamiliar with the standards of medical care established by the World Professional Association for Transgender Health (WPATH)—up to 50 percent of transgender individuals report having to tell their health care provider about the specific care they need. This is marginalizing and does not inspire confidence in health care professionals.

Trans women and men also face other barriers to obtaining care. Almost 30 percent report being verbally harassed in a medical office, and 20 percent report being denied care. Negative interactions can lead to reluctance to seek care. Trans men who have a vagina and cervix may not be established with a provider who can provide cervical cancer screenings or who can diagnose and treat causes of vaginal irritation. As insurance coverage varies, many trans men and women may not have the financial resources to get all the care they need.

Whatever the reason, and there are unfortunately many, 48 percent of trans men and 33 percent of trans women delay or avoid preventative health care.

Trans Men

Vulvar and vaginal changes for trans men

Testosterone for transitioning can produce significant changes in the vulva and vagina. The clitoris will enlarge, from an average length of 1.5 cm to 4.5 cm. As the glans grows, more of it is exposed (the clitoral hood does not grow in the same way), potentially leading to increased clitoral sensitivity. Pubic hair may increase, and the pattern of distribution often changes—more hair on the thighs and possibly also hair that extends from the umbilicus (belly button) downwards.

Testosterone also causes the vaginal mucosa to become thinner and reduces lactobacilli, so the pH becomes elevated. This can start as early as three months after starting testosterone, but the peak effect may not be experienced for two years. Symptoms can include irritation, vaginal discharge, burning, pain with exams, and pain with intercourse for trans men who practice receptive vaginal sex. The lack of lactobacilli and thin vaginal mucosa increase the risk of acquiring sexually transmitted infections (STI) if exposed vaginally.

Treatment for these symptoms includes vaginal estrogen—when dosed correctly, it is not absorbed into the bloodstream and so won't counteract testosterone's effect on other tissues. Some trans men find vaginal estrogen acceptable, but others do not. If the physical aspect of having to place something in the vagina is the concern, a vaginal ring that releases estrogen, which should not be felt when placed correctly and requires changing every three months, may be an option. For trans men who are opposed to the idea of estrogen, vaginal DHEAS suppositories may be an option. DHEAS is a hormone that is converted to estrogen and testosterone in the vagina. More details on the medication and delivery options can be found in chapter 19.

Trans men with a cervix need cervical screening

Not all trans men have a hysterectomy (removal of uterus and cervix), and those who do often pursue that option several years after transition, so cervical cancer screening may be needed for some time. Cervical cancer screening guidelines remain the same for trans men—screening should start at age twenty-one and continue until age sixty-five (screening can stop at sixty-five if the last three tests have been normal). Cervical screening is recommended whether or not sexual activity has started and regardless of the gender of the person with whom you have had sex. A more detailed review of cervical cancer screening can be found in chapter 26.

Trans men are unfortunately less likely to get cervical cancer screening. Even more concerning, they have a ten times greater risk of having an abnormal Pap smear compared with cisgender women (those whose assigned sex at birth corresponds with their gender identity). Trans men are also more likely to have an inadequate Pap smear, meaning the cells cannot be evaluated appropriately. In one study, almost 11 percent of trans men had a Pap smear that could not be appropriately evaluated versus 1 percent of cis women. This is likely due to inflammation from testosterone or discomfort with the test, which may have affected the ability of the health care provider to adequately sample the cervix. The changes in vaginal bacteria may also increase the risk of getting human papilloma virus (HPV), the virus that causes cervical cancer.

Inadequate testing means concerning cells may not have been sampled, and so the test cannot be relied upon for accuracy. Trans men also are more likely to have delays in returning for repeat testing or following up with an inadequate sample or an abnormality because of reduced access or marginalization. Biologically, there is a higher risk for trans men, and societal factors impact access. Not a good combination.

It takes about six months for testosterone to have a negative effect on Pap smears, so if possible trans men should consider cervical cancer screening before starting testosterone. If the results are normal, that gives at least three years before more testing is needed.

Options to reduce the physical discomfort with cervical cancer screening include the following:

- **HPV TESTING ALONE:** This is a vaginal sample and can be done without a speculum. Many studies tell us that self-sampling is as effective as a provider obtaining the specimen, and you may feel more comfortable inserting the swab yourself. Some guidelines only recommend HPV screening alone (meaning without a Pap smear) starting at age thirty, although the American College of Obstetricians and Gynecologists (ACOG) considers HPV screening alone an acceptable option at age twenty-five.
- **VAGINAL ESTROGEN:** When given for 2–4 weeks before a Pap smear, it may reduce abnormal findings and pain with the exam.

It is important for every person to get the HPV vaccine, but especially so for trans men who are at great risk for insufficient screening for cervical cancer and abnormal Pap smears. (For more on the HPV vaccine, see chapter 25.) Trans men considering hysterectomy should have a discussion with their surgeon about removing the cervix (total hysterectomy) versus leaving the cervix (supracervical hysterectomy). While the latter may be technically easier for some surgeons, transition-wise it offers no benefit and means cervical cancer screening needs to continue until age sixty-five.

Menstruation and transition

Trans men who do not take hormones will still have periods. Some trans men opt for a hormone IUD for contraception, as this often leads to lighter periods. Testosterone therapy also affects periods; by two months, they are generally lighter, and they typically stop thirty-six months into testosterone therapy. However, if hormone levels are not monitored to ensure they are in the male range, periods can persist for 16 percent of trans men at six months. For trans men with intermittent access to hormones, periods can return if there are breaks in testosterone therapy. Trans men coming off hormones for fertility reasons will also start periods.

While tampons and menstrual cups may offer more discretion than pads, they can be painful to insert due to the vaginal inflammation from testosterone—especially if the flow is light. We do not have any data on how testosterone impacts the risk of toxic shock syndrome.

Reusable period underwear may be an option for trans men with lighter periods who do not want to use pads, tampons, or cups. While period underwear offers the discretion of no visible pad, if it needs changing when you are away from home the only option is to carry the used underwear around in a plastic bag, which negates a lot of the discretion. See chapter 17 for more information on these options.

Trans Women

Vulvar and vaginal surgery

Surgery can create labia, a clitoris, and a vagina (vaginoplasty). The *glans penis* is used to create a clitoris, and both the new clitoris and stimulation of the prostate with vaginal penetration contribute to sexual pleasure. After surgery, approximately 75 percent of trans women report they are sexually active vaginally, and the ability to orgasm ranges from 70 to 84 percent.

The scrotum is used to create labia, but the optimal technique for vaginoplasty has not yet been identified. Tissue from the penis, colon, and peritoneum (a layer of mucus that lines the abdominal cavity and, among other things, keeps your organs from sticking together) have all been used. Sometimes skin from other body parts is needed as well. Other techniques that are being investigated involve tissue from the mouth (buccal mucosa), amnion (from the placenta), and tissues that have been specifically treated called decellularized tissues. A review of the best technique is beyond this book, but the choice depends on many factors, including underlying health, length of the penis (whether there is enough tissue), and both patient and surgeon preference.

The most common procedure in the United States involves penile tissue with the addition of scrotal or other skin as needed. The average range of vaginal length for cis (cisgender) women is 6.5–12.5 cm—as vaginal length is not related to sexual satisfaction, most surgeons aim for a vaginal length in the mid-range of 9–10 cm. Given the anatomic considerations, there is not always space to create a depth of 10 cm, so what can be achieved may vary. Penile tissue is not self-lubricating, but some people feel that sexual stimulation may be superior, as penile skin is sexually responsive.

A vagina constructed from penile skin is colonized with bacteria routinely found on the skin. Vaginal symptoms, such as discharge and odor, are not related to the same conditions that affect cis women such as yeast or bacterial vaginosis. Discharge is usually due to skin secretions, such as sebum and skin cells.

If discharge and odor are concerns, routine cleaning or douching with water and sometimes a mild cleanser may be indicated, as the new vagina is not mucosa and does not have lactobacilli. Many surgeons recommend douching during the time when dilation is needed daily to remove retained lubricant and the skin cells shed due to the friction. The appropriate management of vaginal odor is not established, but if douching with water has not been sufficient, some recommend douching for a few days with a 25 percent poviodine iodine in water solution. Another option is a course of vaginal antibiotics, typically metronidazole, to reduce odor-forming bacteria.

The advantage of colon and peritoneum tissue is that they are self-lubricating. This requires abdominal surgery, although this can almost always be accomplished with small incisions via the operating telescope (laparoscopically). Discharge can be significant when colon tissue is used for the new vagina.

A vaginoplasty is medically a big procedure. If, for health reasons, someone is not able to tolerate this surgery, then a vulva and clitoris can be created and a small depression made for the vagina. Externally, there is no difference in appearance. This is also an option for trans women who do not want to receive vaginal penetration.

Some important considerations before vaginoplasty include the following:

- **PERMANENT PUBIC HAIR REMOVAL ON AND AROUND THE SCROTUM:** If hair removal is not permanent, it can regrow inside the vagina, causing cysts, vaginal discharge, and odor. Complete hair removal can take up to a year, and electrolysis is the only truly permanent method.
- **STOPPING ALL NICOTINE PRODUCTS FOR THREE MONTHS BEFORE AND AFTER THE SURGERY:** All tobacco products impair wound healing, as they reduce blood flow in small blood vessels. Success of vaginoplasty depends on establishing blood flow, and the use of tobacco can lead to loss of the graft inside the vagina and scarring.
- **DILATION IS NEEDED AFTER SURGERY TO MAINTAIN THE LENGTH AND WIDTH OF THE VAGINA:** For most trans women this will be a life-

long commitment, but it is especially important in the first year after surgery. If there is too much pain to dilate, it is very important to speak with your surgeon immediately. Scarring with loss of width or length can occur very quickly and is surgically challenging to correct.

Pain with sex and dilation can be due to vaginal scarring and/or spasm of the pelvic floor muscles, which are the muscles that wrap around the vagina (see chapters 2 and 34). Pain and/or manipulation from surgery can lead to muscle spasm. In both situations, scarring and spasm, it can feel as if the dilators are hitting a blockage.

STIs after vaginoplasty

If penile tissue is used to create the vagina, it is likely not susceptible to infection with gonorrhea or chlamydia, but the urethra can still get infected due to the proximity to the vagina. Transmission of viral STIs, like herpes, HPV, and HIV, is likely possible, but understudied.

BOTTOM LINE

- Trans men with a cervix are at a higher risk of having an abnormal Pap smear and of inadequate screening for cervical cancer.
- While everyone ages 9–45 should have the HPV vaccine, trans men should consider HPV vaccination and cervical cancer screening before medical transition, if possible.
- Trans men taking testosterone can develop vaginal discharge and pain; it may take up to two years to develop.
- Trans women have different causes of vaginal discharge and odor than cis women.
- Pain with sex for trans women can be due to stenosis of the vagina or muscle spasm (see chapter 34).

CHAPTER 4

Female Pleasure and Sex Ed

IT IS VERY DIFFICULT IN OUR SOCIETY to have non-sophomoric discussions about sex. Because of this, it is women who typically suffer. Female anatomy is erroneously labeled as "dirty," and from an early age, girls are given messages about what a patriarchal society has determined a "nice" girl should and should not do.

Not knowing your anatomy, how it works and how to make it work, is disempowering and puts women at a disadvantage in a sexual relationship. Many heterosexual women learn about sex from male partners, who are often uneducated or undereducated themselves about the mechanics of female orgasms. Every OB/GYN I know has had at least one male partner ask them to point out their partner's clitoris (meaning the clitoral glans) during an exam. On one hand, it's great he is interested. On the other hand, "Come on, dude, you've been together for ten years." Women who partner with women are less likely to have that disadvantage.

Where can women turn for accurate information about sex or to find out if what they are experiencing is normal, a technique issue, or a medical concern? In one study, only 63 percent of OB/GYNs routinely asked about sexual activity, 40 percent asked about sex problems, and 29 percent asked if a woman's sex life was satisfying. This is a problem.

Some doctors, even OB/GYNs, find discussing sex difficult because they haven't received much, if any, training in this type of conversation. For oth-

29

ers, there is a time crunch in the office. Sometimes there are truly no *medical* therapies (think pills or injections) to recommend—some sexual problems are technique- or relationship-related. I'm not defending the lack of questioning from OB/GYNs, just explaining some of the complexities. However, doctors should be asking because then we can refer patients elsewhere when appropriate—for example, to a sex therapist, a marriage and family therapist, or a psychologist. Doctors don't have to treat every condition; referring someone on for help with their sex life should be as natural as referring someone on for a bowel problem or headaches.

The other problem with doctors not asking about sex is women who have medical conditions that interfere with their sex life, typically conditions that cause pain with sex, end up minimized. Many women suffer for years not realizing they have a medical problem that has a diagnosis and treatment.

How Much Sex Are People Really Having?

Surveys tell us that overall satisfaction with sex life is not that high: 49 percent of heterosexual women, 47 percent of lesbian women, and 49 percent of bisexual women state they are happy with their sex life. It's not much higher for men—although the respondents who were the happiest in this study were, no surprise, heterosexual men (but even then, only 51 percent were satisfied).

There is a lot of pressure to say sex is the most important thing. Despite many people saying publicly and privately on surveys that sex matters to them more than almost anything else in life, the reality is that the average amount of time people spend having sex is about four minutes a day. That is probably less time than most people spend grocery shopping or staring into the fridge—and I know which activity I prefer!

The key piece of information here is that dissatisfaction with your sex life seems to be a very common experience.

Why the disconnect?

Why are people having less sex than they desire? It's possible people think they should be wanting more sex due to societal expectations, so they answer surveys with an idealized answer (hey, there are times when I have lied about my weight on an anonymous questionnaire). Admitting a truth to yourself can be very hard. We also all tend to want more of the things we enjoy. Not everyone is in a sexual relationship, and many people are in relationships that just aren't working but they haven't yet figured out a path forward. Most people are not good sexual communicators, and sometimes the sex is just unsatisfying. People also don't prioritize sex, some women have medical conditions that make sex painful, and of course libido waxes and wanes.

Basically, it's complicated.

Sexless relationships are also more common than people think. A sexless relationship, meaning no sex in the past 6–12 months, affects up to 15 percent of couples. There is less data on non-marital relationships. Society almost always lays the blame on the female partner in a heterosexual relationship, but it can often be the man.

The Sexual Response Cycle

Physically, from a pure stimulation standpoint, the clitoris is the most important anatomical structure for female sex. This doesn't mean that some women don't orgasm with nipple stimulation or anal stimulation; this just means the clitoris has specifically evolved for sexual pleasure, and almost always when other erogenous zones are stimulated there is also a clitoral response. Interestingly, the area in the brain that responds to nipple stimulation overlaps with the area that responds to clitoral stimulation.

The classic model of sexual response is a linear progression first presented by Masters and Johnson in 1960. It has four phases: excitement, plateau, orgasm, and resolution. This model has been criticized for not including desire (if you dislike your partner or they turn you off, getting excited may be a challenge). Another model was proposed that added desire to the sequence, but both of these models are male-centric and assume a specific, preset sex drive. This completely neglects many reasons women report wanting sexual intimacy: for example, emotionally connecting with their partner, trust, affection, safety, and respect.

A circular model has been proposed (by Dr. Rosemary Basson in 2000) that endorses the concept that a satisfying sexual encounter does not require starting with a spontaneous sexual drive or desire. This model also incorporates other factors besides physical stimulation that women report contribute to sexual arousal and satisfaction, such as feeling secure, being desired, or a sense of well-being. The circular model accepts that women may not always have a high spontaneous libido and that some women engage in sexual activity initially to feel intimacy or connectedness, and desire kicks in after arousal.

The Basson model supports the idea that sex drive can be spontaneous, but that it can also be the result of a complex interaction of many physical and emotional stimuli and that desire can be spontaneous as well as responsive. It also acknowledges that for many women, intimacy is an important sexual concept.

I often tell women to focus less on the idea of spontaneous libido and more on the idea of satisfaction (emotional and physical)—and, of course, fun and sexual pleasure. Lots of people get hung up on spontaneous libido, which to be honest seems like a response to a specific male fantasy. I prefer to think of sex as a party. It doesn't matter if you received an engraved invitation or were invited by text. It doesn't matter if you took a limo, drove your car, took the subway, or walked. What matters is you were at the party and you had what you consider to be a good time.

Physical changes with arousal and sex

Increased blood flow to the vagina and vulva causes clitoral engorgement, vulvar swelling, and vaginal transudate (wetness or lubrication). The lower third of the vagina may tighten, and the upper two thirds may dilate. The top of the vagina and the uterus elevate or lift slightly.

Orgasm is the rhythmic contractions of the muscles that wrap around the vagina (the pelvic floor muscles). These contractions are a reflex, meaning your nerves and muscles are coordinating the action without conscious input from your brain. This is similar in many ways to having your knee hit with a reflex hammer—your knee moves because a reflex has been triggered, not because your brain is consciously telling your knee to move. Contracting your pelvic floor muscles voluntarily (Kegel exercises) doesn't trigger orgasm, but many women find that purposely contracting these muscles can increase arousal. I sometimes think of this as priming the pump, along the lines of warming up your legs before a run or your car on a cold day. Give it a try!

Female orgasm—the contractions of the pelvic floor muscles—typically lasts 5–60 seconds. The muscle contractions occur at approximately 0.8-second intervals (so one right after the other), and for many women each successive contraction is longer, but weaker. The general range of contractions, number-wise, is 3–15. Orgasm is accompanied by a feeling of well-being and/or release of tension. What is fascinating is that both women and men describe the feeling of an orgasm with almost identical terminology.

For some women, the clitoral glans can be too sensitive to touch directly during foreplay or sex as it has the highest density of nerves. Women who find they can't tolerate a vibrator or direct manual stimulation against their glans may find that a tongue works fine or that they can handle the stimulation if they put a piece of soft fabric between the vibrator or fingers and their clitoris. Fortunately, as the clitoris branches around the urethra, extends into the vagina, and is beneath the labia, it can be accessed for stimulation in many creative ways that don't involve direct contact with the glans. For example, a vibrator with a larger surface area pressed up against the vaginal opening may stimulate the crura of the clitoris. It's fun to look at the size and location of the clitoris and think of different approaches to stimulation.

Some Sex Facts

Lesbian women are more likely to report that they usually or always orgasm during sex (86 percent) compared to heterosexual women (65 percent). This is proof that a penis is in no way required for satisfying sex, nor is it the judge of female sexual satisfaction.

The ideal duration of penile penetration during heterosexual sex according to a survey of U.S. and Canadian sex therapists was 3–7 minutes (1–2 minutes was considered too short, and > 10 minutes was considered too long).

In one study, heterosexual couples reported an average of 11–13 minutes of foreplay and 7–8 minutes of intercourse, and men thought both the foreplay and the penetration lasted longer than the women did. Both men and women reported wanting more foreplay and more intercourse.

What's the deal with vaginal orgasms and the G-spot?

It is hard to overestimate the damage done by Sigmund Freud in popularizing the myth of the vaginal orgasm. Only one third of women are capable of achieving orgasm with penile penetration alone (meaning hands off, penile thrusting only), so the idea that everyone should be having orgasms this way results in two thirds of women believing there is something wrong with their sexual wiring when really they are perfect.

Not orgasming with unassisted penile penetration is not a flaw, it's a feature.

Further supporting this vaginal orgasm myth is the idea of the G-spot, supposedly identified by Dr. Ernst Gräfenberg in 1950. In modern lore, this is a magical spot on the vaginal wall (beneath the bladder) that when touched will drive a woman "wild." Again, many women feel frustrated when they don't have a G-spot.

Digging through the data, we find that Dr. Gräfenberg's original paper did not describe a special spot. His paper is actually called "The Role of the Urethra in Female Orgasm," and he described an "erotic zone" in the front of the vagina that was intimate with the urethra and lower portion of the bladder. Yes, he was likely describing the body, root, and bulbs of the clitoris as they envelop the urethra. As expected, multiple studies have found no macroscopic structure other than the urethra, the clitoris, and vaginal wall in the location of the so-called G-spot. The lower part of the vagina, close to the urethra, will feel great for many women because stimulation here is accessing the clitoris, but it takes the right stimulation—it is not an "on/off switch."

It is not surprising to me when I hear of women who fake orgasms with male partners. After all, they have been led to believe that a female orgasm should be reached with a penis by way of an imaginary spot.

MRI studies looking at anatomy during heterosexual sex reveal that the clitoris can be compressed by the penis, which is why some women can orgasm with penile penetration. Ultrasound studies looking at clitoral swelling during external masturbation and during vaginal penetration indicate that both cause clitoral engorgement. This means that touching externally on your vulva or vestibule or internally with a penis, fingers, tongue, or toys are all producing the same end result—clitoral stimulation. Even nipple stimulation, which many women find erotic, triggers an area in the brain that overlaps with—yes, you guessed it—the area that interprets sensations from the clitoris. The clitoris is the pleasure aggregator and amplifier.

Basically, all pleasure roads lead to the clitoris.

It is best to do away with terms like vaginal orgasm and G-spot, as they are incorrect. The goal is female orgasm, and it can be achieved in so many ways.

Do women ejaculate or "squirt"?

The answer is yes, but not in the way the internet thinks.

If you spend any time looking at online videos of so-called female ejaculation you would come to the false conclusion that some women have a secret vaginal gland that can release a gush of fluid with the right touch. Many of these videos are labeled as "squirting."

For a woman to ejaculate, the fluid must come from the vagina, the urethra, or a specialized gland. For reference, the male prostate releases about 5 ml of fluid with ejaculation, and there is no gland the size of a prostate in the vulva or vagina. So the idea that women can ejaculate a gush of fluid larger than 5 ml is, even without doing the research, rather doubtful.

But I'm me, so I researched it.

There is a pair of glands on either side of the urethra (the tube that drains the bladder) called Skene's glands. These are about the size of a pea or smaller, and they are sometimes referred to as the female prostate because their secretions contain traces of prostate-specific antigen (PSA), a protein found in the male prostate. Skene's glands can secrete a small amount of fluid, perhaps 1–2 ml at most, during sexual activity. It would be medically correct to call this ejaculate, but it will not squirt any distance or have a large volume.

In one study, 38 women masturbated to orgasm (confirmed by monitors that measured pelvic floor muscle contractions), and no ejaculate was seen coming from the vagina or the urethra. However, if the incidence of squirting or ejaculation was 1 in 50, say 2 percent of women, this study might not be large enough to identify them.

Another study looked specifically at a small group of women who reported squirting, meaning they said that they release a large amount of fluid during orgasm. They were screened to make sure they did not have incontinence. The women emptied their bladders and stimulated to orgasm. The amount of urine in their bladder at baseline, while aroused, and after orgasm was measured by ultrasound. Their urine was collected and analyzed before stimulation and after orgasm, and the "squirted" fluid was analyzed as well.

The results? The women's bladders filled remarkably fast during sexual stimulation. There was urine before orgasm and their bladders were empty after squirting. The squirted fluid was identified in the lab as urine.

Why does this happen? It is possible when women report squirting that they are simply having an orgasm strong enough for the pelvic floor muscles to empty their bladder, which is why it is associated with heightened pleasure. It is also possible that a more intense sexual response could result in a faster filling of the bladder.

It is also possible that some women have a lot of transudate—meaning they get very wet—during sex. When they orgasm, that fluid could come out all at once.

I looked at enough squirting videos to categorize most as either women who had inserted water (or another fluid) vaginally and were now releasing it for the video—meaning they were acting—or fluid clearly coming from the urethra and, hence, urine. There were some that showed secretions from Skene's glands, and as expected there were just a few drops of white liquid.

The reason we need to be medically accurate about the source of female ejaculation and squirting is that some women feel they are inadequate if they can't squirt, and there are already enough sex myths that reduce a woman's pleasure to a male metric. If you have urine leakage during sex and it is bothersome to you, then see a bladder specialist (a urogynecologist is a good place to start). If you are having fun and are not bothered, then it doesn't really matter what is coming from where.

A good sexual encounter is not about optics that make a man (it's usually a man in this scenario) feel as if he has achieved something. A good sexual encounter is about pleasure. As long as you are having an orgasm or two, who cares about anything else?

If arousal is partly due to increased blood flow, can special vibrators or medications that increase blood flow help?

Sexual arousal causes increased blood flow to the clitoris. There are several devices on the market that specifically provide suction to the clitoris to draw in blood—think a small suction cup placed over the glans—based on the idea that more blood flow may help physical arousal. There are inexpensive hand pumps, vibrators that fit over the clitoral glans, as well as more expensive devices, like the Fiera Arouser and the Eros Clitoral Therapy Device. Studies on the Eros device are very small, of low quality, and made up of self-selected patients. Having more options for clitoral stimulation and sexploration can be fun and a device that delivers a more suction-like sensation to the clitoral glans—the part of the clitoris with the most nerve endings—may also be an option to try for women who have difficulty achieving orgasm or who have never had an orgasm. However, we don't know if expensive devices like the Fiera and Eros are better for sexual arousal than receiving oral sex, masturbating, or a more traditional vibrator. Everyone is different, and whether these devices appeal could be very personal.

Studies have looked at medications that increase blood flow to see if they improve female sexual response—after all, the class of drugs that includes sildenafil (VIAGRA) works for men by increasing blood flow to the penis. One study indicated that these medications do increase clitoral blood flow for women who report difficulties feeling aroused, but that did not translate into a feeling of sexual arousal. One possibility is the feeling of arousal is not just dependent on blood-flow-induced changes, but the brain needs to perceive that sensation as sexually pleasurable.

What about anal sex?

Anal sex has been increasing since the 1990s, according to surveys in the United States, United Kingdom, Sweden, and Croatia. It is unknown if this is a true increase, meaning more women are truly practicing anal sex, or if more women feel comfortable reporting it due to changes in sexual mores. Currently, 30–46 percent of women report at least one lifetime experience with receptive anal sex, and 10–12 percent report it is a regular part of their sexual repertoire. Reasons women give for engaging in anal sex include pleasing their partner (the most common reason), their own pleasure, vaginal sex is painful, and to maintain their virginity. Some people report seeing anal sex in pornography as a reason to try it, just as some have drawn inspiration from the food scene in the movie 9½ Weeks. Remember, sex in mainstream movies, pornography included, is often as realistic as the driving in car-chase scenes in action movies. According to one study, anal sex featured in 55 percent of scenes in the most commonly viewed pornography, which could lead to false beliefs about its frequency in heterosexual relationships.

Some women report coercion regarding anal sex, as well as so-called "accidental" but actually planned anal penetration by their male partner. It is important when we discuss anal sex as a society that we do not trivialize or normalize this behavior.

Anal sex is often promoted as "better" for men because the anus is a "tighter" orifice. This plays on tired tropes that a vagina is "too loose" for male enjoyment, especially after a woman has been sexually active vaginally or after pregnancy.

Women should try anal sex if the idea appeals to them and they want to explore their sexuality, not because their male partner thinks everyone is doing it or is obsessed with the imagined size of his penis.

WHAT DOES ANAL SEX FEEL LIKE? Studies indicate that approximately 50 percent of women who have anal intercourse find it arousing, although pain is often an issue. At least 50 percent of women report their first episode of anal sex was painful enough that they needed to stop, so it is important to ensure your partner is willing to go slow and abandon the effort if required. Only 27 percent of women who are sexually active anally report little or no pain, so whether the pleasure payoff is worth it for you will be an individual choice.

A good lubricant is essential for anal sex. This will reduce pain, as well as microtrauma to the tissues. Anal sex is the most efficient way to sexually transmit HIV (human immunodeficiency virus), due to the combination of microtrauma and the specific cells in the anus being more susceptible to infection with the virus.

If you are not in a mutually monogamous relationship or there is a concern about HIV transmission, then it is essential to use condoms, whether a male condom for your partner or a female condom in your anus (see chapter 25 for more on condoms). If you plan to also have vaginal sex, you need one condom for anal and another for vaginal penetration. Even if you are in a mutually monogamous relationship, having a condom for anal sex can help you transition between anal and vaginal penetration without needing your partner to clean his penis.

Another reason for using a condom with anal sex is to reduce the risk of transmission of the human papilloma virus (HPV), as this virus also causes anal cancer, and the data is conflicting regarding whether receptive anal intercourse is a risk factor or not. Currently, we have no screening programs for anal precancer and cancer for women, so protection is even more important.

For women interested in anal play, either during masturbation, with a female partner, or with men, there are a multitude of anal toys, such as anal beads and plugs, for experimentation. About 4 percent of women report they used anal plugs and toys regularly in their sexual practice. This is also a good way for women who may wish to try anal intercourse with a male partner to see how they like anal stimulation when they are in control of the situation. An anal vibrator or dildo should have a flared base so it cannot move up inside the rectum. Every general surgeon I know has taken someone to the operating room to remove toys that have become lodged—this can result in very serious bowel injury, so choosing a medically safe anal vibrator is essential.

Some women wonder about anal injury with anal penetration. There is no data to suggest that receptive anal intercourse or anal play can damage the muscles of the anus, but one study (women with an average age of 46) did report that women who had receptive anal intercourse in the past month reported a higher incidence of fecal incontinence—28 percent for women who had anal intercourse versus 14 percent who did not. Whether this was an isolated incident immediately related to the sex or something that happened later on in the month was not described. There was no association of fecal incontinence with anal toys.

BOTTOM LINE

- About 50 percent of women are satisfied with their sex lives.
- A penis is not the most reliable way to achieve female orgasm.
- There is no specific G-spot; the sensitive area that many women describe just inside the vagina is part of the clitoral complex.
- Female ejaculation is tiny drops of fluid, not "squirting" as depicted in most online videos and porn.
- For women interested in anal play or anal sex, starting with a vibrator designed for anal stimulation is a safe, noncoercive way to begin.

CHAPTER 5

Pregnancy and Childbirth

IF A HUMAN COMES OUT OF YOUR BODY there will be physical changes. While I believe that most women understand this intuitively, the magnitude or the reality (or perhaps both) are often a surprise, especially when almost no one talks about the changes they experience after pregnancy. Knowing what to expect after you are finished expecting is very helpful, both so you have a realistic baseline, but also so you know when there is a medical concern and should ask for help.

We don't talk openly about the postpartum period for a lot of reasons. Women are shamed when their body doesn't conform to an impossible ideal set by the patriarchy. Until relatively recently, both society and the medical profession have focused almost exclusively on the baby after delivery. Women also used to stay in the hospital much longer after delivery than they do today and/or they had a home visit from a knowledgeable nurse, so there was someone who they could easily ask about pain, bleeding, or bowel movements without having to figure out how to take a one-week-old to a doctor's appointment.

Pregnancy Changes

Changes to the cervix, vagina, and vulva can start as soon as 4–5 weeks into the pregnancy. Increased blood flow and hormonal changes cause the vagina and vulva to engorge with blood. Consequently, the vaginal mucosa (skin) may look blue due to a change called Chadwick's sign. The skin and muscles soften. The cells on the inside of the cervix proliferate and expand onto the portion of the cervix in the vagina. This is called an ectropion. It can result in more vaginal discharge, and these cells may bleed when touched—for example, after penetrative sex or a Pap smear. Never assume this is the source of any vaginal bleeding, as there are also serious medical conditions that can cause bleeding during pregnancy.

Yeast infections are more common during pregnancy, although the exact mechanisms are unknown. It may be due to the very high levels of estrogen and/or progesterone, the immune suppression during pregnancy, or other factors.

In the third trimester, around thirty-five weeks, a vaginal test for a bacteria called group B streptococci (strep) is performed. The bacteria is normally found in the vagina and/or rectum of 10–30 percent of women. This requires treatment with intravenous antibiotics during labor to reduce the risk of serious infection for the newborn. It should not be treated with home remedies, such as garlic, that you might find suggested online. A pregnant woman with group B strep who does not receive antibiotics has a 1 in 200 chance that her baby will develop the infection, but if she is treated that risk drops to 1 in 4,000.

Sex during pregnancy

It is not uncommon for women to report a decrease in desire in the first and third trimesters. Whether this is due to worries about a complication in the pregnancy caused by sexual activity, a changing body image, discomfort with sex, or back pain is not known. Some women do report an increase in desire.

Some women worry that heterosexual sex during pregnancy could trigger a miscarriage or preterm labor and delivery. Fortunately, we know that women with a low-risk pregnancy who have no symptoms of a vaginal or cervical infection are at no higher risk of having a premature delivery if they are sexually active.

Contrary to urban myth, sexual intercourse close to the due date with a male partner does not appear to trigger labor. Many people talk about exposure to prostaglandins, substances known to trigger labor, from ejaculate, but it is not supported by science. Most studies show that heterosexual sex has no effect on triggering labor or on reducing the risk of cesarean section. The idea that a penis is mighty enough to bring on labor is, to be honest, a bit eye-rolling. Nipple stimulation when the cervix is ripe can trigger labor for some women, but you don't need a penis for that.

It's recommended to avoid sexual activity for women in some higher-risk situations, such as ruptured membranes, placenta previa (where the placenta implants over or next to the cervix), and those who have a high risk of premature delivery (for example, twins or a previous preterm delivery).

Many people have heard about reports of fatal air embolism in pregnancy from both receptive oral sex (cunnilingus) and penile-vaginal sex. An air embolism is a stroke or heart attack due to a large air bubble entering an artery or vein and traveling to the brain, heart, or lungs. The placenta has a direct connection with the maternal bloodstream, and so with enough pressure it is possible for air to travel up through the vagina into the uterus and enter the bloodstream. Air can be introduced by oral sex or with penile thrusting.

Air embolism is described in fewer than one in a million pregnancies, so it is hard to give science-based recommendations. It is best to avoid blowing air into the vagina during oral sex, and some have suggested that the risk of air embolism during penile penetration may be greatest in positions where the uterus is above the level of the heart, but that recommendation is not based on any studies.

Ancient Obstetrical Practices That Should Be Forgotten!

Before I trained as an OB/GYN, shaving, enemas, and cleaning the vulva and vagina with antiseptic were common, but now we know these practices are outdated. This isn't *The Pregnancy Bible*, so I can't go into every question you should ask your provider, but if the person delivering your baby supports a practice that is more than twenty-five years out of date, such as shaving or enemas, I might wonder about the currency of other aspects of their medical care. It's best not to shave yourself before labor either, as this causes microtrauma and may increase your risk of infection.

During delivery, you may have a bowel movement. It is completely normal. Your OB/GYN or midwife should not even notice, that is how routine it is for us. We just wipe the stool away. If it were harmful for the baby, we would not have evolved so the baby's head emerges next to the anus!

Perineal Trauma

Trauma is part of vaginal delivery (it's obviously part of a C-section as well). The vulvar and vaginal tissues have evolved to stretch, tear, and recover—the increased blood flow, how quickly the cells of the vagina are shed and replaced, and the extra folds of vaginal mucosa are very helpful.

Both tearing and an episiotomy (a surgical cut) are collectively called perineal trauma. Many women ask how many stitches they needed, but that is not a reflection of the severity of the injury. A single stitch can be run like a hem and close a large tear. Multiple tiny stitches may be needed to repair a much smaller laceration to achieve the best cosmetic result. What you should ask is the extent of the injury, which is described by OB/GYNs in degrees based on muscle injury:

- First degree does not involve muscle. It is limited to the vaginal mucosa, the vestibule (vaginal opening), and/or the skin of the vulva.
- Second degree extends into muscles and can vary significantly in size, meaning a small partial tear of the muscles beneath the vestibule or all the way through the muscles of the perineal body, stopping just before the anal sphincter.
- Third degree involves all the muscles of the perineal body and the rectal sphincter (it is further subdivided by how much sphincter is involved).
- Fourth degree extends all the way through the anal sphincter into the rectum; fortunately this occurs in only 0.25–2.5 percent of births

First- and second-degree lacerations should be repaired if they are bleeding or if not repairing them would lead to an unsatisfactory cosmetic result. Absorbable skin sutures or surgical glue can both be used. However, third- and fourth-degree lacerations should be repaired surgically (sutured)—if not, there is a higher risk of fecal incontinence. A first- or second-degree laceration has no increased risk of urinary or anal incontinence, but the risk is increased with third- and fourth-degree tears.

Routine episiotomies are not recommended by the American College of Obstetricians and Gynecologists (ACOG). The most recent data tells us that 12 percent of vaginal births in the United States involve an episiotomy, down from 33 percent in 2000. The number of episiotomies should keep going down, given ACOG's policy advising against them. Episiotomy is associated with a larger injury and an increased risk of incontinence. In general, an episiotomy is only indicated in an urgent or emergent situation. I don't know any OB/GYN who practices routine episiotomy, although I have no doubt that a few still do. This is definitely something to inquire about at one of your prenatal visits.

The risk of tearing during a vaginal delivery ranges from 44 to 79 percent—any provider who tells you they can guarantee no tears is not being honest. Most factors that lead to tearing are not within your control, including the size of your baby, whether or not this is your first delivery, and genetics. An epidural has not been shown to affect the risk.

Some interventions that may have a mild to moderate impact on reducing tearing or the need for episiotomies include the following:

- Perineal massage starting at 34–35 weeks. Women or their partners insert one or two lubricated fingers vaginally about two inches into the vagina and apply pressure downward for two minutes, then on each side for two minutes, for a total of ten minutes at least one or two times a week. Coconut oil, olive oil, and lubricant for sex can all be used. For women in their first pregnancy, perineal massage reduces the risk of tearing that requires stitches by 10 percent and the need for episiotomy by 16 percent. What this means in practical terms is that if your risk of tearing that requires stitching is 50 percent, with massage that risk is now 45 percent. If the risk of episiotomy is 12 percent, with perineal massage the risk is now about 10 percent. Perineal massage may also help reduce pain after delivery, although this association is less clear.
- Perineal massage once you are fully dilated (the second stage of labor) may lessen the severity of the tear, but not the risk of tearing.
- Perineal support, putting a hand or a towel on the perineum and applying gentle pressure, hasn't been adequately studied to say if this helps protect from tearing or not.

- Warm compresses on the perineum during pushing may reduce third- and fourth-degree lacerations.
- Delivering on your side may have the lowest risk for a tear, but the studies are not high quality, as requiring a woman to deliver in a position for study is not feasible or ethical.

If you do have a tear that enters into the anal sphincter (a third- or fourth-degree tear), a dose of intravenous antibiotics may be recommended at the time of repair as this reduces complications in the first two weeks (8 percent complication rate with antibiotics and 24 percent without).

Pain Control After a Vaginal Delivery

Swelling, bruising, tearing of muscles and skin, need for stitches, and hemorrhoids can all contribute to pain after a delivery. In general, the longer the labor, the greater the pain because there is usually more swelling. Also, fatigue affects pain processing—if you haven't slept for forty-eight hours and then you pushed for four hours, you will likely have more pain than someone who had a good night's sleep, woke up, and then had a two-hour labor and pushed for five minutes. Other factors that affect pain include the need for a vacuum or forceps and whether this is your first delivery or not. Genetics and previous pain experiences are also important. Another unique factor is how your baby is doing—the stress of a sick newborn may affect how you process pain.

There are so many individual factors involved in how we process pain it is generally not productive to compare one person's pain with another's. You have the pain you have.

Pain after delivery is important to manage *because* it is important to manage. Many guidelines talk about how important it is for a woman to have pain control so she can breastfeed, but to me that ignores the fact that women need pain control because they need pain control. A healthy mother is the best thing for a healthy baby, so I am of the belief that if we focus on the mother then everything else will fall into place.

Topical anesthetics for the perineum are used in many American hospitals, but they have never been shown to be effective at reducing pain after delivery. Benzocaine, the most commonly used anesthetic for this purpose, is a common allergen, and there are rare causes of it being absorbed and leading to a severe blood condition called methemoglobinemia. Also, when someone has stitches for other indications—for example, they accidentally cut their hand with a knife—we don't prescribe or recommend topical anesthetics for pain control. As there is no supportive data for topical anesthetics and there is a risk of causing irritation or even an allergic reaction, give them a pass.

Evidence-based options for pain control after delivery include the following:

- **ICE PACKS:** Reduce swelling and pain, especially when applied for 10–20 minutes immediately after delivery.
- **SITZ BATHS:** Getting in a tub of warm water. You don't have to add anything. You can even empty your bladder in the sitz bath if urine stings when it hits your skin
- **ACETAMINOPHEN AND IBUPROFEN (OR ANY OTHER MEDICATION CALLED A NONSTEROIDAL ANTI-INFLAMMATORY, OR NSAIDS):** These are oral medications. Ibuprofen may be slightly better than acetaminophen. Both are safe for breastfeeding.
- **KETOROLAC (BRAND NAME TORADOL):** An intravenous NSAID that may be especially helpful for women with a third- or fourth-degree laceration.
- **HEMORRHOID CARE:** Options include astringents like witch hazel, topical steroids, and topical numbing gel or creams like lidocaine (anesthetics are okay to use here). If you have a third- or fourth-degree tear, you should not use suppositories in the rectum as this could disrupt the stitches, so only creams, ointments, or gels.
- **PREVENT CONSTIPATION:** Straining will hurt, can worsen hemorrhoids, and can tear stitches. Stimulant laxatives such as Senokot or lactulose are the most effective and are safe for breastfeeding. Ducosate sodium is completely ineffective. No study has shown it works, yet for some reason almost everyone recommends it. The biggest issue with a stool softener is people think they are taking something effective when they are not, and then they wonder why they are still constipated.

If your pain is not well controlled in the hospital, a hematoma (a collection of blood that rapidly expands and causes pain—think massive bruise) must be ruled out. A hematoma may need drainage or even surgery so it doesn't lead to tissue damage or an infection.

It is also important to make sure you can empty your bladder within six hours of delivery. Urinary retention, the inability to empty your bladder, can affect up to 4 percent of women and can injure the bladder if not treated appropriately. Incontinence immediately after delivery is uncommon, so if this happens make sure to tell your doctor or midwife.

If your pain was improving and then takes a turn for the worse, do not assume that it is normal. Check with your doctor or midwife. Potential reasons could be stitches coming apart or an infection.

A word on opioids

Opioids are medications such as morphine, hydrocodone, hydromorphone, or codeine. They are often called narcotics, but that is not a medical term. Some women with a third- or fourth-degree laceration or episiotomy may need a few doses of opioid medications, although it is very important to maximize non-opioid options, as constipation is a known side effect. Opioids are also transferred into the breast milk. An opioid medication is best added in when needed on top of regularly scheduled acetaminophen or NSAIDs.

There is valid concern that opioids are overprescribed to women after delivery. One study tells us that 30 percent of women in the United States received a discharge prescription for opioids after a vaginal delivery, and the number of pills did not vary by size of the laceration or episiotomy. This is overprescribing, and whether it happens because it is a "routine" (not an excuse, just an explanation), doctors and midwives are not educated about other non-opioid medications, women ask for them, or health professionals are trying to prevent follow-up calls for pain is not known.

Studies tell us that 1 out of every 300 women who has never had opioids before delivery will become addicted if she is given a prescription to take home. It takes two doses of an opioid to develop physical dependence, meaning when the medication is stopped, physical symptoms of withdrawal, like feeling unwell and pain, appear. It is easy to mistake symptoms of withdrawal as a false sign that the opioids were helping, and so these symptoms can lead people to restart the opioid medications under the false belief that they need them medically.

Even if you take a prescription of opioids home and never use them, they can still cause harm just by sitting in your medicine cabinet. Children, especially teens, are curious about medications, and taking leftovers found in the medicine cabinet accidentally or on purpose could lead to an overdose or start an addiction.

Lochia

Vaginal bleeding after delivery is called lochia. It starts as bright red and gradually becomes paler in color due to inflammatory cells (a sign of healing in the uterus). Any leftover bits of the lining of the uterus that did not come out with the placenta may also pass with the lochia. Stitches will also add to the discharge as they dissolve.

It is normal to have a heavy, mucusy, blood-tinged, brownish, pretty gross discharge for up to eight weeks after delivery. I remember thinking this was going to go on forever, but it didn't. You shouldn't wear a tampon or menstrual cup for this bleeding until you get the all clear from your provider.

Checking In with Health Care Providers After Delivery

The newest World Health Organization (WHO) guidelines recommend four checkups after delivery. At each one, you should be asked about how your perineum is healing, how your bladder is working, and about your lochia, and any tear or stitches should be evaluated to ensure healing is proceeding as expected. The timing for these checkups is as follows:

- Day one (within twenty-four hours)
- Day three (48–72 hours)
- Between days seven and fourteen
- Six weeks

Healing Process: 6–8 Weeks and Beyond

By eight weeks after delivery, many women are still reporting vulvar and vaginal health issues related to delivery. The most common are hemorrhoids (23 percent), constipation (20 percent), and vaginal discharge (15 percent). However, with time, most issues resolve.

If you think your stitches have come out or your wound is falling apart, do not wait for your six-week checkup. Also, if you have an increase in pain, develop a fever, or have a foul-smelling discharge, call your provider or make an appointment. These can be signs of infection.

When to start pelvic exercises

The French system is often held up as a standard for postpartum pelvic floor therapy—the implication online is that there is a nationwide program for pelvic floor rehabilitation at 6–8 weeks postpartum, although according to the 2016 guidelines by the French College of Gynaecologists and Obstetricians (CNGOF), routine pelvic floor physical therapy is not recommended in the absence of incontinence. This is not shade on the French; they are ahead of many countries in this regard, but there does not appear to be a standardized French technique or timing.

Some recommendations for pelvic floor therapy after delivery include the following:

- Pelvic floor physical therapy should not start sooner than two months after delivery, to allow for the tissues to heal and return to baseline.
- Women who have persistent urinary or fecal incontinence at three months after delivery should be offered pelvic floor physical therapy. At least three sessions with an appropriately trained therapist are recommended, as well as home exercises. This improves the speed of recovery but not the outcome—if you do not do the therapy, you will not be worse off incontinence-wise in the long term.
- If you wish to strengthen your pelvic floor, have no symptoms, and are at least two months from delivery, then home exercises (see chapter 10) are a fine, low-cost way to start.

Pain with sex

Most health care providers recommend waiting 4–6 weeks after an uncomplicated vaginal delivery before resuming sex. The open cervix could theoretically increase the risk of infection (although I'm not sure this has been rigorously studied). Also, the tissues need time to heal.

By six weeks after a delivery, 41 percent of women have resumed sex; 78 percent by twelve weeks; and 90–94 percent by six months. Women with a third- or fourth-degree tear are slightly less likely to have resumed sex by six months (88 percent). Having any kind of tear with delivery increases the chance that there will be pain with sex. If you have pain with sex that persists beyond three months after a vaginal delivery, then you should be evaluated.

The three most common causes of painful sex after a vaginal delivery include the following:

- **LOW ESTROGEN LEVELS IN THE VAGINA:** This is almost exclusively seen in women who are breastfeeding, which can stop ovulation. A small amount of vaginal estrogen cream can solve the problem within a few weeks if lubricant is not sufficient. Once regular menstrual cycles return, your estrogen levels will go up and the vaginal estrogen may be stopped. Using a small amount of estrogen in the vagina is fine while breastfeeding.
- **PROBLEMS WITH THE SCAR OR NERVE PAIN:** Occasionally, the tissues may heal together in a way that creates a web of tissue at the opening, which can cause pain with penetration. Nerve pain in not common, but when tissues tear or are cut, nerves are injured as well. Prolonged pushing can also stretch nerves.
- **MUSCLE SPASM:** The muscles of the pelvic floor can become inappropriately tight after delivery. The cause is unknown, but as it can happen after a cesarian section, stretch or injury to the pelvic muscles does not seem to be a requirement. My theory is the rapid withdrawal of progesterone after the placenta is delivered predisposes women to muscle spasms, as progesterone is a potent muscle relaxant. Specialized pelvic floor physical therapy is the treatment and is highly effective.

IS THERE SUCH A THING AS A HUSBAND STITCH? There are stories that circulate about OB/GYNs who reportedly announce at the delivery that they are putting in an "extra stitch" to "tighten" things up for the male partner. In over twenty-five years in OB/GYN, I have heard one older physician many years ago make a bad joke like this, but I never saw him do it. What I have heard are many male partners joking about this in the delivery room and more than a few asking *in all seriousness* if an extra stitch were possible.

I have asked many OB/GYNs about the "husband stitch," and uniformly they have all recounted almost identical experiences to my own.

It is important not to confuse a repair that has healed incorrectly or one that was not repaired correctly (mistake or error) with one that was sewn too tightly on purpose. There can be a lot of swelling after delivery, and occasionally this can make a repair technically challenging even for a highly skilled physician. Stitches can occasionally come apart a few days after delivery and then the raw edges heal together incorrectly or in a suboptimal way. There is also, unfortunately, incompetence.

Is it possible that some horrible doctors have done "a husband stitch"? Nothing would surprise me. After all, there are rare pilots who show up drunk and rare reporters who fabricate sources. However, the idea that this is common is not something that I can verify. As someone who specializes in pain with sex, I have not seen a case in over twenty-three years of practice.

If a woman feels too tight after a delivery and/or has persistent pain with sex, it is usually the result of muscle spasm. Narrowing of the vaginal opening after a vaginal delivery due to a poorly healed bridge of skin— either due to the way the tissues healed, complications afterwards, or the quality of the repair—does happen, but in my experience, this is less common than muscle spasm.

Long-term outcomes for sexual function

Studies have looked at whether childbirth affects long-term sexual function. A large study of over one thousand women from an ethnically diverse background showed no association between method of delivery or birth complications and long-term sexual satisfaction.

I found this surprising, as some women definitely do have difficulty recovering sexually after a vaginal delivery.

I suspect the answer is both complex and simple. There are so many variables in sexual functioning, but a caring partner who you love and who is a good lover (meaning the kind of lover you need) is probably the most important. Also, pain with sex and difficulties achieving orgasm are very common before pregnancy and can happen to women who have had C-sections and women who have never been pregnant.

Looking specifically at women over forty, this same study tells us that 56 percent of women had lost interest in sex, 53 percent had sex less than once a month, and 43 percent had low sexual satisfaction. The bad news is that is a lot of women. The good news is the method of delivery didn't appear to be the driving factor. Sexual function just isn't about a body part, it's about you as a whole person.

To put it in perspective, changes in libido, sexual priorities, and satisfaction with their sexual relationship also happen to gay men who adopt a baby. Basically, a baby changes things even when there is no pain from delivery and no pregnancy-related hormonal changes postpartum.

BOTTOM LINE

- During delivery, 44–75 percent of women will tear.
- By six weeks after delivery, 41 percent of women have resumed sex.
- Breastfeeding is associated with pain during sex for the first six months.
- Pelvic floor PT is definitely recommended if you have incontinence; in other situations, Kegel exercises are likely as effective.
- The method of delivery may have a short-term impact on sexual function, but not likely a long-term one

Everyday Practicalities and V Maintenance

CHAPTER 6

Medical Maintenance

THE VULVA AND VAGINA DO NOT REQUIRE regular checkups. If you have symptoms or concerns—for example, a pain or an itch, or even questions—then of course you need to be seen, but there is no reason your doctor needs to evaluate your vulva or vagina on a regular basis for disease prevention. Some organs do require screening for health purposes, including the cervix for cervical cancer (see chapter 26), screening for high blood pressure starting at the age of eighteen, and colon cancer screening for otherwise low-risk individuals starting at age fifty. However, not everything requires screening, and the vulva and vagina fall into that category. In fact, yearly pelvic exams are no longer recommended.

Screening vs. Diagnostic Test

A screening test is done when there are no symptoms of a condition—the idea is that finding and treating before there are symptoms will reduce complications and even save lives. As far as the lower genital tract is concerned, the best examples are screening for chlamydia and cervical cancer. Neither of those conditions produce symptoms in early stages, but identifying them early and starting therapy reduces complications, and in the case of cervical cancer, screening can save lives.

Screening can target everyone. For example, all women should be screened for cervical cancer. Screening may also target higher-risk individuals, such as people with multiple sexual partners and STIs.

A diagnostic test, on the other hand, is done to help identify the cause of symptoms. For example, if there is an ulcer on the skin, a swab may be taken to test for herpes or a biopsy may be taken to identify a skin condition. An important concept that doctors don't always explain is that diagnostic tests are also ordered to rule out conditions—so the answer your doctor may be looking for is "not cancer." This can be very frustrating for a patient who thinks they will be getting a definitive answer. A common scenario with the vulva is a biopsy for a persistent itch. A biopsy (a small procedure that removes a 3–4 mm piece of skin) may be recommended to rule out an early cancer. While the biopsy may help diagnose the cause of the itch, many times the results are nonspecific, so the best the biopsy did was rule out cancer (still very important).

Menstrual Cycle Primer

While this is *The Vagina Bible* and not the "Uterus and Ovary Bible," having a good working knowledge of the changes that occur each month with the menstrual cycle will be helpful in understanding a lot of what follows in this book.

Menstruation is the shedding of the lining of the uterus (the endometrium) when a pregnancy has not occurred. The average age of menarche—the first menstrual cycle—is 12–13 years. The first day of the menstrual cycle, or day 1 of your cycle, is the first day of bleeding (so the first day of your period). Menstrual bleeding typically lasts 3–7 days (see chapter 17 for more on the amount of blood).

The menstrual cycle is regulated by several intricate hormonal circuits all working together in harmony. Sometimes I visualize this as three jugglers who occasionally have to throw one of their balls to another while they all continue to juggle. If everything is on point, then the system works flawlessly; however, one late throw or missed catch and everything gets out of whack. The three jugglers in the case of menstruation are the hypothalamus (a part of the brain), the pituitary gland (also in the brain), and the ovaries.

The hypothalamus releases a hormone called gonadotropin-releasing hormone (GnRH) and this process can be easily disturbed by stress, sleep disturbance, and weight loss or gain. GnRH triggers the pituitary gland to release the hormone follicle stimulating hormone (FSH), which tells the ovary to start developing follicles (eggs). The follicles produce estrogen, which makes the lining of the uterus thicken. The estrogen provides feedback to the pituitary gland. When estrogen levels are high enough, the pituitary releases a hormone called luteinizing hormone (LH), which triggers ovulation.

After ovulation the egg heads down the fallopian tube to the uterus, and the tissue left behind (like an eggshell, but soft), called the corpus luteum, produces progesterone. While estrogen thickens the uterine lining (think of it like stacking bricks), progesterone stabilizes the lining (a bit like mortar). The corpus luteum can only produce progesterone for approximately 14 days unless it gets a signal from a pregnancy. Without fertilization, the corpus luteum shrinks and the progesterone is rapidly withdrawn and this causes the lining of the uterus to come out as a period. And we are back at the beginning of the cycle, with day 1 being the day bleeding starts.

Estrogen and progesterone have wide-ranging effects beyond the ovaries, uterus, and vagina. The cyclic changes can affect mood, the immune system, and even sensitivity to touch.

When should I start seeing a gynecologist or other woman's health care specialist?

Some women prefer a gynecologist; however, many prefer their family medicine doctors and nurse practitioners. Even some pediatricians are comfortable providing reproductive health care. Who you see for regular checkups and for symptoms, such as an itch or sexually transmitted infection (STI) screening, may vary depending on a number of factors.

A screening visit regarding reproductive preventive health care is recommended between the ages of thirteen years and fifteen years. This visit could be with any provider who is comfortable talking with teens about sex and reproductive health. This visit is an opportunity to discuss any reproductive health concerns, such as menstrual protection or safe sex. A pelvic exam (meaning checking inside the vagina) is not required unless there are symptoms, and for a teen who has not yet been sexually active a pelvic exam can almost always be avoided.

Screening for STIs should begin whenever a teen becomes sexually active and continue until the age of twenty-four (see chapter 28). Regardless of whether you have or haven't been sexually active, cervical cancer screening starts at the age of twenty-one (see chapter 26). A "get to know you" visit before you may need to get reproductive health care of any kind is never a bad idea. This allows you to get comfortable with the person with whom you will be sharing intimate details before you need to share them. For women who have never been sexually active or never had a pelvic exam, this visit can be especially helpful to familiarize themselves with what the exam might entail and the medical equipment that is involved.

Any woman or teen twenty-four years or younger who is sexually active should be seeing a provider who is comfortable with gynecologic care for annual chlamydia screenings. Screening for other sexually transmitted infections may also be indicated. Urine screening is very effective, so taking a pelvic exam out of the equation often makes this screening easier for many women regardless of age.

What is a pelvic exam?

A pelvic exam has two components: looking inside the vagina with a speculum to see the vagina and cervix, and touching inside with gloved and lubricated fingers of one hand into the vagina (the other hand may press down on the lower abdomen to feel the uterus and ovaries). This second part of the exam may be called an internal exam or a bimanual exam. This evaluates the uterus, ovaries, pelvic muscles, and any masses or irregularities in the vagina or in the pelvis (meaning on or around the uterus and ovaries). Sometimes a rectal exam (inserting a gloved finger into the rectum) may be indicated. Whether an internal exam and/or rectal exam is needed depends on the reason for the exam.

A speculum is a medical tool for looking inside the body. There are many different kinds, and the type used for cervical cancer screening and STI testing is called a bivalve speculum. This is made of two blades (they are not sharp, just slightly curved).

A bivalve speculum is inserted closed, which makes insertion less painful, and then opened once it is deep enough. A screw or similar

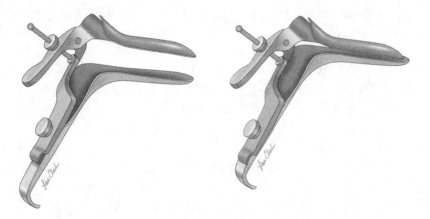

Image 6: Speculum open (left) and closed (right). ILLUSTRATIONS BY LISA A. CLARK, MA, CMI.

device keeps the blades open during the exam. When opened, the speculum allows the provider to see the cervix and the upper vagina. The sides of the speculum are open, and so if the speculum is rotated the vaginal walls can also be inspected.

There are several different types of bivalve speculums, all with minor modifications that can sometimes help make them more comfortable or practical, as every woman is shaped differently. The common speculums are Pedersen, Graves, and Cusco and are named after the men who designed the modifications. A Graves is wider at the tip (this is useful for seeing the cervix for procedures), but is almost never needed for a regular exam. The wider tip can make insertion more painful.

The speculums come in different sizes; a narrow speculum is approximately the width of a finger, and many times this can be used, reducing discomfort significantly. I liken this to trying on clothes at the store—I was always told to start with the smallest pair of pants that I think has a reasonable chance of fitting.

In general, someone who has used tampons or a menstrual cup successfully or who has been sexually active will do well with a speculum and pelvic exam performed by a provider who makes them feel at ease, proceeds at a comfortable pace, and is aware of physical cues that might suggest the exam has become painful and knows to stop and reaffirm that it is okay to proceed or make adjustments as necessary.

A speculum and pelvic exam shouldn't be painful; there may be pressure or minor discomfort, but it should not hurt. If it does, speak up and ask your doctor to stop.

Annual pelvic examinations are no longer recommended, as screening the pelvic organs and vagina this way does not reliably identify any medical condition—in short, it is a poor screening test. If you have no symptoms, your exam is over after your cervical cancer screening.

DOES THE SPECULUM HAVE A RACIST LEGACY? Some women do not like the idea of a speculum because they have been told it was invented by Dr. Marion Sims, known to some as the father of modern American gynecology and to many others, including myself, as a shoddy doctor, a racist, and an all-around terrible man who experimented on enslaved women without consent and who was only in medicine for the money.

It is common medical lore that Dr. Sims reportedly developed the first reproducible surgical technique for vesicovaginal fistulas (a connection between the bladder and vagina due to injuries during childbirth). He did not. Other surgeons had been successful before his time, and reading the work of his peers, it is clear his technique was not easily (if at all) reproducible. Sims also opened the first public hospital for women dedicated to repairing injuries from pregnancy and childbirth. Fistulas were a significant source of distress for women, and Sims hypothesized if he could device a reliable fistula repair technique, he could make a fortune. Sims was eventually asked to leave that hospital for refusing to follow various policies.

Sims did design a speculum for looking in the vagina to facilitate surgery, but this is not a bivalve speculum. Sims was also hardly the first one to design such a speculum. The first speculum may date back to Roman times (one was excavated at Pompeii), and a vaginal speculum was in use by surgeons in 1818, so before Sims's time. In 1825, a French midwife, Marie Anne Boivin, modified the speculum, and what we use today is a version of her creation—a top and a bottom blade that can be opened so the sides (vaginal walls) and top (cervix) can be seen. Sims's device has one blade and a far different sort of handle. It is infuriating that in addition to all the medically unethical and racist things that Sims did to women, he also erased the fact that the bivalve speculum was created by a woman.

While I believe there could be modifications to speculum design to make the experience better for women and provide a better view for providers, for now you can rest assured that the speculum being used by your provider was not designed by Sims, nor based on his design.

WHAT IF SPECULUM EXAMS ARE ALWAYS PAINFUL? There are two reasons: you have a medical condition or your provider has poor technique.

If you only have pain with pelvic exams, then the technique is likely the issue. If you are nervous beforehand or have had a previous traumatic experience, either sexual trauma or a traumatic exam with a provider, those memories can come back during an exam and may make you more likely to have pain during the exam, but they are not the cause.

If you have pain with a tampon or menstrual cup insertion or with sexual activity, then it is possible that you have a medical condition that causes vaginal or vulvar pain, and those may make pelvic exams more painful. However, even in these situations it is best to stop and regroup. Exam techniques can almost always be modified to lessen the pain experience. Many women tell me just knowing their provider cares to minimize their pain matters greatly.

The only situation where a painful exam should continue, and even then this should be with consent, is a true medical emergency—meaning you are hemorrhaging and your provider needs to stop the bleeding immediately to save your life or to prevent other complications, such as needing a blood transfusion. Outside of the emergency department, that is rarely the situation. It does not apply to cervical cancer screening, evaluation of pain with sex, or any other symptoms discussed in this book.

Some women put on a stoic face, others mistakenly believe pelvic and speculum exams are painful for all women, and some women are clearly in pain and ignored by their providers. As I am not one of those providers, I am not sure I have an explanation. All I know is I evaluate women with pain every day, and every day I hear that it was the least painful exam they have ever had. It is better to invest in the outcome and start with a little information, and then as the medical condition starts to improve more evaluation can be done if needed. A lot of testing can be done with just a swab, and so a speculum can often be avoided, with the exception of dealing with vaginitis. However, even then we can start with swabs and build confidence and devise strategies to reduce pain. A narrow speculum, which many women find they can tolerate, is also often all that is needed.

The Potential Downside of Fewer Visits

The annual gynecological exam is really a thing of the past. There are a lot of upsides to avoiding unnecessary testing. Women avoid physical exams that are intrusive and can be embarrassing and/or painful. There is also the benefit of reducing expense as well as worry from false-positive results. In medicine, we have jargon for these incidental yet medically meaningless findings that we are now required to prove are meaningless—incidentalomas.

There is one downside that has not been studied: women who do not see their reproductive health provider annually may have less of a rapport. When you see someone every three or five years, it is a lot harder to bring up intimate concerns than when you see them once a year. It is also true that when annual pelvic exams were recommended, many providers never asked questions about sex, and so these visits involved a lot of frustrating missed opportunities. I am not sure fewer visits will help that.

I often wonder if an annual check-in by phone would be helpful, so a gynecological provider can hear a woman's story and let her know if she needs STI testing outside of the routine screening recommendations, ask about sexual health or other vulvar and vaginal concerns, and provide any age-specific reproductive health advice. Women are exposed to so much misinformation and disinformation that giving women the option of checking in quickly might be something worth studying.

BOTTOM LINE

- Annual pelvic exams are not recommended.
- A pelvic exam should not be painful.
- If a speculum exam is necessary, narrow Pedersen or Cusco speculums are the smallest and are often all that is needed.
- The bivalve speculum used for vaginal exams and Pap smears was not invented by Dr. Sims.
- The only regular evaluations related to vaginal health are cervical cancer and STI screenings.

CHAPTER 7

Food and Vaginal Health

THERE IS AN ONGOING MYTH that food has a direct impact on vaginal health. Over the past twenty-five years, I have been interviewed by multiple reporters on this subject. Many times, I gave a detailed account of why a direct gut-vagina connection is biologically impossible, yet headlines such as "Eat Pineapple for a Sweeter Vagina!" or "Banish Yeast by Ditching Bread!" always appeared. It seems the truth, "Your Vagina Just Wants You to Eat a Healthy, Balanced Diet!" isn't sexy enough.

What's the harm, you say?

This supposed direct connection between food and the vagina is a complete misunderstanding of how the body works, and facts matter. In addition, the idea of eating food to change the way a vagina smells supports the tired and destructive trope that there is something wrong with a normal, healthy vagina. It's simply a different spin on douches.

The other issue with vaginal food fallacies is that they can lead to severe dietary hypervigilance and restrictions—essentially, vaginal orthorexia (orthorexia is an eating disorder with extreme attention to foods perceived as healthy and avoidance of foods believed to be harmful). I have lost track of the number of women who have told me they haven't had a slice of cake or a cookie for years, trying to rid themselves of yeast, and yet they still have their same symptoms. The exasperation in these voices is not insignificant. And really, having a slice or cake or a cookie now and then is nice.

If you have a concerning vaginal odor, you should read chapter 43 and see a doctor or nurse practitioner—the remedy is most definitely not at the grocery store.

Can Fruit Change the Smell of My Vagina?

Vaginal discharge is a combination of epithelial cells from the vaginal walls, breakdown products made by healthy vaginal bacteria (lactobacilli), cervical mucus, and a small amount of transudate (fluid that leaks out between cells). See chapter 2 for a review. The biggest contributors to vaginal scent are substances produced by the lactobacilli, just as body odor is related to skin bacteria breaking down products made by specialized sweat glands.

Food will not kill lactobacilli, make it reproduce, or change the products of lactobacilli metabolism. For food to rapidly change vaginal odor in an eat-this-then-smell-like-that kind of phenomenon, a volatile substance (meaning something that can evaporate and produce a smell) would have to survive digestion or be created by digestion and then make it to the vagina. As only the tiniest bit of fluid from the bloodstream even makes it into the vagina, this would have to be a very potent substance. It would also have to somehow not affect body odor or the smell of urine.

Basically, magic would be required for a food to change the scent of a vagina.

What About Garlic and Asparagus?

There are a few volatile metabolites from food that are known to impact body odors. They have pungent or musty smells, so not sweet or desirable. The best-known example is the smell of urine after eating asparagus. While the actual mechanism is still not known, most researchers think some people metabolize asparagusic acid from asparagus into a sulfur smelling compound that is excreted in the urine. Approximately 40 percent or so of people can smell these unpleasant metabolites. The reason some people can detect the smell as nasty and others cannot may be genetic. Garlic also has volatile metabolites, described as having a garlic-and/or cabbage-like odor, that have been detected in urine and in breast milk. Kidneys and breast tissue actively concentrate certain metabolites, so it makes sense that if you eat enough garlic, a malodorous metabolite could be concentrated in urine or breast milk and impact smell.

The vagina does not concentrate metabolites.

The Sugar-Yeast Connection

There is a relationship between blood sugar and infections, but eating foods high in sugar does not directly impact the vagina.

As we discussed in chapter 2—but it's worth another mention—up to 3 percent of the vaginal fluid is glycogen, a storage sugar. There is also glucose as well. The amount of glycogen and sugar varies depending on the phase of the menstrual cycle, but at times it can be found in a higher percentage than blood.

It is not possible to change the sugar level in your vagina through diet, as the sugar comes from the mucosal (skin) cells. Researchers actually attempted to increase the storage sugar in the mucosal cells by having women eat more carbohydrates, and it was ineffective. In another study, women ingested a load of sugar, equivalent to guzzling two cans of cola, and researchers found sugar levels did not increase in the blood or in the vagina, not even for women with a history of yeast infections.

Your vagina needs sugar, and the levels in your vagina have nothing to do with food.

Yeast infections are a major issue in the intensive care unit. We all have yeast in our bowel, vagina, and on our skin, so when we have invasive procedures that break the skin barrier, the normal, minding-its-own-business yeast can now enter the bloodstream. This is a systemic yeast infection, and it is very serious. Without intravenous therapy, it is fatal. Researchers have looked at diets and nutritional supplements for people in the intensive care unit to try to reduce yeast colonization in an attempt to reduce these serious yeast infections, and to date they have all failed. If diet could reduce yeast colonization, we would already know. A doctor selling a special diet and supplements who has never published research in the area does not have the secret answer to the question of how to reduce yeast colonization. The idea of an anti-candida diet is simply not supported by basic biology or the available research.

There are studies that indicate women with diabetes (a condition associated with higher blood sugars) are more likely to have yeast in the vagina, and that yeast is more likely to overgrow and cause infections. It is also true that this is complex, and the reasons are not fully understood. Recently, data has emerged that points to increased glucose in the *urine* as the cause. When blood sugar levels are high, excess sugar literally spills into the urine. When women empty their bladders, there is a microscopic mist of urine that gets on the skin. While the vagina evolved to tolerate sugar, the skin of the vulva has not, and glucose exposure here can favor the growth of yeast, leading to vulvar yeast infections. Some of that yeast may make it into the vagina, leading to a vaginal infection.

This theory is supported by a safety alert from the Food and Drug Administration (FDA) regarding a serious infection of the genitals (necrotizing fasciitis, also known as the flesh-eating bacteria) associated with a class of medications called sodium-glucose cotransporter 2 (SGLT2) inhibitors. This includes canagliflozin, dapagliflozin, and empagliflozin. The medication is used to lower blood sugar for people who have type 2 diabetes, and it works by helping the kidneys remove more sugar. This could lead to increased glucose on the skin that could favor the growth of pathogenic (harmful) bacteria.

Elevated blood sugars may also impact the way the immune system responds to infections or even the healthy bacteria that helps to keep infections at bay.

So you have read all this, and you are not convinced about the lack of dietary connection between sugar and yeast in the vagina (for women who do not have diabetes) because you feel that you get vaginal symptoms every time you eat sugar.

The answer is what is called a "nocebo effect," which is a negative effect on health due to negative expectations (basically an unpleasant placebo response). It is the result of conditioning, specifically the belief that something negative will happen. This doesn't mean someone with symptoms of irritation after eating sugar is faking or that their symptoms are not real. There are real chemical changes in the brain producing the itch or irritation, but the cause of those changes is a negative expectation, not sugar. Nocebo effects are well studied. Every drug trial that has one group take a placebo, an inert sugar pill, has at least 2–5 percent of people who discontinue the placebo due to serious side effects that are perceived to be drug related. As these people didn't receive an actual medication, their symptoms can only be explained by negative expectations, or nocebo.

Can bread or beer or wine cause yeast infections?

Yeast is used to make wine, beer, and bread, so it is easy to see how the myth of alcohol or bread causing yeast was started. Common sense tells us this can't be so, as the French have been enjoying fine breads and wine for hundreds of years, and French women are not plagued with yeast infections.

Science backs up the common sense. The yeast most commonly used for bread and alcohol is *Saccharomyces cerevisiae*, and this is only *rarely* a cause of vaginal yeast infections (about 1 percent of the time). Sourdough starters scavenge wild yeasts like *Saccharomyces exiguus*, *Candida milleri*, and *Candida humilis* from the environment, which do not cause vaginal yeast infections (they also scavenge *S. cerevisiae*). If that isn't enough reassurance, then consider that yeast in bread, wine, and pasteurized or filtered beer is dead. An unfiltered, unpasteurized beer may have some yeast that is dormant—but again, this isn't the right type.

I understand that a woman claimed to have made bread with a sourdough starter she nourished with her vaginal yeast, and this seems as good a place as any to address this story. First of all, we have no idea if what she grew from her vagina was *Candida albicans* (the most common cause of yeast infections) or even any type of yeast, for that matter. Belief that you cultured something doesn't cut it scientifically. The vagina is filled with bacteria, and any swab not cultured appropriately in a lab may grow all kinds of microorganisms, most of which will not be yeast. Second, her sourdough starter, like all sourdough starters, would have scavenged the wild yeast from the air and surface of the flour, etc., and so even if she did manage to grow yeast from her vagina, it would have added nothing to the baking except temporary internet fame—and, of course, more confusion about yeast. The next time you see this story make the rounds on the Internet, please don't pass it along. Just ignore it.

If you want to prove that vaginal yeast can bake bread, you are going to need to add cultured *C. albicans* directly to the flour as you would any store-bought yeast, but that seems like a thoroughly unnecessary exercise. So let's not.

The Best Foods for Vaginas

There are no bad or good foods, as far as the vagina is concerned. I know this upsets a lot of people, but there are really no good or bad foods in general, with the exception of trans fats, which are modified fats linked with inflammation and heart disease. Avoid these for all kinds of health reasons (this means saying goodbye to icing from a can). There are healthy diets and less healthy diets, and eating well is good preventative medicine, but eating a specific food as treatment doesn't apply to the vagina.

What about cranberry juice for preventing urinary tract or bladder infections? In the early 1900s, before we had modern methods to diagnose bladder infections and before antibiotics, doctors recommended cranberry juice because the hippuric acid that is released as the body metabolizes cranberries makes the urine very acidic. The theory was the acidity would make it harder for bacteria to grow. Cranberries also have a lectin (a protein) that may prevent bacteria from binding to cells in the urinary tract (bacterial adherence to cells is a necessary step in infections). While both of these hypotheses are biologically plausible and worthy of pursuit, multiple studies have looked at cranberry juice and found *no benefit*. In addition, juice has no nutritional value; it's just nature's soda. Cranberry juice, even unsweetened, has a lot of sugar, and some brands can have as much as soda.

Two small studies have linked a high dietary saturated-fat (animal fat, so meats and dairy) intake with bacterial vaginosis, but this is *far* from a certainty. A high-fat diet could also be a correlation, not a cause, meaning women with these diets are more likely to have other risk factors for bacterial vaginosis. How this connection might exist biologically is simply not known. There are other health reasons besides your vagina to try to avoid a diet that is very high in saturated fat.

Eating at least 25 g of fiber a day is the best preventative health advice I can offer vagina-wise, as fiber is a prebiotic, meaning it feeds good bacteria in the bowel. Fiber also draws water into the stool, softening it and helping it move along more quickly, thereby preventing constipation. Constipation can lead to straining, which can cause pelvic floor spasm (potentially causing pain with sex or pelvic pain) and hemorrhoids. The average American only eats 7–8 g of fiber a day, so I recommend a fiber count, meaning writing everything down that you eat for 1–2 days and then checking the fiber count so you know how much you are eating and can make changes if necessary. I'm a little lazy, so I just eat a cereal with 8–13 g of fiber a serving most days, so I know I'm one third to one half of the way there before I've even started my day.

Lots of people ask about fermented foods, such as yogurt, sauerkraut, or kombucha, to help cultivate good gut bacteria. Typically, these foods do not contain the right strains of lactobacilli for vaginal health, although they may have bacteria that is healthy for the gut. Some studies have linked fermented milk products like yogurt with a reduction in bladder cancer, heart disease, gum disease, and cardiovascular disease. Fermentation enhances the nutritional value of vegetables and may increase the iron that is available for absorption. Many women are iron deficient, so this obviously won't hurt.

It is *possible* the bacteria in fermented dairy and vegetables could have a beneficial impact on normal gut bacteria after antibiotics, but we don't have any research on the impact on vaginal health. Having fermented foods if you are on antibiotics is probably not a bad strategy to try to lessen the impact of antibiotics on your gut bacteria (this is a cause of antibiotic-related diarrhea). However, as there are no studies that prove this works, I wouldn't sweat it if you don't like fermented foods and that strategy doesn't appeal to you. Personally, I despise sauerkraut and kombucha, and for me to give them a try there would need to be several very robust studies to show they definitively help protect gut bacteria after antibiotics.

BOTTOM LINE

- Food can't change the vaginal scent.
- There is no anti-candida diet. If you don't have diabetes, what you eat is not going to give you a yeast infection (and even if you do have diabetes, it is more about the urine and immune system).
- No evidence shows cranberry juice prevents bladder infections.
- Eating 25 g of fiber a day will help keep your gut healthy, and indirectly that will help your vagina.
- Fermented foods might (emphasis on might) be useful if you are taking antibiotics.

CHAPTER 8

The Bottom Line on Underwear

ALMOST EVERY WOMAN HAS BEEN TOLD at least once (and often more than once) to wear white cotton underwear as a medical recommendation to prevent yeast infections and other vaginal mayhem. This makes it sound as if vaginas and vulvas are accidents waiting to happen. The vulva can handle urine, feces, and blood, and vaginas can handle blood, ejaculate, and a baby, so this idea that a black lace thong is the harbinger of a vaginal or vulvar apocalypse is absurd.

I love pretty underwear. Perhaps it is from years of my mother buying the kind of underwear for me she thought "nice girls" (i.e., those who only have sex for procreation) should wear—hideously floral and large. It is also possible it's from a lifetime of wearing surgical scrubs, where the only self-expression through clothing could be what was underneath. Regardless, if wearing lace or dyed fabric were bad for the vulva, I would know better than to expose myself to potential infection by wearing them.

Really, white cotton underwear doesn't protect against yeast infections?

The white cotton underwear myth started before we knew about the vaginal ecosystem or the biology of yeast infections. How far it goes back

I am not sure, but it wouldn't surprise me if it dates back to the time when women were advised to douche with Lysol and "lace" meant "loose."

There are low-quality studies that link polyester underwear and panty-hose with yeast infections. These studies interviewed women who did and didn't have a history of yeast infections, and then asked them what kind of underwear they wore. The yeast infections were not proven by culture (the gold standard); rather self-diagnosis was used. This is problematic, for as many as 70 percent of women who self-diagnose with yeast infections are incorrect. When something bad happens, like vulvar or vaginal irritation, people are more likely to remember things they feel could be related than those who have not had the same bad experience. This is called recall bias. Finally, if you have a lot of itching and irritation and you have been told about wearing white cotton underwear, you may have switched and had a placebo effect. More recent studies of higher quality have shown no connection between underwear and yeast infections.

For underwear to cause an issue, it would have to change the ecosystem (perhaps by altering the pH of the skin), trap excess moisture, or cause friction. The combination of moisture and friction can cause microtrauma, which could allow the normal yeast on the skin to cause an infection.

Underwear can't change vaginal pH; that is an inside job. There are a few studies looking at the effects of tight clothing on the vulvar skin, and there was no effect on bacterial colonization or pH. One study evaluated new underwear for athletics (performance underwear), which are not cotton but are designed to wick moisture away from the skin to improve comfort (wet underwear is unpleasant), and there were no health concerns. Thongs also appear to have no negative impact.

The only thing that can change the pH and microenvironment of the vulva is something occlusive—think waterproof, like plastic or latex. This can be an issue for women who have to wear waterproof incontinence underwear daily.

Underwear needs to fit correctly—if you are tugging at your groin or it is digging in or chafing, you could potentially develop skin irritation, but typically that kind of underwear is too uncomfortable to wear long enough to develop a health problem. It is probably also best to not wear underwear made of plastic or latex, as anything that causes you to sweat could be an issue.

What about a bathing suit?

The idea that women sit around in wet bathing suits all day intrigues me. I wonder if anyone promoting bathing suit panic has even seen a modern bathing garment? My suit tends to dry pretty quickly. That *is* sort of the point. Also, a little water against your skin is not going to damage anything. I mean honestly, if it does we have evolved rather unfortunately. Our vulvar skin gets wet a lot, and many humans spend a lot of time in the water. Dampness that dries relatively quickly is not going to cause an issue. If you sit in soaking wet clothes for several hours, you may develop skin irritation called maceration— a superficial skin injury from the combination of moisture and friction. This is why runners put petroleum jelly between their thighs before a long run, to prevent the maceration from friction and sweat. So if you throw on your clothes on top of a soaking wet bathing suit, you could potentially get some chafing, but the comfort factor of soaking shorts or pants is probably going to drive most women to change before they get a superficial skin injury.

Do I even need to wear underwear?

There is no medical reason to wear or not wear underwear. Many women tell me they don't wear undergarments so their "vagina can breathe," but the vulva and vagina don't have lungs. The vagina doesn't like oxygen, or even air. Occlusive garments such as incontinence products can affect vulvar skin integrity, so taking a break from these kinds of products if possible may help the skin, but otherwise the degree of air circulation that comes from wearing nothing is your choice.

Some women find the seams of pants directly against their skin uncomfortable, others don't mind it, and some like how it feels. It's all good. It comes down to comfort, how you feel about underwear, and whether you prefer to wash any vaginal discharge out of your pants, pajama bottoms, or your underwear.

Does it matter how I wash my underwear?

Women are told two competing things about washing their underwear: that they need to practically sterilize them, but also that they should use gentle detergent.

Let's start with common sense. Every time you empty your bladder or bowels there is a microscopic plume of urine and feces that gets on your skin. It is not possible for the vulva to be sterile, and the vagina is full of bacteria. The only way you could make things worse bacteria-wise is if you rinsed your underwear in raw sewage (okay, I am exaggerating a little here for effect). You could wear the same underwear every day for a week, and while they might smell a little ripe from body odor and be a little crusty with discharge, they won't cause an infection.

Clean underwear may matter medically after hair removal, although this has never been tested. All forms of pubic hair grooming (with the exception of trimming) cause microtrauma, and so freshly laundered underwear seems advisable. Remember, most vulvar skin infections start because there was a break in the skin, allowing the normal yeast or bacteria on the skin to breach the first line of defense.

Washing in hot water seems unnecessary with modern detergents. I'm certainly no home economist; however, I do my washing in cold water to save money (energy is very expensive in California) and for the environment. Every bit of electricity we use has some environmental footprint.

Perfumes and fragrances are known irritants (it doesn't matter if they are botanical or lab made), and so it is best to avoid them in products that touch your skin, especially underwear, as the vulva is more prone to irritant reactions. A product can be fine everywhere except your vulva. I recommend using a detergent that is in the "free and clear" category. If you are not having any issues, then the "if it isn't broken, don't fix it" mentality is probably fine, but why needlessly expose yourself to a potential allergen?

If you are concerned that you could be having a reaction to detergent and switching to "free and clear" didn't help, the next step would be a consultation with your gynecologist to rule out other causes. If nothing is found, a visit with an allergist or possibly a dermatologist (sometimes they do skin testing for topical reactions) might be a good idea.

Fabric softener and dryer sheets can also cause irritant reactions, so I recommend avoiding them. A capful of white distilled vinegar in the fabric softener dispenser works well in the washing machine to soften clothes cheaply, and it's likely better for the environment. An added benefit of vinegar over fabric softener is that the latter can apparently increase odor and mildew if you have a front-load washer.

But underwear irritates me...

If it fits right and isn't made of plastic or latex, and you are using the fragrance-free detergent and no fabric softener or dryer sheets, it is unlikely your underwear that's causing the problem. The most common scenario is blaming underwear for unrelated symptoms. Some common causes of pain or irritation with the light touch or gentle friction of underwear are vulvodynia (a nerve pain condition of the vulva), and skin conditions like lichen sclerosus or lichen simplex chronicus (see chapters 33 and 35).

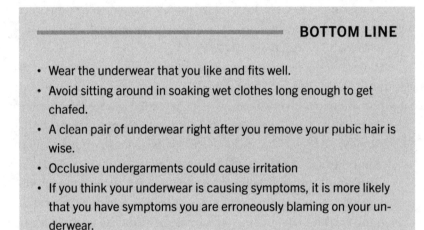

BOTTOM LINE

- Wear the underwear that you like and fits well.
- Avoid sitting around in soaking wet clothes long enough to get chafed.
- A clean pair of underwear right after you remove your pubic hair is wise.
- Occlusive undergarments could cause irritation
- If you think your underwear is causing symptoms, it is more likely that you have symptoms you are erroneously blaming on your underwear.

CHAPTER 9

The Lowdown on Lube

WOMEN REPORT THEY USE LUBE TO MAKE sex more fun, to try something new, and to make sex more comfortable. It's also important to use lubricant with condoms as it reduces condom breakage—and no, saliva does not count, as it's not a great lube. Despite what you may see in the movies, I'd skip honey. I've seen some irritating consequences.

According to a 2014 survey, 65 percent of women reported using lubricant at some point, and 20 percent said they had used lube within the last thirty days.

There are medical conditions that cause vaginal dryness, so if you've never needed lubricant before and all of a sudden you feel like your ecosystem has switched from garden to desert, it is worth checking out with your health care provider. The most common cause is menopause, but other causes of vaginal dryness include a yeast infection, breastfeeding, hormonal birth control that doesn't have estrogen (for example, the Depo-Provera injection and the implant Nexplanon), and muscle spasm around the vagina (the tightness causes more friction, and it can be perceived as dryness).

I hear from women that some male partners "don't like" lubricant or say it affects their erection. It's only a few milliliters of lube (far less than an ounce), so it's not exactly as if his penis is encased in pudding. I'm no urologist, but if he uses this "too wet" excuse, then either he doesn't know what an excited vagina feels like or he could be projecting his medical condition, typically erectile dysfunction, onto you.

Vaginal lubrication is part of the sexual response cycle and can vary from day to day and from partner to partner. The amount of foreplay and penetration will also affect what you need. Sometimes your mind is raring to go and your body hasn't quite caught up yet, so a boost from a bottle can get you there faster.

Whatever the reason, lube is your friend! I think of lubricant in the way I think of glasses—some people have always needed them, some of us need glasses as we age, and some just need glasses for reading. No one is judgy about glasses.

Remember, it's not how you got to the party, it's that you were at the party and had a good time!

The Choices

The lube section at the drugstore or online can be overwhelming, as there are a lot of options—even more so at specialty sex shops. However, at many sex shops you have a lube docent who can provide details on all of their offerings.

There are several categories of lube: water based, silicone, hybrid (silicone and water), oil based, and pure oil (think olive or coconut). Silicone lubricants stay around longer on the tissues versus water-based lubes, so you may need to reapply less and they can be used in the shower or bath. Some people find silicone harder to clean up than water based. Oil also has a lot of staying power and many people prefer the feel, but it can also stain sheets. Water-based lubricants are the easiest to clean up. All of these lubes are fine for anal sex.

Some people really care about the feel of their lube—sensation is very personal. I find there are two main tactile components to consider: the slip and the tackiness. Others are more bothered by the cleanup factor, some find taste an issue, and there are those who don't care as long as it is wet and gets the job done! The great thing about lube is you get to be Goldilocks and try a few so you can figure out your preference.

In addition to feel and cleanup factor, it's also important to make sure your lubricant doesn't irritate the vaginal tissues or negatively affect the healthy bacteria. The World Health Organization (WHO) has guidelines for water-based lubricants. Specifically, they recommend a pH of 3.5–4.5 (the same as the vaginal pH) and an osmolality of less than 380 mOsm/kg (the concentration of molecules in water; low osmolality means fewer molecules and high osmolality means more).

The osmolality of vaginal secretions is 260–280 mOsm/kg. If the osmolality of the lube is higher, it can pull water out of vaginal tissues, potentially causing irritation and increasing microtrauma, and theoretically increasing the risk of contracting an STI if exposed. The WHO recommends against lubricants with osmolality greater than 1,200 mOsm/kg. These recommendations don't apply to silicone and pure oil lubes as they don't have water, so there is no pH (pH is a measurement of hydrogen atoms in water) and no osmolality.

You also want to consider condom compatibility. Specifically, oil-based lubricants can weaken latex condoms. Silicone and water-based are fine. You can use any lubricant with polyurethane condoms. Sex toy compatibility can be an issue, with silicone lubricants potentially degrading silicone sex toys, so always follow the manufacturer's recommendations for lube choice. Silicone lubricants typically have the same basic ingredients: cyclomethicone and dimethicone.

As brands may switch ingredients, it is always important to check the label. There are some specific ingredients that you should know more about in terms of safety:

- **GLYCERIN (WHICH IS GLYCEROL) AND PROPYLENE GLYCOL:** Preservatives in many water-based lubricants. They have a high osmolality, and so the WHO recommends total glycerol content should be less than 8.3 percent. As yeast can potentially use glycerin/propylene glycol as a food source, it is possible they could contribute to yeast infections. High-glycerin lubes can also irritate and be mistaken for a yeast infection.
- **PARABENS:** Preservatives found in some water-based lubricants. They are endocrine disruptors, meaning they can act like a hormone on tissues with a potentially negative effect, although the amount used in lubricant is considered safe. Oxygen can be dangerous for the lungs when it is 100 percent pure (the 17 percent in air is obviously not), so the dose is what matters safety-wise.

For perspective, many plants are endocrine disruptors, like lavender and cannabis (marijuana), and people conveniently forget about those even though studies have raised safety concerns. Parabens have been well tested regarding allergic reactions and are an unlikely cause of irritation.

- **CHLORHEXIDINE GLUCONATE:** Also a preservative. In one study it killed all the good bacteria, so it is best to avoid.
- **POLYQUATERNIUM:** A preservative that may increase HIV-1 replication. There are not enough studies to say this is definitive, but until more data appears, the WHO suggests it go on the pass list.
- **WARMING LIQUIDS, OR COOLING OR "TINGLING" LUBES:** The active ingredient can be a higher concentration of propylene glycol, alcohol, botanicals, menthol, or even capsaicin (what makes chili peppers burn, and this definitely can feel like it burns when it contacts the vagina!). Some of these can irritate and others, like menthol, are untested in the vagina, so we don't know much. "Natural" or "plant-based" does not mean safe.
- **HYDROXYETHYLCELLULOSE:** Part of the "slip" in some water-based lubes. Some organic lubes tout this as natural because it is plant derived, but it's in many conventional lubricants as well, so it is not a special or rare lube ingredient. It can also be used by yeast as a food source.
- **"NATURAL" OR "ORGANIC" LUBES:** Marketing terms. All water-based lubricants contain preservatives, so "natural" does not mean preservative free. One lube even advertises about preservatives that they have "just enough for safety, not enough for harm." I don't think any manufacturer is trying to harm—they don't want bacteria to grow. I personally hate that kind of shade in advertising because it is meant to distract from the fact that the self-titled "natural" manufacturer appears to be offering exactly the same thing as the "conventional" product.
- **OIL BASED:** Contain different oils, such as almond oil, sunflower seed oil, and shea butter. Some have beeswax and vitamin E. Each brand will have a proprietary blend.
- **COOKING OILS:** Such as olive oil or coconut oil. One study linked oils with a higher incidence of colonization with yeast, but another study with olive oil in postmenopausal women revealed

no negative effects. For many years, doctors recommended Crisco, and that seemed well-tolerated, but that contains a trans fat, which is unhealthy (see chapter 7). While it is unlikely to be absorbed, the idea of putting an oil linked with heart disease anywhere in your body seems counterintuitive. While coconut oil has not been studied, I've had lots of patients use it over the years, and I don't remember one complaint.

- **PETROLEUM JELLY:** Has been associated with bacterial vaginosis in at least two studies when used as a lubricant. Give it a pass.

Do I Need a Special Lubricant to Get Pregnant?

Studies in the lab (in vitro studies) have suggested some lubricants could affect sperm function; however, the results are conflicting—sometimes the sperm-friendly lubricant stopped the sperm swimming, and in other studies the same lubricant did not. Some data suggests that glycerin in concentrations higher than 10 percent could be part of the issue, but honestly the data is all over the place. Olive oil, canola oil, and mineral oil have also been studied, and only olive oil seemed to have a negative effect on sperm in the lab. Some people have wondered if the parabens found in some lubes can damage sperm, but there is really no evidence to support that claim.

There are lubricants that advertise as sperm safe; however, a study that followed women attempting to get pregnant found no difference in pregnancy rates between women who used a sperm-friendly lubricant and those who did not.

That's weird, you say! Well, coating sperm with lubricant in a petri dish is quite different from what happens in the vagina. Keep in mind that saliva also reduces sperm motility, and no one is telling couples who want to get pregnant to avoid oral sex.

What should you do? For the average person trying to get pregnant, the science behind special lubricant seems iffy at best, but avoiding a lubricant with a high glycerin content is best for your vagina, so avoid those regardless.

The "sperm-friendly" lubricants are typically more expensive, so you can probably give them a pass unless you are diagnosed with an infertility problem related to sperm function or your fertility doctor makes a specific recommendation—it is possible that even a minor impact from a lubricant might be an issue for sperm with very poor motility.

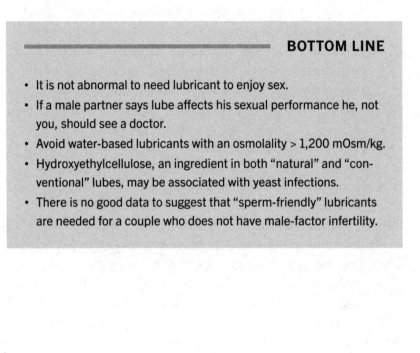

BOTTOM LINE

- It is not abnormal to need lubricant to enjoy sex.
- If a male partner says lube affects his sexual performance he, not you, should see a doctor.
- Avoid water-based lubricants with an osmolality > 1,200 mOsm/kg.
- Hydroxyethylcellulose, an ingredient in both "natural" and "conventional" lubes, may be associated with yeast infections.
- There is no good data to suggest that "sperm-friendly" lubricants are needed for a couple who does not have male-factor infertility.

CHAPTER 10

Kegel Exercises

IN THE 1940S, DR. ARNOLD KEGEL, a California gynecologist, recognized that weakness of the pelvic floor muscles contributed to stress incontinence (leaking urine with coughing or sneezing) and something he called "female conditions" and "ill-defined complaints referable to the genital tract in women." The latter two may be code for pain with sex or difficulties achieving orgasm, although it is hard to know. It is telling about that era of time that even a gynecologist was expected to use euphemisms.

Before Dr. Kegel, the pelvic floor was largely ignored by medicine, mostly made up of male doctors who didn't address sexual function in a meaningful way. Social norms also discouraged women from discussing sexual health issues—women interested in sex were "loose." In addition, most anatomic dissections on cadavers are done on elderly bodies, and muscle mass reduces with age. If my own experience in medical school with the anatomy lab were all I had to go on, I would have probably also thought the female pelvic floor was a minor muscle group.

Dr. Kegel observed that pelvic floor weakness was common after childbirth and made the very astute and commonsensical observation that if exercise strengthened muscles like the biceps, why couldn't that same concept be applied to the pelvic floor muscles?

After much study, Dr. Kegel developed what he called a perineometer, a compressible bulb that went in the vagina attached to a dial, like a blood pressure cuff without the part that goes around your arm. Women inserted the bulb vaginally and squeezed with their pelvic floor muscles, and the dial provided visual feedback on the strength of the squeeze. Dr. Kegel's technique from his original paper has not been modified much, and many of his initial observations have held up to study with modern technology, such as ultrasound and MRI, which were not even close to existence when he was in practice.

Pelvic Floor Refresher

Remember what we covered in chapter 2? There are two layers of pelvic floor muscles: the deeper layer, the levator ani (pubococcygeus, puborectalis, and iliococcygeus) is the hammock extending from the pubic bone out to the hips and back to the tailbone or coccyx, and this is the group involved in Kegel or pelvic floor muscle (PFM) exercises.

Relaxation and injury of the pelvic floor, most commonly tearing of the muscles during childbirth, can lead to incontinence and prolapse, as well as reduced orgasm strength. In addition, we lose muscle mass with age, and this also applies to the pelvic floor, so that is why some of these conditions appear or worsen with age.

Who should do pelvic floor muscle exercises?

Pelvic floor muscle (PFM) exercises can be part of the therapy for urinary incontinence, difficulties achieving orgasm or weak orgasm, pelvic organ prolapse, and fecal incontinence.

Can PFM exercises in your twenties or thirties for women with no symptoms prevent incontinence or other health problems? There is no good data looking at pelvic floor exercises in women who don't have symptoms. Although one study found that women who did these exercises reported that their vagina felt less "loose," but there was no improvement in sexual function.

Whether pelvic floor exercises should be done preventatively is hard to answer; however, common sense suggests that if you are able to do the exercises correctly, you will be better equipped to do them down the road if you develop symptoms of a pelvic floor problem. If you want to see if these exercises improve your sex life, then they may be a fun exercise. If it makes you feel as if you are taking care of yourself by doing them, that is okay, too—as long as you are doing the exercises correctly and you don't get discouraged if they don't make an observable difference.

Kegel exercises can also help women with overactive bladders or urge incontinence get to the bathroom when they really have to go without leaking. This is because a quick set of PFM contractions (called quick flicks) when you are dying to use the bathroom can trigger your bladder to temporarily relax so you can get to the restroom while you are still dry. Not a bad skill to have.

How do I know if my pelvic floor is weak?

Apart from incontinence symptoms, you can ask your doctor, nurse practitioner, or a pelvic floor physical therapist about your pelvic floor. They can insert a gloved finger in your vagina and ask you to squeeze their finger. As some women can have trouble isolating their pelvic floor, a prompt, like asking you to pretend you are out in public and squeezing as if you are trying to hold in gas, can be helpful.

There is a formal scoring system for pelvic floor strength. You don't really need to know, but if you like to track those things it is a five-point scale: 0 = no contraction, 1 = flicker, 2 = weak, 3 = moderate, 4 = good, and 5 = strong. You do not have to make your pelvic floor strong enough to lift a surfboard or rocks, what the internet apparently calls "Vaginal Kung Fu"—I do not make up these terms, I just explain the science. Hoisting heavy objects with your pelvic floor could potentially lead to tearing the muscles and seems rather unnecessary. It is not as if you need to crack a walnut with your pelvic floor.

Ultrasound and biofeedback devices (a sensor that you squeeze with vaginal muscles that provides visual feedback on a screen, much like Dr. Kegel's original device) can be used to measure the contraction, but these are generally not necessary for an initial evaluation. They do add a wow factor, but they also add expense. An ultrasound can be helpful for women who are unable to do pelvic floor exercises despite extensive coaching, as it may identify a muscle that has been torn.

As the pelvic floor muscles function outside our conscious control (for example you don't think about emptying your bladder or having an orgasm), many women can't contract them on demand without some training. Even after an exam with an assessment and instruction more than 30 percent of women still have difficulties. The most common error is tightening the gluteal muscles (buttocks), the hip adductors (squeezing the thighs together), or tightening the abdominal muscles instead of the pelvic floor. Breath holding is also not uncommon, and some women strain or bear down (as with a bowel movement). Other factors besides technique that contribute to difficulties working the pelvic floor muscles include tears in the muscle and nerve damage.

Issues with learning to use the PFM exercises correctly could be part of the reason why they have not shown to be preventative care for women without symptoms, as in many studies correct technique was not checked by a qualified expert.

Pelvic Floor Muscle Exercises: Getting Started

The first step is learning to isolate the muscles. Some tips include:

- Envision the movement as picking up a marble with your vagina.
- Put a mirror between your legs and look at the vaginal opening while you are first doing the exercises or when you wish to check form. The vaginal opening should be lifting and drawing upwards.
- Try to stop the flow of urine while you are on the toilet. If you slow or stop your stream, you are using the right muscles. Remember how it feels, but only do this once or twice, as this is for show, not practice. This is because urinating is a complex reflex, and if you mess around with it too much, it could stop working the way you want it to!
- Pretend you are in a crowded elevator and squeeze the muscles you would to stop a fart. You should feel a pulling sensation into your body if you are doing it correctly.
- Place a lubricated tampon in your vagina and tighten the pelvic floor muscles as you gently pull on the string. You should feel resistance. This is a form of simple biofeedback.
- Place one or two fingers in your vagina and tighten your pelvic floor muscles. You should feel a squeeze.

- During intercourse, practice on your partner's penis or on their fingers and ask if they can feel the squeeze.
- If you are unsure you are doing it correctly, then you should probably see your doctor, nurse practitioner, or a pelvic floor physical therapist.

Pelvic Floor Muscle Exercises: The Actual Exercises

Once you feel comfortable identifying the muscles, move on to the exercises. When you are first starting, lay down with your knees bent and take deep, relaxing breaths. You want to make sure your belly (abdominal wall), buttocks, and inner thighs are always relaxed. This will help you isolate your pelvic floor correctly.

There are two types of exercises—sustained contractions and quick flicks:

- **A SUSTAINED CONTRACTION:** Involves holding the squeeze or contraction. Start by squeezing your pelvic floor for five seconds, then relax completely for ten seconds (or two breaths if that is easier). Each contraction and relaxation is one repetition. Do ten repetitions three times a day. Build up the length of time of sustained contractions to ten seconds, so ten reps of ten seconds three times a day.
- **QUICK FLICKS:** A simple contraction and release and should take 1–2 seconds—five quick flicks are one cycle of quick flicks. Do five cycles of quick flicks with a 5–10 second rest afterwards (so twenty-five quick flicks) for one set. Do one set of quick flicks three times a day.

If you know you are going to cough or sneeze, try to do a sustained contraction right before, as it will help prevent leakage of urine. If you have an intense urge to urinate and are worried about leaking, do a set of quick flicks. It will temporarily relax the bladder muscle and give you time to calmly walk to the toilet.

It will take 6–12 weeks to see improvement. Like all exercises, consistency is the key. After 4–5 months of daily practice, you will have achieved the most benefit. At this point, you can back off to three days a week.

Kegels Are Not Working for Me—Help!

If you are having difficulty mastering the technique, or after a few months you are not seeing any change, consult a gynecologist with experience in the area and/or a pelvic floor physical therapist who can help correct technique and rule out any medical reasons the muscles may not be contracting, such as a muscle tear or nerve damage. If you are not doing the pelvic floor exercises correctly, you could develop a pain condition— never mind the frustration of doing something every day and not getting benefit. A medical professional can also rule out conditions that may be masquerading as pelvic floor weakness.

Many women will benefit from a specialized physical therapist. Often it is just a few visits, but keep in mind that your progress will depend in part on how often you do the home exercises. Without daily home exercises, progress can be slow. Physical therapists also have other tools, like biofeedback machines and even electrical stimulation, which delivers a small, painless current to the pelvic floor muscles to increase blood flow and make them contract, helping your brain learn to isolate the muscles.

Pelvic Floor Training Devices and Apps

A low-tech approach is vaginal weights, which were first introduced in the 1980s, and are typically medical-grade silicone or stainless steel cylinders or balls. The original study used a set of nine weights from 20 to 100 g, but they now they come in a variety of "sets" (typically four or fewer weights). While inserting the weight does create some motor activity (meaning it stimulates the pelvic floor muscles), the method is primarily about the muscles working to retain the heaviest weight against gravity while standing for fifteen minutes, twice a day. Many women don't use weights correctly, as it is possible to contract your buttocks or thighs or abdomen and retain them vaginally, so you have to be mindful of technique. Weights with a string can be inserted vaginally, and while laying down you can tug with the string and contract your pelvic floor to retain the weight, although this method has not been studied.

A review of data shows that the weights are no more effective than doing PFM exercises without them. However, if they motivate you or you like the idea, as some devices can also be incorporated into sexual play (for example, the company Lelo makes vibrating balls that can be inserted vaginally), then weights may be an option for you.

Another option is a home machine to provide feedback. There are probably still some low-tech devices floating around on the market like Dr. Kegel's original perineometer, a compressible pump for the vagina attached to a dial. The harder the squeeze, the more the dial moves.

There are now Bluetooth-enabled vaginal devices, and the dial that provides the feedback is your smartphone. Two devices are Elvie and PeriCoach. Despite Elvie's endorsement by the International Urogynecological Association (IUGA), there are no published clinical trials as of 2018. I emailed the company for confirmation. It is discouraging to hear celebrities mention products like these as part of their exhausting, product-filled vaginal regimen, but then have no studies to corroborate the claims.

Low-tech pelvic floor trainers don't seem to offer any benefit over simply doing the exercises, so without data it is hard to make recommendations about these newer and expensive Bluetooth devices. If a product like this really appeals to you and that motivates you to do your exercises, then perhaps the $130 or so may be worth it for you. If you use all the functions on your smartwatch on a regular basis, then maybe a high-tech pelvic floor trainers will appeal to you. However, if your bathroom scale sits unused in a corner, ask yourself: how will this be any different?

Regardless of the device, be it pelvic floor weights or a Bluetooth-enabled trainer, make sure it can be cleaned appropriately. Don't choose Goop's infamous jade egg, touted as a secret sexual practice of ancient Chinese empresses and concubines. There is no evidence they were anything of the sort, and the idea that these jade eggs are somehow known to a for-profit business in California yet unknown to scholars is, shall we say, somewhat suspect. Smartphone apps are another option. They provide technique advice, education, and reminders, although they cannot tell you how well mechanically you are doing the exercise. One study looked at the free app Tät (UMEA University) and found the women who used it had greater progress than those who did not.

As of early 2019 there were more than one hundred exercise apps on the market, so how to choose? A 2018 study found 32 PFM training apps in English for nonpregnant women that required no device and evaluated the apps for content, ease of use, and privacy. Some apps collect data that could be sold to a third party, and considering the intimate nature of that data, some women may prefer to opt out.

The two apps rated the highest by the experts, Kegel Trainer and Kegel Trainer Pro, also had the highest user satisfaction ratings and are both endorsed by the IUGA.

BOTTOM LINE

- Pelvic floor weakness can contribute to incontinence, prolapse, and a weaker orgasm, and pelvic floor muscle (PFM) exercises can be helpful.
- There is no good data on how well PFM exercises work as preventative care for women without symptoms.
- PFM can be hard to do, biomechnically speaking. Even with instruction many women will contract the wrong muscles.
- Many women will manage just fine with home exercises after appropriate instruction.
- No study has shown that a device or even expensive trainers have any additional benefit. One study shows an app may be helpful.

Skin Care and Cleansing

CHAPTER 11

Vulvar Cleansing: Soaps, Cleansers, and Wipes

THE VULVA, LIKE MOST OF THE BODY, medically requires very little, if any, cleaning. I know this is a shock to many people, but how much you wash is personal, based on how you were raised, your preferences, where you live, how much dirt you get on your body, and how much you sweat. The only parts of your body that medically need regular cleaning are your teeth and your hands. When we open doors or shake hands or prepare food, we are at risk of transferring virus or bacteria from our hands to our nose, mouth, or eyes. We don't shake hands, eat, or cut raw chicken with our vulvas.

Also, the vulva evolved to cope with semen, blood, feces, and urine long before the Romans mixed a paste of fat and ash to create the first soap.

Vulvar Cleanliness 101

The main reasons women report that they wash their vulvas are odor prevention and to "feel clean." It is important to remember that the concept of female cleanliness has largely been driven by a male-dominated society that for centuries, if not longer, has decided normal female genitals and secretions are "dirty."

Another driving force is the multimillion-dollar-a-year feminine cleaning product industry. Don't kid yourself: they are not here for your health. They are here to make women feel their normal anatomy is dirty, and that "feminine freshness" is the feeling of "confidence, comfort, and cleanliness." Yes, that is from an advertisement for a popular product. Many of the ads for these products are barely updated versions of the Lysol douche ads from the '30s and '40s.

I smell vulvas (and vaginas) all day long. That is actually part of my job, as some vaginal conditions are associated with odor. Healthy vulvas don't smell any more than any other body part. I see women who have not showered the day they see me or who have come right from the gym, and there is no odor.

Some women are aware of groin odor from their apocrine sweat glands, the specialized sweat glands in the groin and around the anus. This is the genital tract equivalent of armpit odor. Apocrine sweat glands are located deep in the hair follicle and secrete sebum, a thick oily substance that becomes part of the acid mantle. Skin bacteria can break down these oils, releasing volatile chemicals with a distinct odor. Menstrual blood also reacts with lipids on the surface of the skin, oxidizing the iron molecules in the hemoglobin and producing the distinct metallic smell of blood. Other factors to consider regarding odor and how often you wash are incontinence, leftover ejaculate, lube, and whether or not you have a skin condition, as topical ointments and creams may not all be absorbed and the residue can sometimes have a medicinal odor.

Washing is most important for women with moderate to severe urinary incontinence and fecal incontinence. Urine and feces can damage the acid mantle of the skin and lead to skin inflammation and injury, so cleansing skin that has become soiled in this way is important to limit the damage.

Where to Wash

Let's start with where NOT to wash. The vaginal opening or vestibule (so inside the labia minora) is mucosa, meaning it is the same tissue as the inside of the vagina and does not need to be washed. The labia minora do not have odor-producing apocrine sweat glands, and the skin on the labia minora is the thinnest on the vulva and is the most susceptible to irritation. A good basic rule is to not put any cleaning product between the labia minora, but water is fine. The groin, labia majora, mons, and around the anus can be washed with product.

Water vs. Soap vs. Cleansers

Vulvar cleansing has never been studied. That is interesting, considering the array of products that claim to be gynecologist tested or approved.

What I advise has largely been extrapolated from studies that look at the best way to clean the diaper area of premature and term babies. Obviously, it's not a direct comparison, but as the labia minora have thinner skin than the rest of the body and urine and feces are involved, I think this is the best proxy.

Water may not completely remove sebum and feces, so some women may want to use something more; however, some have skin conditions or such sensitive skin that they find everything irritates and they can only use water. I care for many women with these conditions, and as long as they do not have fecal incontinence, there seem to be no health issues.

Some women will want use a cleansing product daily, others a few times a week, and some just after sex or during their period to remove the smell of ejaculate or oxidized blood. Some women will be fine with just water. Just keep in mind you're not removing baked-on food and you don't have to nuke the influenza virus, so nothing harsh or bactericidal is needed.

There are two different types of products to consider: soap and cleansers. Soap strips away part of the acid mantle—the natural oils and bacteria that are an important part of the skin's defense. If a product is called soap, I don't care how gentle it claims to be—it can dry the skin, which can leave you feeling irritated and possibly more susceptible to microtrauma. The other issue with soap is it undergoes a chemical reaction when mixed with water that increases the skin pH to 10–11. Remember, the pH of the vulvar skin is acidic, around 5.3–5.6.

Cleansers are not soap; they are synthetic surfactants and other chemicals designed to strip away dirt and leave the acid mantle intact. In general, cleansers are better for your skin than soap. I use cleansers only except on my hands, which get alcohol-based sanitizer or soap. I use the same cleanser for my face, body, and vulva because I am lazy, and the idea of keeping several products on hand seems like a dreadful chore. I also only have so much room in my bathroom.

Do I need a special "feminine" wash?

No, but let's unpack this a little, as many women use them.

Some of these washes make claims they can reduce bacterial vaginosis (BV). They can't. An external wash cannot possibly impact the inside of the vagina, and washing internally with one of these products (some women do that—please don't) could definitely increase your risk of BV by killing good bacteria or irritating the vaginal mucosa. If an external product claims it can regulate vaginal pH, then the manufacturers have already provided one misleading claim, so I always wonder what other false claims they are making.

Many "feminine washes" have fragrance, even the ones advertised for sensitive skin. Fragrance is a common source of irritation and allergy.

These products also have destructive messaging. One well-known company has an advertisement that suggests women might detect an odor after crossing their legs!

I mean, come on.

What are the best products?

As companies change formulas, it is hard to make specific recommendations. In addition, pH isn't always listed. With those conditions in mind, here are some general recommendations:

- **IF IT'S NOT BROKEN, DON'T FIX IT:** If you've been using the same product for years and have no issues, what you are doing is probably fine as long as you are not cleaning the inside of your vagina. Skin loses moisture with age, so if you are using soap you may want to think about a cleanser as a preventative measure.
- **AIM FOR A PRODUCT WITH A PH BETWEEN 5.3 AND 7.0, BUT CLOSER TO 5.3–5.6 (THE PH OF VULVAR SKIN) IS LIKELY BETTER:** Regular exposure

to a pH of 7.5 or higher can damage the lipid layer in the skin. A study looking at cleansers found the pH of Cetaphil Restoraderm was 5.93, Eucerin Gentle Hydrating Cleanser was 5.30, and Eucerin pH 5 Bar Cleanser had a pH of 5.81. Most cleansers and soaps don't list the pH (although for Eucerin pH 5, it is part of the name).

- **AVOID PRODUCTS WITH NATURAL AND SYNTHETIC FRAGRANCE ADDITIVES:** These are common sources of irritant and allergic reactions.
- **AVOID METHYLISOTHIAZOLINONE (MI) AND METHYLCHLOROISOTHIAZOLINONE (MCI):** these are common irritants and allergens. Other common irritants/allergens are formaldehyde, lanolin, and tea tree oil.
- **THE TERMS "MILD," "BABY," "PH BALANCED," "DERMATOLOGIST TESTED," AND "GYNECOLOGIST TESTED" MEAN NOTHING MEDICALLY:** They are marketing terms. One study looking at soaps and cleansers marketed for babies and children found 35 percent had a pH over 7.0!
- **IF IT IRRITATES, DON'T USE IT:** Really, you don't need to get used to it. The corollary is that you can develop an allergy to a product at any time, even after twenty years of use. Also, companies don't mail warning cards when they change ingredients.
- **IF YOU PREFER SOAP TO A CLEANSER:** Use an unscented product. One option is liquid castile soap (one option is Dr. Bronner's unscented baby soap), and that seems to be well tolerated. I have also had patients do well with a pure glycerin soap, like Pears.

Should I Use a Hair Dryer on My Vulva?

No, most definitely not. The moisture in the vulva skin is a protective mechanism, and a hair dryer can damage the acid mantle and overdry the skin, even on a cool setting.

A Word on Wipes

Up to 40 percent of women in North America have used wipes externally on the vulva. It is easy to see how they have become so accepted; they seem to be in every drugstore, some celebrities champion their use, and they are for babies, so they must be gentle and safe! The widespread promotion of these products is based on the idea that normal female anatomy needs additional cleaning after using the bathroom compared with men. Why could women possibly need more anal cleaning than men after a bowel movement? That's misogyny.

Wipes are useful to remove fecal material and urine from the genital skin as the chemicals, enzymes, and bacteria in feces and urine, as well as the wetness, can damage the acid mantle, leading to irritation and skin breakdown. That is why wipes are useful for babies who are incontinent and wear diapers, which are occlusive and keep the stool smushed against the skin. A washcloth and cleanser work just as well; however, the practicalities of using those outside your home and even in the home can be challenging. If you have fecal or urinary incontinence, then wipes may be handy outside the house and for occasional use at home when a washcloth is not an option. Another excellent option is a bidet.

What's the problem with wipes?

They are a common cofactor in contact dermatitis in the vulva and anal area. The vulva is fifteen times more likely to be irritated by these products than other areas. Instead of intimate wipes, they should be called irritant wipes.

Looking at all the wipes on the market, there are over a hundred potential allergens to consider. The most common allergens in wipes include fragrance ("natural" or synthetic) and the following preservatives: methylisothiazolinone (MI), methylchloroisothiazolinone (MCI), propylene glycol (PG), bronopol (2-bromo-2-nitropropane-1,3-diol), and iodopropynyl butylcarbamate.

A recent review of the potential allergens in wipes identified products with the fewest known allergens. Here are the ones on the list made by companies that do not also sell douches (I try not to send any business to companies that sell a product that we know harms women):

· Equate Baby Everyday Clean Wipes, Fragrance Free

- Ladygroomer Woman Wipes, Fresh Scent, Flushable Moist Wipes Designed for Women
- pjur Med Clean Personal Soft Cleaning Fleece
- PureTouch Individual Flushable Moist Feminine Wipes
- Swipes Lovin Wipes, Unscented
- Up&Up Extra Large Cleansing Washcloths

You should not interpret this list as risk free, irritation-wise. Ingredients change, and repeated exposure can lead to sensitization and allergic reaction. As manufacturers get rid of ingredients that cause irritation and allergic reactions, they may make substitutions that could potentially be equally as bad or even worse.

Every time I wipe I see stool, so I have to keep wiping; wipes help me clean those nooks and crannies effectively

I know this is a long header, but I hear this all the time. This is as good a place as any to review wiping.

When you have a bowel movement, you may not completely empty your rectum, or even if you do, stool that is higher up simply moves down to the rectum. The rectum is a storage pouch that sits just above the anal canal. Rubbing or stimulating the external anal sphincter—with aggressive wiping, for example—triggers a reflex that causes the sphincter to relax, and a small amount of stool will be released from the rectum. You may see that on the toilet paper and mistakenly believe it was because you have not wiped enough. So you get more toilet paper or a wipe and dig around again, and a little more stool comes out. And again. And again. The more you wipe, the more you irritate the skin, all the while thinking you are irritated because there was stool on your skin.

The areas that are okay to wipe are outside on the perineum and around the anus. Once you get directly on the external anal sphincter (the opening), this is a no-wipe zone; blotting is preferred. The other option is a bidet.

BOTTOM LINE

- Overcleaning can be a source of irritation, as it can damage the skin's acid mantle.
- Cleansers are preferred over soap.
- Give feminine washes a pass, as they are more likely to contain irritants and allergens and they have a destructive, patriarchal message.
- If you don't have incontinence, save your money and your vulva and don't buy wipes.
- Wiping aggressively over the anus can paradoxically cause you to have more stool on the toilet paper.

CHAPTER 12

Vaginal Cleansing: Douches, Steams, Sprays, and Potpourri

YOUR VAGINA IS A SELF-CLEANING OVEN.

If vaginas don't need any help with cleaning or maintenance, why a chapter? Many women clean vaginally with at least one method (sometimes more than one), so medicine is not doing a good job of presenting the harms of vaginal cleaning in a relatable way. That, and the patriarchy is a relentless foe.

My hope is that if you are someone who uses these products, I can convince you to give them up. If you are someone who doesn't, maybe knowing more about them might help you start a conversation with a friend or family member who does.

The History of Vaginal Cleaning

Vaginal cleaning has a complex history, and undoing centuries of misinformation and misogyny is hard.

The idea that a healthy vagina is unclean and/or requires some kind of prep for men is a great example of the dangers of ancient medical beliefs.

Many cultures have long-standing practices of vaginal astringents and antiseptics to dry the surface of the vagina so men can enjoy "dry sex." Historically, women used a variety of products, like fruit acid or oak galls, to desiccate the surface of the vagina. The increased friction from dry tissue and/or the obvious discomfort of their partner was apparently a turn-on for some men. I have often wondered if normalizing a practice that made sex painful for women was an invisible chastity belt. I have heard from some women who partner with men who have erectile dysfunction that these men say they are more likely to lose their erection with lubricant, and so it is possible that some women prioritize their partner's pleasure and endure painful sex. It would not surprise me if the "ancient" practice of vaginal drying was also normalized for male partners with erectile dysfunction. It is also possible that many men throughout history have been as phobic of normal vaginal discharge as some are today.

Another belief that has historically contributed to douching and still does today is the mistaken idea that attempting to wash out sperm from the vagina could be a contraceptive. It's not. By the time you've grabbed the douche, enough sperm has already made it past the cervix and is well on its way to the fallopian tubes. Douching also doesn't make it past the cervix.

Women today primarily say they douche or do intravaginal cleaning in search of "freshness," something that has no medical or even cultural definition.

Medicine also has a bad track record with douches and vaginal cleaning. Many doctors, even as late as the 1970s and possibly the '80s, recommended douches. It was likely seen as an easy solution for a myriad of female health concerns, like pain with sex or low libido. Many doctors, almost every one of them a man, would have promoted douching to our mothers and grandmothers. When generation after generation of women have been told their vaginas are dirty or a source of marital distress by both the medical profession and society, it is easy to see how it may take more than two generations to undo.

Another time I hear women say they perform vaginal cleaning is after sex with a man, as some women don't like the idea of ejaculate inside their vagina or running down their leg. Women are also inserting wipes vaginally to scoop out ejaculate.

There are some new wrinkles in the vaginal cleaning saga. Big Feminine Hygiene (BFH) are companies selling washes, sprays, wipes, or any odor-control or cleansing products for the vagina. The douche manufacturers are still there, but there are various new products. In addition, Little Feminine Hygiene (LFH) is getting in on the act. Celebrities like Gwyneth

Paltrow and an ever-growing number of spas market practices like vaginal steaming, which are based on the idea that there are "toxins" or "impurities" to remove. Same destructive messaging, different packaging. Any company that promotes articles about vaginal steaming profits from this disinformation, as these articles tend to get a lot of traffic. And of course, many small businesses are getting into Little Feminine Hygiene, selling vaginal tightening sticks or homemade herb balls on Etsy or Instagram for "cleansing."

There's a lot of money in vaginal shame.

What Do You Mean by Intravaginal Cleaning?

The most common method is douching, which is flushing the vagina with a "medicated" solution. There are small, handheld devices that push fluid into the vagina under some pressure, and others that allow it to flow in via gravity. In North America, most women buy premade douches, in which the most common "medicated" solutions are vinegar and iodine, but some women make them at home.

Douching is not the only method women use to clean. Besides douching, women insert feminine wipes vaginally, they use feminine washes even though the products say "for external use only," and they use deodorant suppositories and even deodorant sprays.

While not reported in studies, many women tell me they insert their fingers vaginally to scoop out discharge. Not quite douching or wipes, but definitely not needed. The discharge comes out when it is ready. There will always be some discharge, and it might look weird or sticky on your fingers and lead to you believe that it is abnormal when it is not.

Other methods of cleaning are vaginal steaming, either at a spa or at home, with various herbs or plants (vaginal potpourri), and even ozone (very, very dangerous).

How Many Women Are Cleaning Vaginally?

It depends on the population surveyed, as there is a lot of regional and cultural variation. In North America, up to 57 percent of women have cleaned vaginally in the past year. Other studies say 12–40 percent of women douche regularly (at least once a month), and 6 percent of women regularly use either "feminine" or baby wipes to clean vaginally.

Among women who douche, about 20 percent are doing so at least once a week. Women who douche also tend to start young, with 80 percent starting before they are twenty years old. They are also more likely to use other products for vaginal cleaning.

Where Are Women Getting Their Messaging About Douching and Vaginal Cleaning?

Most women report learning this practice from their mothers, but some learn it from the media or friends, and many say they simply taught themselves. Given all the products on the shelves, the constant articles about vaginal maintenance, social media posts and YouTube videos, as well as the fascination with celebrity vagina prep regimens, it is easy to see how a woman who never heard about vaginal cleaning at home could quickly come to believe that vaginal neglect is a thing. It is likely that women who didn't learn about douching at home can't specifically remember where they heard about it because the messaging is everywhere.

More than 50 percent of women who clean intravaginally report they are encouraged to do this by their sexual partner. Younger women are more likely to succumb to partner pressure; in one study, 77 percent of women aged 18–25 said they washed inside their vagina because that was what their partner wanted.

The Dangers of Vaginal Cleaning Regimens

Multiple studies tell us that douching is harmful. It damages the healthy vaginal bacteria and the protective mucus layer. This makes a woman more vulnerable to bacterial vaginosis (a bacterial imbalance in the vagina) and increases her risk of getting gonorrhea or HIV if exposed. Paradoxically, killing the good bacteria may actually increase vaginal odor.

The dangers of wipes inserted vaginally, hygiene sprays (these are meant for the vulva, but about 1 percent of women report using them vaginally), and odor-control suppositories have not been studied, but many of them contain products that irritate and are potential allergens. Almost all of them contain fragrance. Wipes, sprays, and odor-control suppositories could very easily kill good bacteria and irritate the mucus and the lining of the vagina in the same way as douches. Every one of them also has damaging messages on the packaging, such as "effectively masks natural odors" and "wonderful tropical scent."

It's a vagina, not a piña colada.

Studies tell us that vaginal washing with soap increases the risk of HIV transmission by almost four times—whether this is due to damaging the lactobacilli or protective mucus or irritation and microtrauma is not known. Even washing vaginally with water increases the risk of getting HIV if exposed by 2.6 times!

Natural or botanical products are no better. Herbs, lemon and lime juice, astringents like oak galls (basically nests for wasp larvae), and other tightening products have a high risk of killing healthy vaginal bacteria and damaging the mucus layer, as well as irritating the vaginal tissue, causing microtrauma. Just like douches, these products could paradoxically increase vaginal odor and increase the risk of irritant reactions and allergies, and increase the risk of sexually transmitted infections.

"Vagina steaming" involves sitting over a pot of steaming herbs. The most common one is apparently mugwort, a close relative of the potent allergen ragweed, but various plant products are recommended. The idea behind it, according to Gwyneth Paltrow (an apparent devotee), is that the steam "cleanses" your uterus. This is physically impossible, as steam cannot make it through the cervix and into the uterus (for something to do that, it needs to be under a lot of pressure or be able to swim well, like sperm). Also, the uterus does not need cleaning. If any vapors even made it to the vagina, they could irritate—and of course, steam can burn. If air is introduced along with the steam, that could favor the growth of dangerous bacteria.

Most of the steam probably just hits the vulva, but that is not a great place for allergens either. It has no benefit, promotes a serious misunderstanding about anatomy and physiology, and has the potential to harm. In short, it's a scam.

In some countries, women can get ozone blown into the vagina. This could definitely be hazardous, as ozone is a highly dangerous gas. In addition to damaging the vagina, if any escapes into the room and you breathe it in, it could cause serious lung damage. Stay away from ozone!

If vaginal cleaning is so dangerous, why do women keep doing it?

Studies tell us that most women who douche or use other products made by Big Feminine Hygiene believe they are safe—because otherwise why would stores sell them?

Stores also sell cigarettes.

While studies tell us a significant percentage of women report vaginal cleaning, in my experience very few women admit to the practice. My concern is that women underreport to medical professionals because they don't want a lecture (we shouldn't lecture, we should inform), or they don't believe it is harmful in general or for them specifically. It is also possible that some truly believe it is harmful, they just prefer to use a douche, and finally that there are likely women who are told by male partners that it is a requirement—it is implied, a direct request, or even an order.

More than 90 percent of women who report douching say they have no intention of giving it up, so there are probably a variety of complex social, relationship, and cultural reasons.

BOTTOM LINE

- Your vagina is a self-cleaning oven.
- Anyone who suggests vaginal cleaning or tightening is recommended is wrong.
- Vaginal cleaning will damage the good bacteria and mucus, increasing a woman's chance of odor, bacterial vaginosis, and sexually transmitted infections.
- Vaginal steaming, ozone, and "ancient" tightening products are equally as harmful as anything from a drugstore.
- Wipes should not be inserted vaginally.

CHAPTER 13

Hair Removal and Grooming

PUBIC HAIR HAS A PURPOSE, a fact that some women and men seem shocked to hear. It develops during puberty, and its function is likely protecting the vulva by providing physical protection, trapping microscopic dirt and debris, and maintaining humidity (if you remember, the vulvar skin has a high moisture content).

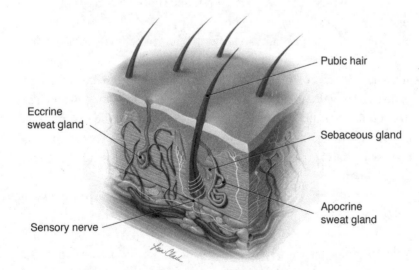

Image 7: Pubic hair and sweat glands. ILLUSTRATION BY LISA A. CLARK, MA, CMI.

Two different glands, the sebaceous and the apocrine glands, empty onto the pubic hair shaft, secreting sebum and oils that track up the pubic hair to the surface and become part of the acid mantle, the protective oily layer on the skin.

Pubic hair may also play a role in sexual pleasure as tugging or traction on pubic hairs stimulates touch receptors (each hair is attached to a nerve ending). It is also possible that pubic hair has a role in odor dispersal and spreading or trapping pheromones.

Pubic hair is different in many ways from the hair on your head. The hair follicles are spaced differently (this is why you can't get pubic lice on your head—they need hair follicles a specific distance apart). Pubic hair may also be a different color from the hair on your head. Unlike the hair on your head, pubic hair won't keep growing indefinitely (that would present a physical challenge to reproduction) and doesn't change during pregnancy or after delivery. The amount of pubic hair and the thickness of each hair does decrease with age, and it also grays.

The Culture of Pubic Hair Removal

Currently, pubic hair removal is very popular, and college-age women are more likely to remove or groom their pubic hair than older women, although the practice is widespread. In one study, 83 percent of women ages 18–65 reported removing pubic hair partially or completely. Complete removal of pubic hair varies, but 76 percent of college-aged women in the United States and Australia have removed all of their pubic hair at least once. Approximately 60 percent of men indicate they prefer a female partner with no pubic hair, whereas only 23 percent of women say they prefer their male partner to be hairless. Despite the vast numbers of women who report they remove their pubic hair, only 4 percent report discussing hair removal techniques with their doctor—hence the need for this chapter!

Pubic hair removal has been around for a long time. In ancient Egypt, pubic hair is represented as an inverted triangle, and razors intended for pubic hair removal have been found in tombs. In the past, many women removed pubic hair as a way to reduce lice. Some even wore pubic hair wigs called merkins to hide this fact and to cover genital ulcers from syphilis that would now be more visible in the absence of pubic hair. Pubic hair removal is also a practice in some religions.

Women's pubic hair is typically not depicted in ancient Western sculptures or works of art—artwork almost exclusively produced by men. This absence isn't because these artists didn't know how to render hair—the women almost always have exquisitely detailed hair on their head. Ancient Greek sculptures often show pubic hair for men as well as anatomically detailed penises (albeit on the small side, as sexuality was at odds with intellect and a great brain was the ideal), but the statues of women never have labia or pubic hair, but a mound. Whether the absence of pubic hair in Western art was due to the fact that this was a beauty ideal, showing pubic hair was improper or scandalous, or because of the association with lice (although you also get lice in your head hair) is not known. The first depiction of female pubic hair in Western art wasn't until Goya's *The Naked Maja* in the late 19th century, and this was apparently outrageous even though just a few wisps are barely visible.

Visible pubic hair was often the definition of public nudity, so burlesque and erotic dancers removed their pubic hair as a way to show more skin. There is also the almost ubiquitous absence of female pubic hair in women's magazines, lingerie and bathing suit advertisements, movies, and mainstream pornography. It isn't known whether this culture of hairlessness is a result of market pressures to cater to a strong male preference, a carryover from previous beliefs that pubic hair is risqué, celebrity endorsements (e.g., pubic hair laser removal being featured on an episode of *Keeping Up with the Kardashians*), or the fact that the internet allows us to see more images of naked bodies.

Pubic hair and "cleanliness"

With this history of pubic hair removal across multiple cultures, it is easy to see how both women and men have come to think of pubic hair as "dirty." Medicine has not, until recently, been helpful in dispelling this myth. For years, doctors insisted that women be shaved before vaginal deliveries in the name of "cleanliness."

The vulva has been exposed to blood, feces, urine, and seminal fluid long before the ability to remove hair or wash with soap existed. If the absence of pubic hair was beneficial, bacteria-wise, then we simply wouldn't have it.

Pubic hair removal is a cause of injury—over 50 percent of women who have removed pubic hair report at least one complication such as lacerations, burns, rashes, and infections. Almost 4 percent saw a health care provider for the injury. Of all genital injuries in the emergency department, 3 percent are due to pubic hair removal. Surgical intervention related to a grooming injury, including draining an abscess or stitches, is not uncommon. Injuries are more commonly reported by women who remove all of their pubic hair.

One study reported a razor injury was the most common pubic hair–related injury to send women to the emergency room, and another suggested women who wax reported fewer injuries. However, waxing is done less frequently than shaving, and burns from waxing have been reported, so it is not possible to conclude that waxing (or sugaring, for that matter) is safer. Women who have their partner perform their grooming on them are more likely to experience injury.

Can you prevent infections? This has not been studied, but using an antibacterial wipe or washing with an antibacterial soap is probably a good idea before any method of hair removal. This is the one exception that I have for soap. Removing skin bacteria in surgery has been shown to reduce infections, and so the same principle might logically apply here.

Women with diabetes who have elevated blood sugar and women who have a suppressed immune system should skip hair removal, as any injury is much more likely to develop into a serious infection.

Pubic hair removal is also associated with an increased risk of sexually transmitted infections (STIs) in some studies. In one study, 8 percent of non-groomers versus 14 percent of groomers (so almost double) reported a history of an STI—people who removed all of their pubic hair were the most likely to report a history of an STI. The study controlled for age, the frequency of sex, and the number of partners to find that grooming was associated with a higher rate of STIs.

People who removed all of their pubic hair were four times more likely to report a history of a skin-to-skin contact STI like herpes or human papilloma virus (HPV) compared with those who did not. Another study linked pubic hair removal, especially complete removal, with HPV infection, precancer, and cancer of the vulva.

While these studies don't prove a cause and effect, and there could be other factors involved, the hypothesis that the microtrauma of hair removal is a potential portal of entry for HPV or herpes has merit. Another possibility is the lack of pubic hair could change the ecosystem—for example changing the acid mantle or humidity in a way that favors STIs.

Other reasons for pubic hair removal

Approximately 40 percent of women report they remove their pubic hair before going for a pelvic exam. Please don't!

Attractiveness, confining to social norms, improving sexual function, hiding gray hair, and enhancing femininity are also given as reasons for pubic hair removal. There is data that says the first naked genitals that you see prime you to consider them as your baseline for "normal" or typical. So given the almost complete absence of pubic hair in art since the beginning of time and now in pornography, it is easy to see how the absence of pubic hair has come to be accepted as the social norm.

There is no data that suggests pubic hair removal enhances sexual function. It is possible women may feel better about their body or feel sexier and as your brain is your most powerful organ for orgasms, this could be an indirect effect. Given that pubic hair is attached to a nerve, the hypothesis that removing hair reduces sexual sensation seems more valid. Tugging of pubic hair may also increase sexual stimuli. However, sensation with and without pubic hair has not been studied.

Regarding the lack of pubic hair being associated with femininity— well, that is an interesting social conundrum. The appearance of pubic hair is part of puberty, the transition from childhood to being a woman. Pubic hair is literally a biological sign of womanhood.

Main Types of Hair Removal

There are two main types: depilation and epilation. Depilation involves removing the hair at the surface or just below the surface, and epilation involves removing the entire hair shaft and bulb. Depilation typically lasts two weeks, depending on how fast your hair grows, but as epilation involves removing the entire shaft and the bulb, it may last 6–8 weeks. The hair is attached to a nerve, so this is why epilation may be painful.

We know the most about shaving, mostly because of men and facial hair. Thanks, dudes, but also *sigh*. It angers me that we have no data to inform women accurately about meaningful medical differences between methods. Much of the information women receive is anecdotal or marketing from salons or companies that sell razors or waxes or devices.

A Rundown on Methods: Pros and Cons

The safest medical recommendation is a trimmer, which cuts the hair above the skin surface and should not cause trauma when done correctly. However, many women still wish to remove their pubic hair, and simply saying *do not remove your pubic hair* is neither practical nor helpful advice. Women get to choose what they do with their own bodies, and if the small risk of injury or a potentially increased risk of STIs are worth it personally, then they are worth it. We all have our own risk-benefit ratios.

As noted, women who have a compromised immune system—for example those on chemotherapy—and women with diabetes who have elevated blood sugars should avoid hair removal. Both situations are associated with an increased risk of serious infections. Women who are at increased risk for STIs may wish to avoid grooming or groom at least a week before a sexual encounter to allow any microtrauma to heal.

Studies that have looked at injury report the highest risk with shaving; however, those studies may not be accurate if shaving is the most common technique.

Depilation techniques

Shaving is the technique of using a razor to cut the hair at or just below the skin surface. There are no studies on pubic hair shaving, so the advice that I have is adapted from the recommendations for men with pseudofolliculitis barbae (basically, chronic ingrown beard hairs from shaving). Technique generally revolves around minimizing trauma (razor burn is a painful rash due to skin trauma) and not breaking or cutting the hair below the skin surface, as this increases the risk of ingrown hairs. Some important points regarding technique:

- **THE BEST TIME TO SHAVE:** The best time is after a short shower, as the moisture causes the hair follicles to swell, making the cut cleaner.
- **USE A PRODUCT TO PREP YOUR SKIN:** This means shaving cream, not a quick pass with a bar of soap in the shower. This minimizes microtrauma.
- **SHAVE IN THE DIRECTION OF THE HAIR GROWTH:** This reduces the risk of the hair shaft breaking beneath the skin's surface.
- **USE A RAZOR WITH A SINGLE BLADE:** With a double blade, the first blade pulls the hair up and the second cuts it, but the lower the cut, the deeper the hair shaft retracts into the hair follicle—and the greater the risk of an ingrown hair.
- **DON'T PULL THE SKIN TAUT WITH ONE HAND:** This also increases the chance the cut will be below the skin surface.
- **CHANGE YOUR RAZORS REGULARLY:** Make sure you don't use the same razor for a year (not that I have ever done that, or anything).
- **CONSIDER AN ELECTRIC RAZOR AND USE AS DIRECTED:** These typically don't give quite as close a shave as a blade.

Chemical depilatories are usually made of calcium hydroxide and sodium hydroxide. These are applied to the skin, and they disrupt the disulfide bonds of the hair's protein structure, which dissolves the hair shaft so it can be wiped sway. The biggest issue is local irritation to the skin and allergic reactions. Exercise caution and avoid getting them on the more delicate skin of the labia minora.

Epilation

Waxing and sugaring both involve applying a substance that adheres to the hair follicles and, when pulled off with enough force, pulls out the hair along with it. Wax can be hot (there is a risk of burns) or cold, and sugaring is also hot. Hot wax can be hard or soft. Both are applied with a wooden stick—hard wax is peeled off with fingers, and soft wax requires applying a strip of muslin. Sugaring involves caramelizing sugar until it looks a bit like sticky toffee. It is applied with a stick as well and is typically then pulled off with fingers. With waxing, the hair can be pulled in any direction because it sticks so well. Technique is more important with sugaring because it isn't quite as adhesive, so hair must be pulled in the direction of growth to minimize breakage.

If sugaring is less adhesive, might it be less traumatic to the skin? No one has ever studied that; however, if it is adherent enough to pull hair out, then it is obviously causing microtrauma to the skin surface. Whether wax takes off more layers of skin cells than sugaring is unknown, so I took it upon myself to get one side of my bikini done with hard wax and the other via sugaring (both techniques without muslin to reduce the variables). I also asked a gentleman friend to compare the smoothness afterwards, without telling him which side was which. The waxing and sugaring were equally painful, and both sides seemed equally smooth. If you prefer one over the other, it is likely a personal choice or what works best for your skin.

If you get waxed or sugared at a salon, specifically ask if they use individual wooden sticks for each pass, as you do not want them double dipping, which can add skin bacteria to the warm wax or sugar they are using on you and everyone else. The pain of pulling the hair out can be lessened somewhat by applying a hand firmly and immediately to the area after removing the wax. Some salons advise applying numbing medication, like lidocaine, before. I would not do this with hot wax or sugar, as you need to know if it is too hot so you don't get burned.

Home epilators are devices that grasp hairs and pull them out. Think of them as tweezers on steroids. There is very little data on them, and in studies looking at the risks of grooming they must be lumped into the "other" category. They are painful, like waxing.

Laser hair removal is a technique of applying energy in the form of light to damage the hair follicle. The melanin in the hair absorbs the light, so a specific wavelength is needed because melanin absorbs light in the range of 690 to 1200 nm. White and blond hair is the hardest to treat, as there is less melanin to absorb the light. The lasers that are used include the ruby, alexandrite, diode, Nd:YAG, and intense pulsed light. Success rates one year after treatment can be as high as 80 percent, but results vary. Laser is not technically considered a permanent method, as the hair follicle can recover. Different lasers are better for different skin colors and types of hair, so I recommend seeing a board-certified dermatologist or plastic surgeon with a large cosmetic practice—they have the most experience, and you want someone who has more than one kind of laser. If all they have is a hammer, everyone could look like a nail. Laser hair removal can help some women with hidradenitis suppurativa, a chronic inflammatory condition of the skin (often called acne inversa in Europe) that affects hair follicles.

Electrolysis is the only truly permanent form of hair removal. This procedure involves inserting a tiny probe into the hair follicle and passing an electric current to damage the follicle so the hair cannot grow back. There are three types of electrodes: galvanic, thermolysis, and a combination or blend method. Galvanic takes longer to treat each follicle (up to three minutes, versus seconds for thermolysis) and is more painful, but is also more likely to result in permanent hair removal. The blend techniques seems to be the most effective for balancing the efficacy and treatment aspects. As hair is removed one by one, it is a slow process. Complications of electrolysis include scarring and pigment changes due to inflammation. Electrolysis is recommended before bottom surgery for trans men, as it is the only permanent form of removal.

Ingrown Hairs, Razor Burn, and Infections

Ingrown hairs occur when the hair breaks just below the surface and inflammation or trauma blocks the opening of the follicle or causes a hair to bend back on itself and grow into the skin. Very curly hair has the highest risk, as it is predisposed to curling back on itself—this is why you likely never get ingrown hairs on your legs, but you do in your bikini area. Shaving may have the highest risk, as the sharp, cut edge of the hair is more likely to penetrate the skin. Genetics also probably influence hair follicle shape and sebum production, making some women more prone than others.

The inflammation of the hair under the skin can lead to a painful bump. If bacteria is trapped as well, infection can result.

Strict attention to technique to minimize breaking the hair shaft is the most important thing to consider, but all epilation involves removing hair from below the skin surface, so there is no way to completely remove risk. If one method works better for you, then that method works better for you. Many aestheticians recommend exfoliating before waxing or sugaring to help the wax adhere. This may improve technique. It is also

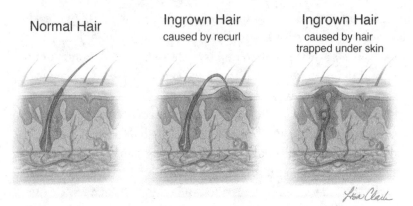

Image 8: Normal hair; ingrown hair—hair recurl, hair trapped. ILLUSTRATIONS BY
LISA A. CLARK, MA, CMI.

possible that removing dead skin cells may reduce blockage of the hair
follicle afterwards.

As for the salon recommendations of using expensive products with
alpha hydroxy acids, such as glycolic and salicylic acid? These products
are supposed to loosen sebum, so theoretically they could prevent ingrown hairs, but there is no data on their safety for the genital area. If you
want to try these products, that is your call; however, they do sell very inexpensive, disposable salicylic acid wipes for acne, and these would be
useful for targeting specific spots or precise application at a fraction of the
cost. The wipes come in 0.5–2 percent concentrations. It is always best to
start with the lowest concentration.

Ingrown hairs typically work their way out. If you can see the bump
well and it is not right next to your labia minora or anus, you can apply
some 5 percent or 10 percent benzoyl peroxide cream to dry the area and
reduce inflammation and bacteria. If you see the hair poking above the
surface you can pull it out with clean tweezers, but don't break the skin
to remove it, as that can introduce bacteria and lead to serious infections

Irritation of the hair follicle can cause inflammation, called folliculitis.
These are small, irritated bumps. Mild inflammation may resolve on its
own, but if it doesn't, a low-potency topical steroid can be used.

Cuts, abrasions, and ingrown hairs can lead to infection. If there is redness that extends from any bump onto the skin, pus, or significant pain,
you should consult with your health care provider. If you regularly get

large nodules and draining lesions that look like terrible acne and you are attributing them to hair removal, it is a good idea to get screened by your doctor to make sure that you don't have the inflammatory skin condition hidradenitis suppurativa.

A Gynecologist's Personal Approach to Hair Removal

I'm going to tell you what I do and why. This doesn't mean that you should do it, as my technique has never been studied. However, like many women, I've struggled with ingrown hairs and razor burn over the years, and I have tried a variety of measures and settled on several that work for me. I accept that pubic hair removal has risks, but I prefer that it doesn't stick out of my underwear.

My first strategy is to not remove pubic hair on my labia majora or around the anus. The closer you get to mucosa, the greater the risk of irritation. Perianal dermatitis (chronic inflammation and redness) can be very challenging to treat, and I do not want to potentially increase my risk by causing microtrauma in the area. Also, full hair removal has the highest risk. I trim over my labia majora.

I don't shave. Not because of the increased reports of injuries: I can't trust myself to keep the right skin prep product in my shower, and I know I will drag a razor over dry or barely prepped skin. I also know I have had the same razor longer than many boyfriends. Because of that, I wax. Sugaring was okay, but for me it didn't offer anything over waxing, and I found all the digging and pulling required (there is much more than wax) annoying.

I prep my skin for hair removal in many ways like we do before surgery. If this reduces infection after surgery, it seems intuitive that it would also reduce infection after shaving. I clean the area a few hours before with an antibacterial skin wipe. This could irritate the vagina and anus, so I would not use them on the labia minora or around the anal area. We put clean dressings on surgical wounds for twenty-four hours after surgery, so I take clean underwear to the salon to wear afterwards. I use a salon that doesn't double-dip with the wax sticks, and I ask the aestheticians to test the wax temperature on my inner thigh first.

I avoid cleaning or trauma to the area for the rest of the day. The next day, I start using my moisturizer (coconut oil) and cleanser again on my vulva, and a week later I start using salicylic acid pads every few days to loosen sebum and prevent any occlusion of hair follicles.

BOTTOM LINE

- Pubic hair removal or grooming is very common. Most women report doing it at some point, and many report doing it regularly
- Only 4 percent of women get guidance from medical professionals; however, there is very little data on how to advise women of the safest techniques.
- Removing pubic hair does not improve cleanliness, and there is emerging data that it is associated with an increased risk of infections like HPV and herpes, although the exact mechanism is not known.
- Strategies to minimize breakage of the hair shaft below the skin surface are the best way to prevent ingrown hairs.
- For laser hair removal, seek the opinion of a board-certified dermatologist or plastic surgeon.

CHAPTER 14

Moisturizers, Barriers, and Bath Products

THERE IS AN EVER-GROWING MARKET of special vulvar moisturizers, and it seems that bathing products, especially bath bombs and soaks, are everywhere, and some are specifically targeted for vulvar or vaginal "health." The way some of these products are promoted makes it sound as if it is a miracle the vulva has made it this far.

There are some benefits to moisturizers and a lot of pleasure to be had in bath products or fancy jars on the bathroom sink. We all define self-care differently. My pleasure item is shoes, but I can see how, for other women, indulgence could be a bathroom sink that looks like a steampunk apothecary. When using any product, it is important to be mindful of your reason. There are medical benefits, and then there is joy. It is not wrong for pleasure to be a motivator, I just don't kid myself that my fancy shoes are good for my feet.

What Is a Moisturizer?

A moisturizer is a topical substance that increases the hydration of skin by protecting and repairing the skin's outer layer, the stratum corneum. The main active ingredients in a moisturizer include one or all of the following:

- An emollient, which lubricates and softens. Examples include glycol, glyceryl stearate, and oils.
- An occlusive agent, which coats the skin and acts like a protective barrier to stop water loss. Examples are petrolatum, dimethicones (silicone derivative), and oils.
- A humectant, which pulls water out of the atmosphere and brings it to the skin. Examples are glycerol and hyaluronic acid.

Commercial products may also have emulsifiers (to keep the oil and water components from separating), preservatives, and other ingredients like fragrance. Some commercial products also have water, which has only a very passing effect on hydration.

Does the Vulva Need a Moisturizer?

The vulva has more moisture than other skin. Pubic hair and the acid mantle are defense mechanisms that protect against moisture loss. Aging, skin irritation from incontinence, soaps, wipes, pubic hair removal, and using a hair dryer on the vulva (don't do this!) can all negatively affect skin moisture. Moisture loss in the vulva skin can lead to symptoms of dryness, irritation, and increased susceptibility to microtrauma.

Moisturizers help protect the skin, and they can treat xerosis, the medical term for dry skin. They can reduce redness, itchiness, and fissures. Whether you need a moisturizer depends on your symptoms, such as vulvar itch or irritation, and your risk of developing dry skin— for example, if you remove pubic hair and/or use soap regularly instead of a cleanser.

Some factors that lead to dryness are modifiable. For example, you can stop hair removal or give up perfumed soap, although some women prefer not to do this. Aging, which is a huge moisture suck, is not possible to reverse, no matter what any self-described anti-aging expert claims. Medications can also lead to dry skin and may not be possible or practical to stop, including chemotherapy for cancer or oral retinoids for severe acne. As the vulva is more sensitive to moisture loss, the first symptoms (and sometimes the only symptoms) may be on the vulva. Medical conditions that damage the acid mantle, like incontinence or skin conditions, can be challenging to treat, and so stopping the cause of the skin barrier dysfunction may not be possible.

If your vulva feels dry and/or itchy, trying a moisturizer may be a good idea. However, if there is no improvement after a week or two, then an appointment with your health care provider to rule out any medical conditions is recommended.

Should I use a moisturizer preventatively?

We don't know if a moisturizer is helpful skin maintenance for women who feel fine but are looking for preventative care. It seems medically intuitive that it may not be a bad idea to try, especially if you are in your forties or older, or if you chronically remove hair or can't give up irritants like soaps or wipes. It is also probably useful if you have incontinence or a skin condition that affects your vulva, such as lichen simplex chronicus (an eczema-like condition) or lichen sclerosus. If you have a skin condition that affects your vulva, it is always a good idea to discuss a moisturizer with your health care provider before you start.

I started a moisturizer when I hit menopause, and my vulva started to feel more supple after a few weeks. I didn't realize how accustomed I had become to the dryness and how much I look forward to the "ah" moment that immediately follows application. If you don't feel dry or use any regular products on your skin that irritate, a moisturizer is probably one of those things to try, see how you like it, and go from there.

Are there downsides to moisturizing?

Some products can block pores and lead to folliculitis (basically acne on the vulva). There is also the risk of irritation and allergic reactions and the hassle of using something chronically. I understand some women love applying creams or ointments as a beauty regimen, but for me it seemed like one more thing I was going to forget, so it took some dedication to get a regimen going. Maybe it just made me feel old to have to start to use a moisturizer? I'm over it now, but it took a few weeks.

What Is the Best Moisturizer?

No moisturizer has been specifically studied for the vulva, so this is an area where I can only offer general guidance. Here are some common products and the available data:

- **COCONUT OIL:** This has been studied on the skin of premature babies with no ill effects, and it performed better than mineral oil in preventing water loss from the skin. Lipids from the oil coat the skin, and it may have beneficial anti-inflammatory activity. It also has only one ingredient, so if it irritates there is no big mystery to solve. It is cheaper than many other options, absorbs well, and smells nice. Some researchers have suggested virgin coconut oil, obtained without chemicals or heat, might offer even more anti-inflammatory activity, but there is no good data to support that hypothesis. Coconut oil is both an emollient and an occlusive agent.
- **OLIVE OIL:** This has been studied as a vulvar moisturizer for breast cancer survivors who could not use estrogen and was well tolerated. It is also an emollient and has occlusive properties.
- **BABY OIL OR MINERAL OIL:** These are by-products of distilling petroleum. While I hate the term "natural," it would not be wrong to say mineral oil is every bit as "natural" as coconut oil, as both come from nature. A petroleum derivative sounds scary, but it has been used for a very long time and has a long safety record. Cosmetic-grade mineral oil is safe for external use. Outside the U.S., mineral oil is often called liquid paraffin or *paraffinum liquidum*, which to be honest sounds a bit like a magic spell. It is both an emollient and an occlusive agent.
- **PETROLEUM JELLY OR PETROLATUM:** A combination of mineral oils and wax, it is a refined product, not fabricated in a lab, so it, too, could be classified as "natural." It functions as an emollient and as an occlusive coat. It is very good at stopping water loss and very well tolerated. Again, keep external.
- **ANY DIAPER RASH CREAM OR OINTMENT:** They typically have a combination of emollients, occlusive products, and humectants. Ingredients may include lanolin, petrolatum, cod liver oil, mineral

oil, paraffin, aloe, wax, and dimethicone as well as preservatives. Anecdotally, I would say that A+D seems well-tolerated, but it has lanolin and some women can be allergic.

- **VMAGIC, A SPECIFIC BRAND MADE OF OILS (OLIVE, AVOCADO, AND SEA BUCKTHORN), BEESWAX, AND A PROPRIETARY BLEND OF HONEY AND PROPOLIS (A KIND OF BEE GLUE):** It's more expensive than just buying oils, and no studies indicate avocado or sea buckthorn oils add anything more than the olive oil or coconut oil in your kitchen cabinet. If a pricey product gives you pleasure, that is great. The product claims to be "chemical-free," which is disingenuous as nothing is chemical free, not even water. In some advertisements, I have also seen their advertising use the "feeling fresh" trope, which is the hill I am always willing to die on.

- **VITAMIN E:** This comes in capsules, and some women like to break them open and use the oil. I give this product an asterisk, safety-wise. While unstudied topically, when taken orally in doses of > 400 IU/day, vitamin E increases the risk of death from any cause. I'm not worried about topical vitamin E being absorbed and killing anyone, but the hypothesis behind vitamin E and increased risk of death is the antioxidant properties may help cancer cells grow faster than healthy cells. With that in mind, could it favor the growth of precancerous cells infected with the human papilloma virus (HPV)? We don't know what we don't know, and since there are other oils to use, it is hard to recommend vitamin E.

Products to avoid

Do not use creams and ointments with salicylic acid or retinol (common in face creams) as they could be irritating. Avoid any product that claims to brighten the vulva—0.5 percent of women report they currently or have previously used these. Topical skin lightening products work by affecting the production of melanin, the pigment that produces skin color. They typically contain one or more of the following: ascorbic acid (vitamin C), retinoic acid, alpha hydroxy acid, or salicylic acid. Hydroxyquinone is available in the U.S., but it is banned in Europe. These products have not been tested for the vulva, and many of them are irritants. Another concern is there is a robust market for illegal skin whiteners, and dangerous ingredients like mercury have been found in products from Europe and Asia.

Melanocytes and melanin are part of your immune system, and so there could be ramifications beyond the irritation of the products. If you have dark patches that bother you, see a health care provider and get the right diagnosis. If the issue is a generalized but mild darkening of your labia and/or around the anus, the most likely cause is changes from chronic hair removal.

Where Should I Apply a Moisturizer?

The labia majora, the perineum (between the vaginal opening and the anus), and on the skin around the anus. Try not to get it in the vagina or anus, although it is fine if coconut or olive oil find their way to those areas.

Any Other Issues?

Any product with an oil is not compatible with latex condoms. We have no data to say how long you should wait after application of an oil so you don't compromise the integrity of a latex condom. A few hours is probably fine, but that is a best guess and should not be taken as gospel.

If you do use coconut oil, make sure everyone in the house knows the coconut oil in the bathroom is for bathroom use. A good friend was eating some cookies one night that her fourteen-year-old daughter had made. When she asked about the ingredients, her daughter replied that she had used coconut oil. There was a pregnant pause as my friend mentally calculated that the location of the only remaining jar of coconut oil was in her bathroom. She was now faced with a moral dilemma: should she tell the family they were eating vulva cookies or not?

Bath Bombs and Bubble Bath

Bath bombs and bubble baths give a lot of people a lot of pleasure. They are pretty, smell nice, and add an extra element of self-care. Many of these products are sold under the guise of wellness, meaning the promise of something medical. The smell and the softness of the water may be pleasing and help you relax, but the skin softness and emollient properties offer no lasting benefit. The reason to use these products is simply joy. That is how I think about wellness: does it bring you joy?

There is at least one bath bomb that makes the claim that it is beneficial for vaginal pH. That is the biggest warning against using it, as the company must think the vagina fills with water during a bath. When you bathe, you do not get a douche. Then there is the fact that no topical product can alter vaginal pH any more than temporarily, and attempts to alter the pH are typically damaging to the vagina.

Bath bombs and bubble baths typically have fragrance, and if they have cool colors then they have dye. Some even have glitter (a big favorite in my house). I'm currently a bath bomb aficionado, as one of my sons is an addict. I'm amazed that society focuses on the nonexistent smells of the female genital tract while largely ignoring the greasiness of the male adolescent, many of whom seem as averse to water as the Wicked Witch of the West. If bath bombs are what get my teenage son to rinse the testosterone-fueled sebum-fest off his skin, then bath bombs it is!

Whether these products are synthetic or botanical does not change their risk for irritation or allergic reactions. Irritation and allergies aside, there is no convincing evidence that bath bombs or bubble baths cause urinary tract infections, although an irritant reaction on the vulva could easily be mistaken for a bladder infection, as the symptoms overlap significantly. Before puberty, girls are at higher risk of irritant reactions, as their labia are very small and don't cover the vestibule (vaginal opening), and the mucosa at the vaginal opening doesn't have estrogen. So for some younger girls, these bath products can be irritating.

Bubble baths that produce fantastic bubbles are essentially diluted liquid soap, and (as we have already reviewed) soap strips the protective fatty layer off the skin and can paradoxically leave the skin drier. If you are going to use them, keep in mind that it's probably best not to indulge daily. They usually have a surfactant like sodium lauryl sulfate, or SLS, which can cause allergic reactions for 3–5 percent of people.

If you find the softness or feel of the bath products soothing, but want a fragrance-free and dye-free alternative that is unlikely to be irritating at all and are willing to give up bubbles, you can consider these two options:

- **EPSOM SALT, WHICH IS MAGNESIUM CITRATE:** These have been used for years, so it has an extensive track record. They don't add anything health benefit-wise; however, they also appear to have no health risk. You can also add some olive oil or avocado oil to the water if you like. Your skin will feel temporarily very soft. It's pleasing, but not medically beneficial.
- **OATMEAL (THE REGULAR FIVE-MINUTE CEREAL STUFF, NOT THE STEEL CUT):** Put a handful in a pantyhose sock with the top tied in a knot, and then throw it in the bathwater. The pantyhose stops your tub from getting disgusting with oatmeal mush. Oatmeal has anti-itch properties. It's not lasting, but it can be soothing while you are in the water and temporary relief from itch can sometimes break the cycle. I used this when my children had diaper rash.

If you want a homemade bubble bath (won't have big bubbles), here is a recipe:

- 2 tablespoons olive, avocado, or almond oil
- 2 tablespoons honey
- ¼ cup liquid castile soap (fragrance fee)
- A drop or two of vanilla extract or any essential oil that doesn't irritate your skin, if desired

If you want huge bubbles, you need to go commercial. If it doesn't irritate or leave you feeling dry, then the joy factor is probably worth it. If your skin is broken or irritated, then bath products may increase your risk of irritation. The vulva is more sensitive to irritants, so a bad reaction to one of these products could simply be vulvar itch or irritation.

BOTTOM LINE

- Mosturizers can be useful on the vulva, especially during menopause, for dry skin, and with incontinence.
- Expensive moisturizers have no obvious advantage over inexpensive products such as coconut oil, olive oil, or petroleum jelly.

- Bubble baths don't cause bladder infections, but for some women, especially girls before puberty, they can irritate the vestibule.
- If you love bath bombs or bubble baths and you don't get irritated, then the joy is probably worth any potential risk.
- There are some cheap, homemade options with a lower risk of irritation for those who can give up big bubbles.

Menstrual Products and Mythology

CHAPTER 15

The Truth About Toxic Shock Syndrome

I AM OLD ENOUGH TO REMEMBER the peak fear of toxic shock syndrome (TSS) in 1979 and 1980. I had just started my period, and soon after, stories about flesh-eating bacteria lurking in the vagina seemed to be everywhere. TSS scared many women away from tampons, and that fear has been exploited by those who wrongly suggest that a woman is somehow ruined if she inserts a menstrual product vaginally before some theoretical future husband's penis. Fear of TSS also sells magazines, gets page clicks, and has been weaponized by those who advance the idea that "natural" menstrual products are somehow better. Add in cultural taboos about menstruation and the ridiculous societal squeamishness about periods, and we have a breeding ground for misinformation.

Fortunately I have the antidote. Facts.

What Is Toxic Shock Syndrome?

Toxic shock syndrome, or TSS, is a severe response to a toxin that has entered the bloodstream. A toxin is a substance made by an organism—bacteria, plants, and animals can all make toxins. A good example is snake venom.

Two types of bacteria can produce a toxin capable of causing TSS: Group A strep, the same bacteria that causes strep throat, and *Staph aureus*. Group A strep doesn't thrive in the vagina, so it doesn't cause menstrual TSS, or mTSS. (Group B strep is found in the vagina, but it isn't a toxin producer.) Most cases of mTSS are due to a toxin called TSS-1 made by the bacteria *Staph aureus*. TSS is defined as menstrual if it occurs during or within 2–3 days of the end of a period. Nonmenstrual TSS affects women and men equally and typically happens after surgery or an injury, like a burn. It affects about 0.3/100,000 people a year.

The symptoms of mTSS are fever, a sunburn-like rash that peels, low blood pressure, vomiting, and diarrhea. Organs can shut down, and lack of blood flow to limbs can even lead to amputations (fortunately, this is very rare). The average duration of hospitalization is six days, and some women are sick enough to need intensive care. With good medical care, the risk of death is less than 4 percent. Survivors can have recurrences, memory loss, and serious health problems. It is a serious illness.

Between 1979 and 1980, there were 1,264 cases of mTSS in the United States and 72 women, 6 percent of those affected, died. The risk of mTSS has dropped and now affects approximately 1/100,000 women of reproductive age. In 2015, the last year we have full data, 47 women in the U.S. had TSS (most of those were likely menstrual related, but the data doesn't distinguish between mTSS and nonmenstrual TSS).

The Complexity of Menstrual TSS, or mTSS

The bacteria *Staph aureus* is a colonizer, meaning many of us carry it on our body but it doesn't cause any problems under typical circumstances. Approximately 10 percent of women of reproductive age are colonized vaginally with *Staph aureus* (wearing tampons does not increase the risk of colonization) and 1 percent of women have a strain capable of making TSS-1. These are the only women at potential risk for mTSS.

The amount of *Staph aureus* in the vagina increases during menstruation when iron from blood increases TSS-1 production. Fortunately, the body has natural defense mechanisms against TSS: 80 percent of women have protective antibodies that can neutralize the toxin (this is why younger women have the highest risk of mTSS: they have had less time to develop antibodies), and some women lack the receptor on their vaginal tissues needed for the toxin to attach to cells and gain entry to the bloodstream.

As 70 percent of women have used tampons at some time, 1 percent of women have TSS-1 producing bacteria, and less than 0.01 percent of women of reproductive age a year get mTSS, these defense mechanisms are generally very effective.

The Rely Tampon:
An Important Menstrual History Lesson

In the 1970s, Procter & Gamble wanted to get into the tampon market with a game-changing product that would disrupt the competition. Until that point, all tampons had the same basic construction: a cylinder of cotton, cotton-rayon, or a cotton-viscose blend that primarily expanded length-wise. Procter & Gamble's answer was the Rely tampon. It was made of polyester foam in cubes and chips plus carboxycellulose (a gelling agent, also used in food like pudding, a good example to remind everyone that just because you can eat something does not make it safe for the vagina!) in a teabag-like pouch. The slogan was, "It even absorbs the worry." I tried Rely when I was fourteen years old, and the tampon absorbed so much blood that getting it out was like giving birth to a giant peach! I had not had sex before, and I have no doubt I caused microtrauma during removal.

Menstrual products in the U.S. are regulated by the FDA (Food and Drug Administration) as medical devices, and any product that differs substantially from what is on the market needs to submit studies for review or they cannot be marketed. Technically, menstrual products are reviewed, not *approved*, by the FDA. The FDA application for Rely was started before this policy was enacted, and so it was grandfathered in without review. An aggressive marketing campaign followed, and by the late 1970s about 25 percent of American women were using Rely.

And then the cases of mTSS started to appear.

Rely was problematic in its design. The foam cubes had more surface area for bacteria to grow and introduced more oxygen than a standard tampon. The cellulose (thickener) was a good growth media for bacteria. Some other manufacturers added polyacrylate, an absorbent material, to tampons to compete with Rely, likely compounding the mTSS problem.

Rely was pulled from the market on September 22, 1980, and cases of mTSS started to drop. Polyacrylate was removed from tampons in the U.S. in 1985.

Keep the Rely tampon in mind every time you see a new "disruptive" tampon or menstrual cup technology hit a crowdfunding platform, because bold new designs are not always safe. If a product differs in any significant way from a traditional tampon or menstrual cup, safety studies and an FDA review are required.

With Rely off the market, how does mTSS still happen?

All tampons, the contraceptive sponge, diaphragms, and menstrual cups increase the risk of mTSS. How this happens is not well understood, but the major mechanisms appear to include some or all of the following:

- **INTRODUCTION OF OXYGEN AND CARBON DIOXIDE WITH INSERTION:** Both help bacteria grow. Menstrual cups may introduce more oxygen with insertion than tampons.
- **ALLOWING GROWTH OF BACTERIA THAT DOESN'T PRODUCE TSS-1:** Other bacteria produce carbon dioxide (it is a by-product of bacterial respiration), and that can help *Staph aureus* grow.
- **SPECIFIC TAMPON FIBERS FAVORING GROWTH OF BACTERIA:** Older studies suggested cotton was less likely to favor growth than rayon or viscose; however, a newer study that replicates the low-oxygen environment of the vagina tells us that the growth of both *Staph aureus* and TSS-1 may be greater with cotton-only tampons. Do not assume cotton is safer.
- **MENSTRUAL CUPS MADE FROM SILICONE AND THERMOPLASTIC ELASTOMER CAN ALLOW BIOFILMS:** This is a protective coating that allows bacteria to avoid detection and destruction by the vagina's defense systems. One study suggests that menstrual cups made of thermoplastic elastomer may induce less biofilm than those made of silicone.
- **ABSORBENCY:** The greater the absorbency of tampons, the greater the risk.
- **TRAUMA FROM INSERTION OR REMOVAL:** This can introduce the toxin

of TSS directly into the bloodstream, bypassing the normal defense mechanisms.

Practical Advice for mTSS Safety

It is impossible to bring the risk with vaginal products to zero, but considering how many women use tampons and how few get mTSS, the risk is low. In the U.K., the risk of mTSS is now less than the risk of TSS from other causes. To put it in perspective, the risk of getting mTSS each year in the U.S. is about the same as the risk of dying after being hit by lightning. Some women will view this as low risk and others as high risk, although I always remind women that we do many things every day that are far more dangerous than wearing a tampon or a menstrual cup. For example, almost 6,000 pedestrians a year are killed by cars, and yet we don't tell women not to go for walks. Women can get abscesses and other serious infections from pubic hair removal. Every intervention has risks, and only you can assess your own risk-benefit ratio

The risk of mTSS is the highest for younger women. That doesn't mean fifteen-year-olds shouldn't use tampons; it is just information to use when you make decisions about your body. Even for women under twenty-four, the risk of mTSS is still less than 2 per 100,000 women per year.

Practical tampon advice:

- **USE THE LOWEST ABSORBENCY:** Some manufacturers make boxes with a range of sizes. If all you have is a large or a super plus (women over the age of forty know what I am talking about), then you are likely using a tampon that is too absorbent on lighter days (should you have those).
- **DO NOT ASSUME ALL-COTTON TAMPONS ARE SAFER:** The latest study suggests rayon blends are safer. Whether the lab study translates to real life is not known.
- **BE MINDFUL OF TRAUMA WITH INSERTION AND REMOVAL:** Using a less-absorbent tampon on lighter days may help.
- **THE RECOMMENDATION TO CHANGE A TAMPON EVERY EIGHT HOURS IS NOT BASED IN HARD SCIENCE, BUT IT SEEMS THE BEST "EXPERT" ADVICE FOR NOW:** Changing more frequently won't reduce your risk. In

fact, it could even increase risk, as more insertions mean more oxygen and carbon dioxide in the vagina and more trauma.

Practical menstrual cup advice:

- **DO NOT ASSUME THEY HAVE A LOWER RISK THAN TAMPONS:** One study showed they are more favorable for growth of *Staph aureus* and TSS-1 than tampons.
- **CHOOSE THE SMALLEST CUP THAT GETS THE JOB DONE:** This could mean having cups of different sizes for light and heavy days.
- **HAVE TWO CUPS, AS THE MANUFACTURER INSTRUCTIONS FOR RINSING BETWEEN EMPTYING ARE NOT SUFFICIENT TO KILL TSS-1:** The cups should be boiled between insertions, so keeping a clean one on hand is likely best.

Sea sponges

A sea sponge is an aquatic organism made of spongin. They have no specialized organs (no lungs, heart, kidneys, etc.); rather, they breathe and feed by filtering seawater though their tiny chambers, which gives them a lot of surface area. Sponges are very absorbent—about two thirds of a sponge is empty space and able to retain fluid. In addition, the spongin swells to prevent liquid from leaking back out. Sponges also expand in all directions. Essentially, they sound like nature's version of the Rely tampon—lots of surface area for bacteria, lots of air pockets, super absorbency, and swell width-wise that could potentially cause micro-trauma during removal.

Cleaning a sponge appropriately is also a challenge. When they are used in the kitchen, they need to be washed on hot in the washing machine with detergent and bleach to kill bacteria, but no one has researched how to clean the sea sponge to kill *Staph aureus* (the bacteria that causes TSS) or the TSS toxin. I tried boiling one for an hour, and the sponge hardened, shrank, and changed color.

A study from 1982 tells us women who use sea sponges have significantly more bacteria in their vagina during their periods, including *Staph aureus*, than women who wore tampons or pads. Between periods there was no difference, so the big bump in potentially dangerous bacteria seemed to be sea sponge related. We have no idea how sponges affect production of the TSS toxin. Evaluation of sea sponges by the FDA in the 1990s revealed the nooks and crannies were filled with microscopic dirt and debris (not surprising, as they filter the ocean).

It is illegal to sell sea sponges for menstrual use in the United States, and the FDA has sent warning letters to several retailers. There is no data to say they are safe, and anyone suggesting they are is, in my opinion, unethical.

Polyester foam products

In some countries, there are menstrual sponges made from the same polyester foam as the Rely tampon. This is also the same foam used for the contraceptive sponge, which carries a risk of mTSS. Some women use polyester makeup sponges as a "period hack."

While we don't know specifically how the polyester foam in Rely contributed to mTSS, it seems counterintuitive to use a product that is made with some of the same material as the tampon with the highest risk of mTSS. I can't find any safety studies on polyester foam (tampons or makeup sponges); however, I did put a polyester foam makeup sponge in water, and it released an impressive amount of air compared to a super plus tampon, which is not reassuring. I'd personally give polyester foam products a pass.

Crocheted or knitted tampons

I've heard some women make their own, and of course you can buy them on Etsy (I've spent many hours down the rabbit hole that is "vagina Etsy"). These tampons are typically made from cotton. No one has submitted these products to the FDA for approval and there is no data on how they could irritate vaginal tissues or affect the growth of bacteria or production of the TSS toxin.

Even though these tampons are reported to be 100 percent cotton, that does not make them similar to commercially available cotton tampons. I bought three, and I was struck by how loosely they are knit—a lot of air could potentially be introduced during insertion, and that is a key mechanism in TSS toxin production. It is also unclear how to clean them to kill bacteria and neutralize the TSS toxin.

The other issue—not that you really need one—is absorbency. None of the three that I tested absorbed more than 5 ml, which is less than a regular-sized commercial tampon.

Give knitted or crocheted tampons a pass.

Could tampons or menstrual cups be safer?

Consider the hundreds of thousands of women in the United States who use tampons and cups. The risk of mTSS is approximately 1/100,000 women a year. So a study to prove a product is safer than what already exists on the market would be a challenge. Rare events are very hard to study, prevention-wise, although it doesn't mean companies shouldn't try. Lab data that shows a product inhibits production of the TSS toxin might be a good start. Safer designs might also look at materials that resist biofilms, introduce less air with insertion, and minimize trauma with insertion and removal.

There is no test to predict who is at risk for mTSS and who isn't, and no test for early mTSS. Another area of research might involve knowing who carries a toxin-producing strain of *Staph aureus*, testing the presence of protective antibodies, or testing for early detection of mTSS, as early intervention improves outcomes.

BOTTOM LINE

- Only 1 percent of women are at risk of developing mTSS, as they carry the strain of *Staph aureus* in the vagina capable of producing the toxin.
- The key mechanism in mTSS seems to be introduction of oxygen, but other factors may be involved.
- Do not assume menstrual cups are safer than tampons.
- All-cotton tampons do not appear safer than those with cotton and rayon or cotton and viscose.
- Don't use sea sponges.

CHAPTER 16

Are There Toxins in Tampons and Pads?

LEARNING ABOUT MENSTRUAL PRODUCTS outside of scientific sources is challenging because a lot of people are invested in period panic. One of the most common myths I am asked to debunk is "toxins" in pads and tampons. Fear sells.

A Word About Regulations

In the United States, the FDA regulates all products for menstrual hygiene. These products (pads, tampons etc.) are not FDA approved; rather, they are registered and given clearance for marketing. Being registered with the FDA means these products are subject to manufacturing oversight, and complaints and adverse events must be tracked. At any time, the FDA can ask to see this paperwork, and if it is not in order production/sales could be shut down and additional enforcement action taken.

Unscented pads and scented pads using materials that have been studied and previously cleared by the FDA are Class I medical devices, meaning new studies are not required as long as the product is not materially different from what has previously been approved. The product is registered and goes to market.

Scented pads using new materials and any device inserted vaginally (for example, tampons and menstrual cups) are Class II medical devices. Tampon manufacturers are required to submit paperwork that proves their products are similar to a product currently on the market or, if they have a novel design or material, they must provide safety studies. Menstrual cups have an expedited process and can go straight to market without a go-ahead from the FDA, but the product still has to be registered.

Perusing the FDA site, I found letters from the FDA to companies about concerns regarding the manufacturing processes and cleaning recommendations for menstrual cups, which shows the expedited process for menstrual cups is not a "Get Out of Jail Free" card.

What About Hidden Toxins?

Myths about hidden toxins and dangers with tampons and menstrual cups predate "Big Natural." They even predate Google! I remember being asked about tampons and asbestos by women in the early 1990s. There isn't any. There never has been any. Another pre-internet myth is that menstrual cups cause endometriosis. There was even a petition to the FDA to get them banned. There is no link between the two.

Pad and tampon manufacturers in the U.S. are not required to list ingredients on the package or on their website, and so this is often offered as a reason for concern. While I agree every product should have all ingredients listed, I've researched many tampons and pads for this book, and each one had the ingredients listed. I checked several "Big Company" and "Natural" products with their FDA applications and they matched.

Why "Natural" manufacturers are not lying about their ingredients but "Big Companies" are has never been explained to my satisfaction.

What About Residues?

For a tampon to be approved, the manufacturer must demonstrate that is it free of herbicides and pesticides, or if they are present how the manufacturer determined they are present in acceptable levels for human use.

The most prevalent myth surrounds dioxins, which are known carcinogens for animals and probably carcinogenic for people. No one wants to put a probable carcinogen in their vagina! Older methods for bleaching cotton and in the manufacturing of rayon produced low levels of dioxins. Bleaching methods were changed (the culprit was elemental chlorine), but there still are traces of dioxin in tampons, pad, and disposable diapers, even those made of 100 percent cotton. Not because of problematic manufacturing, but because dioxin is everywhere in the raw materials, be it cotton or wood pulp, due to pollution.

Exposure to dioxins in tampons is thousands of times less than what you are exposed to in your food, and there is no difference in dioxin levels in 100 percent cotton "health food store" tampons versus "conventional" cotton/rayon blends. Interestingly, in one study the tampon that had the highest level of dioxins was from an "organic" company. According to one study, "exposures to dioxins from tampons is approximately 13,000–240,000 times less than dietary exposures." So even if you use 12,000 tampons in a lifetime, you are not approaching the lower level of dietary exposure, and there is no evidence that 100 percent cotton products offer a lower exposure.

Another internet myth is that "conventional" tampons contain glyphosate, an ingredient in some herbicides, like Roundup. The WHO lists glyphosate as a possible carcinogen; however, there is a lot of science that disagrees with that conclusion. The glyphosate tampon "data" (I struggle to call it that) is unpublished, which makes it as valuable as hearsay. Glyphosate works by binding to an enzyme that humans do not have and is not absorbed across skin or mucosa, found in the vagina, so tampon-wise it seems like a nonissue.

What about other substances? There are groups that claim to have found carcinogens, irritants, and other harmful chemicals in tampons and pads. The problem is this analysis is not published in peer-reviewed journals, so experts can't tell if the results are valid or not. The testing methods may not be accurate, either. For example, one group tested pads by burning them and measuring the off-gassing, but that is not an appropriate testing method. I don't like this tactic. I agree we should have transparency about residues, but there are experts in environmental health who could do this testing in a way that would let us know if the results are valid or not.

An important point that is constantly overlooked is that no tampon manufacturer has published their analysis of chemical residues for peer review. A company can claim they are free from whatever residue they want, but if it is just on their website and not published, it is an unverifiable claim.

In my opinion, the best answer would be for the FDA to have a standardized method of residue detection for tampons and to release the results publicly. That would also be the cheapest way to go.

BOTTOM LINE

- Ingredients/components don't have to be listed on pads and tampons, but every product I checked matched the FDA submission.
- The FDA requires tampons be free of herbicide/pesticide residue (or have such low levels that they are not medically relevant)—no manufacturer makes this raw data available about their product.
- Dioxin levels are the same in 100 percent cotton organic tampons and rayon blends.
- There is no data indicating there is glyphosate in tampons. Glyphosate is inactive in humans and not absorbed through the vagina.
- Most so-called "organic" tampons have not submitted their own safety data; they are cleared for use based on tampons that have already been cleared by the FDA.

CHAPTER 17

Menstrual Hygiene

DOCTORS LEARN VERY LITTLE ABOUT MENSTRUAL PRODUCTS in training. We are taught how to manage a stuck tampon and that tampons have a role in toxic shock syndrome, but we learn nothing practical on how to advise women about their choices. I've often thought this to be odd. After all, ophthalmologists learn some practical information about glasses and contact lenses, and they have opticians to help.

As a gynecologist, I became very interested in menstrual hygiene. Part of this was spurred by toxic shock syndrome—I studied infectious diseases, so I made learning about menstrual products a priority. I've been blogging for over eight years on women's health, and I've had to research so many products and regulations that I now feel like both a gynecologist and whatever term we would use for the optician equivalent for menstrual products. Maybe a "menstrutician"?

Some Menstrual Basics

The average menstrual fluid loss is 30–50 ml a day (1 to almost 2 ounces). Over a period, which typically lasts seven days or fewer, a woman loses an average of 80 ml of blood, but it can range from 13 ml to 217 ml. Women with medically heavy periods (menorrhagia) can sometimes bleed up to 400 ml per period, which is a lot!

It is important that women choose the product that works best for them, because studies tell us what women find most distressing is not the volume of blood, but the fact that the blood has leaked onto their clothes. Sometimes leaking can be a sign of a heavy period, but sometimes it indicates the wrong product choice.

It is interesting that there is no correlation between the number of pads used during a menstrual cycle and blood loss—how often women change their menstrual product is more a personal preference than a my-pad-is-soaked problem. In one study, the range of blood on a pad before it was changed varied from 14 ml (a completely soaked overnight pad) to less than 2 ml (a small spot on a nighttime pad). A common metric that health care providers use to gauge the heaviness of menstrual flow is how many pads are used per hour or two hours—by this we mean a completely soaked pad. It is important to have the same language about just how soaked a pad actually is, because 14 ml is very different from changing a pad with only 2 ml. When you speak with your doctor or provider make sure you explain how soaked or stained a pad is when you are changing it and the size of the pad (overnight, heavy flow, medium flow, or light flow).

Menstrual blood has venous blood (what you normally bleed when you are cut) as well as vaginal discharge and cells from the lining of the uterus (called the endometrium). It can look like blood, it can look like red mucus, it can be almost black, and it can be clotted—none of that is abnormal medically. Sometimes menstrual blood can even look so much like tissue, it could be confused with a miscarriage. This medical phenomenon is called a decidual cast, which occurs when a large portion of the endometrium comes off at once. Period blood is normally liquid as the individual cells of the endometrium are not stuck together. However, imbalance between the hormones progesterone and estrogen can cause the cells to come off in sheets as opposed to individually (think a hundred Lego blocks attached together versus individual blocks). A common cause is hormonal contraception, as many women are progestin (a synthetic form of progesterone) dominant versus estrogen dominant. It is not medically harmful.

U.S. women spend about $3 billion per year on sanitary protection. In many countries these products are taxed, which is ridiculous, as they are essential. The right product can reduce discomfort, give peace of mind, and may even reduce hysterectomies. This is because excessive menstrual blood loss is often defined as soiling clothes, not volume of blood. If a woman is leaking blood onto her clothes because she is using a product that is ill-fitted or not designed for her blood loss, she may think she is bleeding heavily and seek medical and even surgical intervention (like a hysterectomy), when really what she has is a product problem. In addition, girls and women without access to menstrual protection miss days of education and work.

Doing the right thing aside, governments would probably save money if they made menstrual hygiene products less expensive, because it would reduce medical expenses and days off from work for heavy bleeding that was really due to the wrong choice of menstrual product.

Disposable Menstrual Pads

In the U.S., about 12 billion disposable pads are used each year, making this the most common product choice. Disposable pads have a layered design with the following components:

- **THE TOP SHEET:** Lets moisture through but keeps the skin dry. More moisture leakage back to the skin could increase irritation and potentially raise the vulvar pH, changing the environment for skin bacteria. The top sheet can be cotton or a synthetic fabric, like polypropylene/polyethylene, which is the same kind of material in some athletic wear. Synthetics allow less moisture leakage back to the skin—some as little as 5 percent. Perforated top sheets may help reduce wetness by allowing some airflow. Practically speaking, if you don't feel wet, then your pad is likely working well for you. Some pads also have an emollient in the top sheet, and a study has not identified it as a source of irritation, although the study was funded by the manufacturer. Whether an emollient could help or irritate women who are more prone to skin issues is unknown.
- **THE COTTON-LOOKING STUFF:** Usually cellulose based, but may be a combination of cotton, cellulose, rayon, and polyester.

Absorbent wood cellulose has been used in pads since the 1920s. It was introduced because it was cheaper and more absorbent than cotton.

- **A GEL OR FOAM ABSORBENT CORE:** Increases absorption capacity significantly and allows incredibly thin pads to really bring their A game. The gel is a little slower to absorb than the cellulose or other materials, but it holds on to the blood better. Not every pad has an absorbent core.
- **WATERPROOF BACK SHEET:** Typically a plastic to keep the blood from leaking through. Some have wings to wrap around your underwear to hold the pad in place and catch side leaks. I personally feel wings are one of the greatest inventions of the 20th century, but I know some women despise them.
- **ADHESIVE:** Usually similar to craft glue.
- **WRAPPER:** Some are compostable and some are not.

Pads are typically well tolerated. In post-marketing surveillance of a new pad with some of the most high-tech synthetic ingredients, there was one health complaint per 1 million pads shipped.

No product that touches skin is going to be complaint-free, but the very low number of formal complaints with pads is reassuring. There is a myth that Always pads are more irritating, but the study that I just quoted regarding consumer complaints about a new pad design was about a new Always pad with an absorbent core. I am not here to defend or promote Procter & Gamble, but there really seems to be no data to say one pad is better tolerated than another. It is possible that one brand of pad may irritate you and another may not. Sensitivities, unlike allergies, are hard to define and hard to study. Also, touch and feel are very personal. You like what you like, and what irritates you may not irritate someone else.

Pads with odor control may have fragrance or absorbent mineral particles in the core that trap volatiles. Fragrance in any part of the pad that touches your skin can lead to irritation for some women. I recommend against all menstrual products with fragrance. Pads can also be a source of irritation, either due to a sensitivity to the materials or friction from an ill-fitted pad.

Some pads are compostable, and that can impact purchasing decisions.

Pantyliners

Pantyliner use is very common—about 50 percent of women in North America and Europe wear them either as backup support for a tampon or menstrual cup or exclusively on light days, and 10–30 percent of women wear a pantyliner daily. We all have discharge, and so it is a personal choice whether you get that discharge on your underwear or a pantyliner.

Many women worry that daily pantyliner use can affect their skin. Vulvar skin issues usually arise when moisture is retained against the skin for extended periods of time—as from a soaking wet pad or underwear. While most women try to change wet pads or garments quickly, some have wondered if a plastic back sheet could increase moisture and/or change pH of the skin with daily use. Most studies tell us this is not an issue with menstrual pads, but that reflects intermittent use, not months at a time.

Pantyliners do have a small but measurable impact on skin temperature and surface moisture (so-called breathable pantyliners don't mitigate this), but it doesn't seem to be clinically relevant for women without skin conditions. Four studies have looked at the impact of pantyliner use for healthy women and found no association with any health problem. One study looked at 10–12 hours of pantyliner use daily for seventy-five days compared to a control group who only wore underwear and found no change in yeast, vaginal pH, inflammation, or other health concerns. Some lower-quality retrospective studies linked pantyliners with vaginal infections; however, if you have an infection, you are likely to have recall bias and remember things you feel may be associated. In addition, infections can change discharge or irritation, two symptoms that might prompt a woman to wear menstrual pads, so this could be correlation, not causation.

This data only applies to women with healthy skin. Women with skin conditions could potentially find pantyliners irritating, as the microenvironment on the skin surface may be more vulnerable to subtle changes in moisture or skin temperature.

If you prefer daily pantyliners and have no vulvar concerns, there is no data to suggest they will cause harm. I would advise against fragrance, as, given the thinner nature of the product, it could contact the skin. If you develop any kind of chronic irritation or vaginal discharge, it is probably worth giving up pantyliners until you have the issue controlled.

Reusable Menstrual Pads and Liners

In many countries where disposable pads are not available, washable pads dramatically improve the quality of life for girls and women, allowing them to attend school or work and reducing complications from skin irritation. Some women also prefer these products for tactile or environmental reasons.

There are no studies of cloth versus disposable pads. Looking at cloth versus disposable diapers as a proxy, disposable diapers tend to be associated with less bacteria on the skin and fewer irritation issues, but urine and feces really can't translate to menstrual blood.

There is also a "feel" factor involved in comfort. Some women prefer the feel of fabric, and others find fabric pads are too damp as there is no top sheet to keep wetness from flowing backwards.

If what you are using is not causing irritation, then it is probably just fine. Some women hate the feel of disposable pads, other women prefer washable pads for environmental reasons, and some women find a washable pad is more wetness than they like.

Period Underwear

This is not your ruined, nasty underwear from that time you had a critical tampon event, but underwear that absorbs blood, replacing pads, tampons, or menstrual cups. The claim is a pair of this underwear can absorb at least a tampon's worth of fluid, but what a tampon can absorb varies based on its, well, absorbency. The range for period underwear absorption-wise is anywhere from 5 ml to 25 ml.

Period underwear has absorbent layers of synthetic microfibers and apparently a polyurethane (plastic) component, but the companies say their material is proprietary, and so it is not possible to know. They are expensive, and if you generally use three or four tampons or pads a day, you might need three pairs of underwear just to get through your day. You'll also need a plastic bag to take your soiled underwear home, because at $40 to $50 a pair, you don't want to throw them away. You also can't slip them off like a pad, so if you are wearing pants or tights you have to take those off first, which can sometimes be a chore in a public restroom. If you want to wear them two days in a row, you may need more pairs or to be willing to do more laundry.

An in-depth review from the site Wirecutter (affiliated with *The New York Times*) tested multiple brands and rates Dear Kate and Thinx as their top picks. If you are interested in this underwear, I would suggest looking that review up on your favorite search engine.

Given the expense and absorbency, they are probably best suited as backup for a tampon or menstrual cup or for light days. They may also be a good option for younger girls who are just going through puberty and may have unpredictable periods and trans men who may be on hormones and have lighter periods.

There is no reason to think there are major health issues with these garments. The material that touches your skin seems similar to the top sheet in many pads, and a version for incontinence (same basic fabric and design) has been tested in a few published studies with no skin irritation.

Thinx also makes a large absorbent towel for period sex. It is $369. I think you can buy a lot of navy blue towels for that price.

Tampons

Women have used a variety of vaginal products for centuries, but the first U.S. patent for a tampon was in 1933 for Tampax, the name a combination of tampon and vaginal pack.

The standard tampon design is two parts: the pledget, which is the absorbent part, and the string. Modern tampons absorb primarily lengthwise; if they absorbed width-wise, they could cause pain and potentially microtrauma with removal. In the U.S., any wrapping and applicator is considered part of the tampon, and all components must be submitted to the FDA for clearance before marketing.

Originally, tampons were all cotton, but rayon (a fiber synthesized from wood pulp) was added as it was cheaper than cotton and more absorbent.

Tampon absorbency is standardized by the FDA (see Table 1 on p. 150)—1 g of blood is approximately equal to 1 ml of blood.

What a tampon can hold in the lab may be different from what it can hold in a vagina without leaking. One study looked at Tampax to establish

Table 1: Standard Tampon Absorbency

ABSORBENCY	VOLUME OF BLOOD
Slender/light	< 6 g
Regular	6–9 g
Super	9–12 g
Super Plus	12–15 g
Ultra	15–18 g

real-life absorbency, and a completely soaked regular, super, and super plus each came in below or at the lower range of absorbency.

Other Tampon Tidbits

When a tampon is positioned correctly, it shouldn't be felt.

Tampons should not be worn during sex. That could be painful for you and—if you have a male partner—painful for him. It could also lead to trauma. Tampons are fine to wear during oral sex.

There is no increased risk of pulling out your IUD if you wear tampons.

Rogue tampons

Tampons can be left behind. Sometimes people can't get their tampon out and are too embarrassed to go to the doctor, and sometimes people forget. It happens more than you think, so please do not be ashamed about it. I've accidentally inserted a second one and not realized for several hours until I stopped to think what was bugging me. There is more room than you think at the top of the vagina. Alcohol use is also a cofactor for forgetting about tampons.

The most common sign of a forgotten tampon is a foul-smelling discharge, as the tampon becomes a perfect place for bacteria to overgrow. If you find a forgotten tampon at home and remove it on your own, it is probably a good idea to see your doctor for an exam. If you are in the emergency room or doctor's office and they pull out a tampon that was left behind, do not be embarrassed by the smell. It happens a fair bit, and we just want to help you feel better and are prepared. Forgotten tampons are common enough that every office or emergency room I have worked in has an informal protocol for disposing of them in the most odor-free manner possible.

What's the deal with tampon applicators?

They were originally designed because women were believed to be too squeamish to touch themselves, although this seems to be primarily a North American phenomenon. Tampons without an applicator do require that you insert your finger inside your vagina, so an applicator will reduce contact with blood but won't eliminate it. An applicator also doesn't give you better placement. Tampons with applicators are less common outside of North America.

First-time tampon tips

If you have had insertional sex with a penis or finger play, it may be a little easier, but everyone is different. Squatting or standing with one foot on the toilet seat are both good positions to try, as they open your pelvic floor. If you are tense, the pelvic muscles can contract, and you will feel as if you are hitting a wall and the tampon may not go in or may come right back out.

If you are nervous at all or this is the very first time you have inserted anything into your vagina, I recommend the slimmest tampon with a plastic applicator. Plastic applicators have rounded tips and are smoother than the tampon itself or a cardboard applicator. You can also apply lube to the plastic, and if you need to fiddle a bit or it takes you a while to take the next step, the applicator won't start to weaken like cardboard can when it is wet.

If you can't get the tampon in, try sliding your finger inside your vagina—if it goes in no problem, then try with the tampon again. If that doesn't work (and you are feeling up to it, and nothing hurts), I recommend lying on your bed with your legs flopped open (like a frog) and placing a pillow under your hips. Take some slow, deep breaths and try again. If this doesn't work, then see your doctor or nurse practitioner. Chances are everything is fine and it is a technique/nervousness/muscle spasm issue, but women can have a septum (extra hymenal tissue in the vagina) that is blocking the path. If insertion is painful at any point, then stop. It is better to get some advice from a woman's health care provider. Painful experiences are simply not necessary, and you want to rule out any medical conditions.

Menstrual Cups

I am sure almost everyone has seen a pad or tampon applicator washed up on a beach, so it's no wonder more women are turning to menstrual cups, which are reusable and more environmentally friendly. Menstrual cups are made of silicone, latex, or a thermoplastic elastomer, which is a polymer made from rubber. In general, it is considered safe for latex-allergic individuals; however, always follow the advice on the package and ask your own doctor if you have a latex allergy.

Cups and toxic shock syndrome were covered in chapter 15—do not assume they are any safer than tampons, I recommend having two so you can properly clean before reinsertion (unless you want to use a backup method while you are cleaning).

None of the cups on the market have published any safety studies. Menstrual cups were in use long before the FDA changed the rules on submissions. For example, the Tasette was a menstrual cup from the 1950s, and it looks exactly like the cups of today. A 1959 paper describing the benefits of tampons and cups states menstrual cups were a modification of diaphragms, and so it seems they were originally cleared for use based on similarity to diaphragms.

Published data on menstrual cups is sparse. In general, there is more safety data on tampons. This doesn't mean cups are unsafe, but I do find it ironic that many consumer advocates rail against the big manufacturers of pads and tampons for lack of data and transparency yet there is next to nothing about menstrual cups. There are no studies looking at the response of vaginal tissues to wearing a menstrual cup several days in a row. I've never seen any issues, but it simply hasn't been studied.

In the FLOW study (Finding Lasting Options for Women—some study acronyms are the best!), 91 percent of women who tried a menstrual cup said they would continue to use it and would recommend it to others. In another study where women used pads or tampons for three cycles and a menstrual cup for three cycles, women typically found cups superior for comfort and collection of menstrual blood. Irritation and difficulties with insertion were most common in the first two cycles, by the third cycle few problems were noted (this is a similar ease-of-use trajectory to that found for the female condom). There appears to be no increased risk of vaginal infections or bladder infections for cups versus tampons.

The insertion technique for menstrual cups is very similar to that of a tampon, but as a cup is larger, you need to ensure it is in far enough that you don't feel it while sitting. It can take a few uses to get the hang of removal without making your bathroom look like a crime scene. Removal is best done sitting on the toilet so you can dispose of the blood. I am highly adept at putting things into and removing them from the vagina, and I made a mess the first two times I tried. I recommend trying your first insertion and removal in the privacy of your own bathroom.

There are so many cups on the market (more than twenty manufacturers, many with more than one type of cup and cups in different sizes) that making a specific recommendation is hard. There are also no studies on fit. Most manufacturers post the dimensions, but given the number, that is a lot of information to slog through. There are sites where women have compiled all the available cups and sizes for comparison, so for a cup novice that might be a place to start. One site with lots of aggregated information is putacupinit.com.

One study that provided 101 women with the same-sized cup did not report more failures among women who had previously been pregnant or by age—although in fairness, that wasn't the purpose of the study, so they may not have looked at the data in a way that could answer the question. Some cup manufacturers refer to the age thirty in their size recommendations, but you don't wake up on your thirtieth birthday with your vagina magically expanded. Without studies, it is hard to understand how that is a medical recommendation versus a wild guess. We used to think diaphragm size mattered, but there is data to suggest that the model size (70 mm) diaphragm is as effective as one fitted by a physician. A cup should be comfortable to insert, and when you are wearing it, you should not feel it and should be able to empty your bladder without difficulty.

Some cup manufacturers don't recommend using a cup with an IUD due to concerns about pulling the IUD out with the cup. I have a friend who pulled her IUD out with a tampon (there was some excessive alcohol consumption involved, so her judgement about what she was grasping and how hard she was pulling may have been impaired)—however, it doesn't seem common with either cup or tampon use.

Disposable menstrual cups

There are two products currently on the market in the United States, Flex and Softdisc. They have a firm ring, and a clear, plastic-wrap-looking material forms the cup. Both are made of "polymer," which is a molecule made up of smaller units. Both products are now owned by the same company. Before they merged, I emailed them and was told by one company that the ingredients were proprietary, and the other did not reply. Failure to be transparent with products is not limited to pads and tampons.

The devices on the market are cleared for use based on their similarity to the first disposable cup made by Ultrafem in the 1990s. Ultrafem was approved based on being similar to other materials. As far as I can tell, no one has ever published studies on disposable menstrual cups. This doesn't mean they are unsafe—they are similar enough to diaphragms—but this means we don't have data.

I've heard claims that disposable cups are "the only internally worn product not linked to TSS," which is true but also not true. Technically, TSS related to disposable menstrual cups has not been reported, but they have a tiny share of the menstrual market, and there are fewer than fifty cases of TSS a year, so there are likely not enough users to assess risk. TSS has been reported with diaphragms, so the risk is there and to insinuate otherwise is disingenuous.

Disposable menstrual cups are often touted as a product for mess-free period sex. Obviously, sex is messy to begin with, especially if ejaculate is involved. Blood is harder to clean out of sheets, and some women have such heavy flow that it can affect what they feel. I've tried these cups for sex (there is no better road test for any period product than those special, heavy periods of your forties) and they were just okay. Sometimes they leaked, and sometimes they didn't. It wasn't enough of a wow factor for me to keep buying them, but they might work for some women. I just went back to my old standby, a navy blue towel.

Another use for disposable cups could be women who love cups but are going to be in a situation where cleaning is a challenge, like travel or camping.

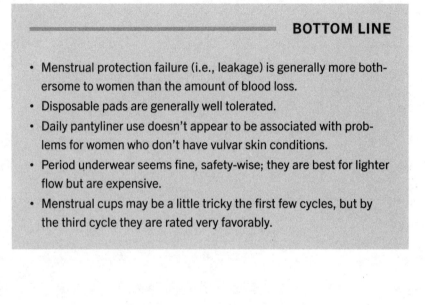

BOTTOM LINE

- Menstrual protection failure (i.e., leakage) is generally more bothersome to women than the amount of blood loss.
- Disposable pads are generally well tolerated.
- Daily pantyliner use doesn't appear to be associated with problems for women who don't have vulvar skin conditions.
- Period underwear seems fine, safety-wise; they are best for lighter flow but are expensive.
- Menstrual cups may be a little tricky the first few cycles, but by the third cycle they are rated very favorably.

Menopause

CHAPTER 18

Menopause

OVER 60 MILLION WOMEN IN THE UNITED STATES are menopausal, meaning they are one year from their last menstrual period or they have had their ovaries removed before the onset of menopause. The average age of non-surgically-induced menopause is fifty-one years. The age a woman goes through menopause is unrelated to the age she started her menstrual cycle (what we in medicine call "menarche"). The one exception is when the menstrual cycle starts at the age of 16 or older; then menopause may be slightly delayed.

The hallmark of menopause is the dramatic reduction in levels of the reproductive hormones estrogen and progesterone.

A Menstrual Cycle Review

Each menstrual cycle is a complex interaction between the brain, the ovary, and the lining of the uterus (endometrium). A hormone called FSH (follicle-stimulating hormone) triggers the development of follicles in the ovary, the follicles produce estrogen, and with ovulation, the egg releases for potential fertilization. With age, the ability of the follicles to produce estrogen declines, so the brain produces higher levels of FSH in an attempt to stimulate the ovaries (a bit like raising your voice when you know someone is in the next room and you can't hear if they are replying to your question or not).

Without sufficient estrogen to provide feedback to the brain, FSH levels remain elevated. (In a way, it's as if the brain keeps shouting at the ovaries to produce estrogen and there is no mechanism for the ovaries to reply, "Sorry, we've had the going-out-of-business sale, the shop is closed.") Levels of FSH over 30 ng/ml are typical with menopause, but hormone levels are generally not needed to make the diagnosis of menopause. One exception is a woman who has had a hysterectomy, as focusing on the last menstrual cycle is obviously not reliable. If signs of menopause appear before the age of forty, the diagnosis of ovarian insufficiency (a condition we used to call premature menopause) should be suspected, and hormone tests are recommended for confirmation. This should not be thought of as an early menopause; rather, it is a distinct medical condition.

The transition to menopause in the forties and early fifties can be a meandering descent with years of unreliable menstrual cycles or a precipitous crash—think regular periods like clockwork and then nothing. Some women have terrible symptoms, and others do not. Interestingly, symptoms aren't linked to hormone levels; rather, they are a complex recipe of genetics, tolerance, and how much estrogen is produced in adipose tissue (fat), as that can convert other hormones into estrogen using an enzyme called aromatase.

Genitourinary Syndrome of Menopause

We used to call the vulvar and vaginal changes of menopause atrophy, as the vaginal tissues become thinner and can shrink. There are some issues with this terminology. Atrophy is only part of the picture; there are many other changes. While the lower third of the vagina and vestibule (vaginal opening) are rich with estrogen receptors and consequently can be significantly impacted by menopause, there are estrogen receptors in the clitoris, labia, urethra, and bladder, and so the symptoms and physical changes are not confined to the vagina. Atrophy is also synonymous with shrinkage. Women are already diminished by society as we age, and so using a term that evokes that for our genitals is not ideal.

The new terminology, genitourinary syndrome of menopause (GSM), is more encompassing and keeps everyone thinking of the vulva and bladder as well as the vagina. I'll admit GSM isn't a catchy acronym, but it is far more accurate and inclusive—and not pejorative.

How Menopause Affects the Vulva

Estrogen increases blood flow to the tissues and helps maintain tissue strength and elasticity. As levels drop, the tissues can become more fragile and lose the ability to stretch. The skin can also become thinner and feel dry, and there can be redistribution of fatty tissue. The labia majora can shrink or change shape. The labia minora can reduce in size, and the ability of the vaginal opening (vestibule) to stretch can become impaired. The amount of erectile tissue in the clitoris also decreases with age. Whether this is an estrogen-related phenomenon or simply part of normal aging (muscle fibers shrink with age) is not known. We also do not know if the loss in clitoral volume has a role in the sexual difficulties some women experience during and after menopause.

Pubic hair graying is age-related and not hormone-related. It is due to a loss of melanin production. The studies on pubic hair color and aging are sparse. One study found no graying of pubic hair before the age of forty-five, although it was only a sample of sixty-four women. My anecdotal experience from years in practice and talking with girlfriends supports the idea that gray pubic hair before forty-five is uncommon. While there are no studies on pubic hair graying versus the head on your hair, anecdotally I can tell you the two do not seem related, so if the hair on your head grays early, that doesn't mean your pubic hair will or vice versa. With age, pubic hair can reduce in amount.

How Menopause Affects the Vagina

The lack of estrogen affects glycogen deposition in the vaginal mucosa. The cells lose volume and there is less glycogen to feed lactobacilli, so they begin to die and different populations of bacteria can be established. Consequently, some women may notice a change in vaginal odor. There is also a reduction in cervical mucus and less transudate (fluid that leaks from blood vessels into the vagina). Given the change in bacteria, cervical mucus,

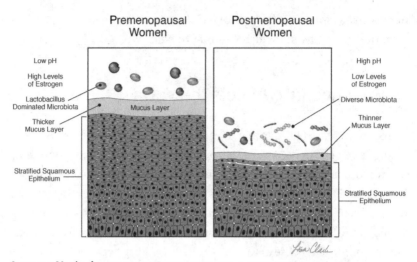

Image 9: Vaginal mucosa. ILLUSTRATION BY LISA A. CLARK, MA, CMI.

and transudate, the vagina can feel drier and lubrication during arousal is reduced. The vaginal tissues become thinner and the ability to stretch is reduced. For some women, the size of the vagina, especially the width, can shrink. Over time, some women can experience a shortening of their vagina. The combination of reduced discharge and thinner, less elastic tissues can lead to microtrauma and even visible trauma with sexual activity.

Loss of tissue support can cause cells of the urethra to protrude and become irritated—this is called a caruncle. It can look very disturbing, and many women are concerned it is a cancer (that's how bad it can look). Caruncles are usually less than a centimeter in diameter and are red and beefy in appearance. The change in vaginal bacteria and the lack of estrogen to support the bladder and urethra can increase the risk of urinary tract (bladder) infections. This may also contribute to the high percentage of menopausal women—50 percent—who report some kind of urinary leakage (incontinence)

Symptoms of GSM

Vaginal dryness is the number one symptom, but others include a sandpaper feeling in the vagina, vaginal irritation, a change in discharge, decreased lubrication, pain with sex, bleeding after sex, burning on urination, increased urgency (need to empty your bladder urgently), and bladder infections.

As many as 15 percent of women report symptoms during peri-menopause, and by three years after menopause as many as 50 percent of women experience GSM. Of those women affected, 50 percent report that symptoms interfere with their sex life, which is 25 percent of all menopausal women! Women who are 45–64 years of age are most dis-tressed by these symptoms. It isn't known if the symptoms of GSM truly reduce over time, if women give up seeking care for their symptoms be-cause they have been dismissed or ignored too many times, if women become less bothered because other medical conditions become more important, or if priorities shift due to a lack of a sexual partner or a part-ner capable of having sex.

What we do know is that most women do not attribute their symp-toms to menopause—in one study, only 4 percent thought they could be menopause related. No one wants to believe they have age-related symp-toms (I'm fifty-two years old, I get that), but for women there is another cultural barrier—the uniquely terrible way that society treats aging women. Talking about sex is hard enough for many people, but the idea of an older woman daring to be sexual? There is a culture of silence about aging vulvas and vaginas. Society wants us to be doting grandmothers and eccentric detectives. So it is harder for women to gain knowledge about symptoms of menopause than it is for other very common condi-tions associated with aging, such as lower back pain or arthritis.

Women are also failed by medicine. Most women with GSM don't seek medical help. Many who do seek care are not asked about their sex life or sexual difficulties. Self-advocacy is important, but there are so many barriers.

Tissue Changes During GSM

Approximately 50 percent of women have changes during GSM when a sample of cells is evaluated microscopically. In a study that looked at mi-croscopic changes in GSM, women with more severe changes were more likely to report difficulties lubricating with sexual activity (as expected), but tissue changes of menopause could not predict who was having pain with sex. This doesn't mean tissue changes don't cause pain with sex; rather, pain is complex. Consider back pain—60 percent of people with no back pain have abnormal findings on MRI. With medicine, it is always important to put things in personal perspective. Some women will have severe symptoms of GSM and minimal microscopic changes, and some women will not be bothered by symptoms and yet have severe microscopic changes.

A study that looked at over 800 postmenopausal women found that the most protective factor for microscopic changes in the vaginal tissues (apart from using hormones) was being overweight—medically, this can be explained by the fact that adipose tissue converts other hormones into estrogen. A known factor that increases the risk of both symptoms of GSM and microscopic changes is cigarette smoking, as it has an anti-estrogen effect.

This same study also reported that African American women had fewer severe changes from GSM under the microscope. The reason is not known. There could be genetic factors, differences in the vaginal microbiome (the bacterial makeup), or other factors. One study found higher circulating estrogen levels in African American women versus white women. However, the fewer microscopic or even macroscopic (visible) physical changes should not be confused with a lack of symptoms.

Is "If You Don't Use It, You Lose It" True?

This is the theory that women who are not sexually active after menopause risk severe vaginal and vulvar changes that can lead to vaginal scarring and permanent closure of the vagina. This sounds very scary, but once you go digging you find there are a lot of assumptions, an outdated article, and (of course) the mythology that a penis is the cure for everything.

The idea that sexual activity with a penis preserves the vagina from GSM always sounded biologically preposterous and devoid of common sense to me, in addition to ignoring the experiences of women. After all, if sex prevented the painful changes of menopause, why do women stop having sex because of pain when they become menopausal? While I risk a TMI moment, and I admit this is anecdotal, sex did not protect my vagina. I went through menopause at the age of forty-nine, and regular heterosexual intercourse offered no protection. Within a year, I needed pharmaceuticals.

The main theory is that the local trauma of sex keeps the tissues healthy, possibly due to increased blood flow (the body's response to injury is to send more blood to the injured site). Also, repetitive pressure can stretch tissue. For example, if you pull on your labia regularly, they will get longer, although the tissues do not become more elastic.

The idea that sex with a penis keeps the vagina healthy appears to have originated with the sex researchers Masters and Johnson, who evaluated fifty-four menopausal women and found only three became aroused with sexual stimulation—these women were the only ones having sex. Of course, it was entirely possible that none of the other women were having sex because it hurt too much or there were other factors involved. This is a great example of how an observation does not imply cause and effect.

A study in 1981 attempted to look at the "use it or lose it" connection and evaluated twenty-four menopausal women having sex and twenty-one not having sex (very small numbers for this kind of study). They found the women not having sex were also cuddling and masturbating less. There were no statistically significant differences in the vulvar changes (there was a trend, but that doesn't count—especially not with such small numbers), and no vaginal tissues were examined microscopically! There was an increase in male hormones among the women having sex, but to conclude that sex or masturbation is protective involves taking several leaps of faith to conclude those hormone changes were due to sexual stimulation and that they were protective. I just don't understand why people cite this paper as proof that sex is protective.

As we discussed earlier, a more recent (2017) study looking at over 800 women and the net effect of menopause on the cells of the vagina found no difference in cellular changes between women having sex and those who were not. If sex were tissue-protective, women who were having sex would have fewer changes. This study mirrors what I have seen over the years. Vaginal symptoms of menopause lead to sexual difficulties for many women, but certainly not all.

In incredibly rare cases, there can be so much inflammation from menopause that women can develop some vaginal scarring that needs specialized treatment. If a woman is not sexually active, she may not realize this is happening. In this situation, regularly stretching the vagina, with dilators or a penis, could have prevented the scarring by mechanically stretching the tissues, not by causing changes at a cellular level. This extreme inflammation of menopause leading to scarring is uncommon. I can count on one hand the number of cases that I have seen over the past thirty years, and pain with sex is one of my specialties. What can happen is the extreme pain of GSM can lead to spasm of the pelvic floor muscles that wrap around the vagina (this is a condition called vaginismus—see chapter 34). This spasm can narrow the vaginal opening and feel like a roadblock, making pain with sex worse and giving the sensation that the vagina has closed.

Do Changes of Menopause Get Worse with Age?

The 2017 study I referenced earlier found the severity of tissue changes didn't correlate well with age, but another older study (also of high quality) did find an association. However, both of these studies just looked at women at one point in time. Until we have a study that follows women over years with vaginal swabs, we won't have a definitive answer.

Some women present with their first symptoms of GSM ten or more years after their last period, and others have problems before their periods even stop, so clearly there are many factors involved. While some may be biological, meaning individual hormone levels and pain thresholds, it can also take a long time for women to get good information, to feel comfortable speaking up, or to find someone who will listen. So how much of it is a delay due to accessing care and how much to the fact that symptoms truly don't develop for ten years or more is hard to know.

Medication-Induced GSM

Medications that stop estrogen production or block the effects of estrogen on the tissues can also cause GSM. The most severe symptoms come from medications called aromatase inhibitors. These are medications used to treat women with certain kinds of breast cancer. Aromatase inhibitors block the production of estrogen in every tissue because they block the enzyme aromatase, a necessary step in estrogen production. While most estrogen comes from the ovaries, there are other sources, such as adipose tissue, so blocking all sources of estrogen results in a rapid and drastic drop in estrogen.

Another medication that reduces estrogen levels dramatically is the class of drugs called GnRH agonists (gonadotropin-releasing hormone agonists, used in the treatment of endometriosis and breast cancer)—they interfere with how the brain communicates with the ovaries. The impact can be severe for many women, but as it doesn't block estrogen production in adipose tissue there may be some circulating estrogen, so some women may be spared symptoms of GSM.

Tamoxifen, another breast cancer medication, blocks the effect of estrogen on tissues. Tamoxifen acts like an antiestrogen on some tissues, and on others it can act like an estrogen. For example, it is an antiestrogen in the breast (which is why it's used for breast cancer), but in the uterus it acts like an estrogen. The impact on the vagina is variable, and some women will develop GSM symptoms while others do not.

Some chemotherapy drugs stop ovarian function. This depends on the type and dose of chemotherapy, the duration of treatment, and age—women over forty are at greater risk. The mechanisms are unclear, but it is believed some of these medications trigger the death of follicles in the ovary. For some women the effects will be permanent, meaning all the follicles are depleted, and for others there are remaining follicles that are able to recover over time, restarting estrogen production.

BOTTOM LINE

- Physical changes of menopause affect the clitoris, labia, vagina, urethra, and bladder.
- Symptoms related to genitourinary syndrome of menopause, or GSM, are experienced by 50 percent of women.
- The most common symptom of GSM is vaginal dryness.

- Sexual difficulties related to menopause are reported by 25 percent of women.
- Most women are not asked about symptoms of GSM, so self-advocacy is important.

CHAPTER 19

Treating GSM

Symptoms of GSM (genitourinary syndrome of menopause) affect approximately 50 percent of women. For more information on the vulvar and vaginal changes associated with menopause, head back to chapter 18. Here we will focus on treatment.

The most common symptoms that lead women to request medical help are dryness, pain with sex, and irritation. Other bothersome symptoms include a sandpaper-like feeling, vaginal burning, vaginal discharge, and a change in vaginal odor. Some women become more prone to bladder infections.

The average age of menopause is fifty-one years, but hormone levels start to drop beforehand. When women develop symptoms can vary, but if your periods have stopped or have begun to space out and you are forty years of age or older, then GSM should be considered for any vulvar or vaginal symptoms.

The pain and increased microtrauma associated with GSM can also aggravate preexisting conditions of the vulva and vagina, such as skin conditions and vulvodynia, a nerve pain condition of the vulva. It can be hard to know which symptoms are due to GSM and which are due to other causes, so it is very reasonable to start with treatment for GSM and then reevaluate after 6–8 weeks to see what bothersome symptoms remain.

Many women with GSM go undertreated or even untreated, and so they suffer. In the previous chapter, we addressed issues with women and/or their providers not suspecting GSM or women having their concerns dismissed. There are unfortunately other barriers to therapy, including the following:

- **PRICE:** The cost of products might prevent some women from getting the ones that could be most beneficial to them.
- **DISSATISFACTION WITH THE OPTIONS OR INCONVENIENCE:** Some women are bothered by the mess of vaginal products, find the products irritating, or do not want to use something daily.
- **NOT UNDERSTANDING HOW LONG IT TAKES TO SEE RESULTS:** Usually the minimum is six weeks, but many women stop sooner, thinking their therapy has been ineffective.
- **FEAR OF HORMONES:** Many products have scary warnings on the packaging.

Attention to Vulvar Care

Regardless of your symptoms, good vulvar skin care is an important foundation, as the loss of moisture associated with aging can aggravate symptoms of GSM. Some recommendations include the following:

- **USE A CLEANSER, NOT SOAP:** As we discussed in chapter 11, soap is drying.
- **LIMIT INTIMATE WIPES TO MANAGING INCONTINENCE WHEN YOU ARE OUTSIDE THE HOME:** As you age, your skin may be more prone to irritation from these products.
- **IF YOU HAVE URINARY INCONTINENCE, USE INCONTINENCE PADS, NOT MENSTRUAL PADS:** The average episode of incontinence is often more volume of liquid than an overnight pad is designed to hold. The fluid also comes out all at once, not over twenty-four hours. Wearing menstrual pads may keep your skin wet with urine, increasing irritation and skin breakdown.
- **CONSIDER A DAILY VULVAR MOISTURIZER:** See chapter 14. Coconut oil, olive oil, and petroleum jelly are good low-cost alternatives.

- **IF YOU REMOVE YOUR PUBIC HAIR, CONSIDER SWITCHING TO A TRIMMER OVER YOUR LABIA AND MONS:** Pubic hair increases humidity and hence traps moisture against the vulva.
- **IF YOU SMOKE, DO YOUR BEST TO QUIT:** Smoking has antiestrogenic effects.

Vaginal Moisturizers

Vaginal moisturizers are supposed to rehydrate vaginal tissues and replace lubrication. They are used regularly, not just during sex. Studies tell us vaginal moisturizers are typically well-tolerated and can improve symptoms, especially the sensation of dryness. Moisturizers are most effective when there is one main bothersome symptom. They are unlikely to treat odor, as they do not replace the lactobacilli (good bacteria).

Vaginal moisturizers have a temporary effect on vaginal pH—meaning the physical presence of the product lowers the pH, but does not cause lactobacilli to grow as it does not increase glycogen (the storage sugar). Under the microscope, moisturizers do not dramatically improve the appearance of tissues.

Moisturizers can be water based (glycerin is a common ingredient), silicone, oil, or hyaluronic acid based, or a combination. Hyaluronic acid is a large molecule that is found in and around skin cells that lubricates and hydrates cells.

Vaginal moisturizers are formulated so the active ingredients adhere to the vaginal mucosa, so they stay in place for several days. Most of them are meant to be inserted vaginally every 2–3 days. These products are fairly effective when used regularly. They are often the placebo arm in studies of vaginal hormones, and sometimes they perform as well or almost as well as low-dose estrogen. When stopped, the symptoms will return.

Many of the water-based vaginal moisturizers on the market do not list their pH or osmolality, so assessing long-term safety for vaginal tissues, especially for women who may be exposed to HIV, is not known. The few studies that exists are short term—meaning twelve weeks of use. Whether a product with a high osmolality could irritate over time, say twelve or twenty-four months of use, is not known. Keep in mind that

Table 2: pH and Osmolality of Common Vaginal Moisturizers (2018 data).

PRODUCT	BASE	PH	OSMOLALITY
HYALO GYN	Hyaluronic Acid	N/A	N/A
K-Y Liquibeads	Silicone	N/A	N/A
Moist Again	Water	5.68	187
Replens	Water	2.98	1491
Vagisil ProHydrate Natural Feel	Hyaluronic Acid	N/A	N/A
YES VM Natural Vaginal Moisturizer	Water	4.15	250

companies can change their recipes, so the osmolality and pH of products could change without notice. If you are not at risk of STIs and your product is not irritating, then whatever you are using is likely fine.

Lubricants are discussed in detail in chapter 9. There are unfortunately few studies looking at lubricant choice specifically for postmenopausal women. One small study suggested that for women who could not use estrogen, a silicone-based lubricant was more effective in reducing pain than a water-based product.

Topical Estrogen

Vaginal estrogen is considered the gold standard for GSM. Of all the options, both pharmaceutical and over the counter, vaginal estrogen is by far the most well studied.

When the data on vaginal estrogen was reviewed a few years ago, over 1,800 studies were identified, although only forty-four were of good enough quality that they were considered worthy of reviewing. In medicine, forty-four studies is still a lot, but it is a good snapshot of the dismal quality of many medical studies.

Vaginal estrogen works by increasing glycogen in the vaginal tissues. Glycogen is a source of nutrition for the lactobacilli, which then produce lactic acid that lowers the pH. Estrogen also increases blood flow, tissue elasticity, and the production of collagen (a protein that strengthens tissues). The net result is an increase in lubrication, vaginal discharge, tissue elasticity, and resilience. Studies show estrogen is very effective for treating all of the symptoms of GSM, may improve symptoms of urinary incontinence, and may reduce the risk of urinary tract infections.

There are two hormones used in pharmaceutical-grade vaginal estrogen in the United States: estradiol and conjugated equine estrogens (CEE). Estradiol is the main hormone produced by the ovary and is synthesized in a lab from another steroid hormone. Some people market estradiol as plant based; while technically that is true, the actual process involves cholesterol being extracted from a plant in the lab with chemicals, and then the cholesterol is exposed to chemicals to convert it to estradiol. This is definitely not ground-up yams. CEE is extracted from the urine of pregnant mares, hence the trade name Premarin: PREgnant MARe's urINe.

Vaginal estrogen (as of 2019) comes in a variety of formulations: cream, rings, vaginal tablets, and gelcaps. The dosing ranges vary widely, from 8 mcg a week to 400 mcg a week. Vaginal CEE only comes in a cream. The advantage of estrogen creams that is the dose can be tailored. The ring, tablets, and suppositories each come in one dose.

If the main bothering symptom is pain with sex, the data suggests starting with more than 10 mcg of estradiol twice a week. It isn't wrong to try the lowest doses; however, if you don't have the benefit you want in 6–8 weeks, then increasing the dose is likely indicated.

For all of the estrogen regimens, with the exception of the ring, the dose is nightly for two weeks and twice a week after that. One study suggests women could start with a twice a week regimen—it may take a few weeks longer to get relief, but some people do find regimen switches confusing and it may be easier to start with twice-a-week.

Vaginal CEE can't be compared directly with the estradiol regimens, as there is no direct conversion. The starting dose is typically 0.5–1 g vaginally a night for two weeks and twice a week after that.

There could be a transient increase in blood levels of estrogen in the first few weeks, especially with the cream (which has a higher dose of estrogen), as the inflammation of GSM may allow more of the drug to be absorbed initially. This may be why some women report breast tenderness in the first few weeks. Once the estrogen treats the vaginal inflammation, the levels drop. Elevated levels have not been reported with the tablets, capsules, ring, or the lowest dose of the cream (0.5 g twice a week).

Risks with the topical estrogen products are low. There is no increased risk of breast cancer, heart attack, or stroke, despite the package labeling. All estrogen products come with a "black box warning," required by the FDA, that lists possible side effects as the following (in capital letters): "WARNING: ENDOMETRIAL CANCER, CARDIOVASCULAR DISORDERS, BREAST CANCER, and PROBABLE DEMENTIA." Pretty scary, right? This warning is based on an older study that suggested a very small increase in these risks when estrogen is given systemically (meaning delivered to the bloodstream, for example with a pill or a patch). This has never been shown with vaginal estrogen, but the FDA rules require that if the risk is seen with one form of the drug, it must appear on the labeling for all forms.

Systemic Estrogen

Estrogen can be taken by a patch, a pill, a ring, or a topical lotion for general symptoms of menopause like hot flashes or to prevent osteoporosis. When taken this way, it is called systemic therapy because it enters the bloodstream. Systemic estrogen therapy can help many women with GSM, although it may not be quite as effective as topical application. This route is generally not recommended if GSM is the only bothersome symptom as there are small risks—for example, an additional 1 in 1,000 women per year who take systemic hormone therapy will get breast cancer (for perspective, this is also the risk of drinking one glass of wine a day). In addition, women who have a uterus must also take the hormone progesterone to protect them from developing endometrial cancer (cancer of the uterine lining).

A full discussion of the pros and cons of systemic hormones for other symptoms of menopause are well beyond this book. Perhaps my next book should be *The Menopause Bible*?

Vaginal DHEA

Prasterone is DHEA (dehydroepiandrosterone).

The body makes sex hormones, including testosterone and estradiol, from cholesterol. DHEA is an intermediate hormone in this process. The

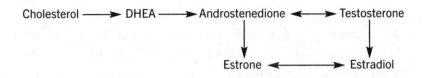

Image 10: Production of testosterone and estradiol from cholesterol.

two-way arrows in image 10 mean production can occur in either direction, so estradiol can be made into estrone and estrone into estradiol. Testosterone can be made into estradiol, but the reverse is not possible.

This process happens inside any cell with the enzyme aromatase, and vaginal tissue has aromatase. With intravaginal DHEA, the hormone is absorbed by the vaginal mucosa, where it is converted to testosterone and estradiol, although the exact hormone that exerts the effect on the vaginal mucosa is not known. Blood levels of testosterone and estradiol do not increase, so it appears that all the hormone that is produced acts locally. The uterine lining does not have the enzyme aromatase, so it is not at risk of developing hyperplasia (precancer) or cancer.

Prasterone is effective when given daily; when used twice a week it is less effective, but that may be enough for some women who prefer this product but do not want the mess of daily use. The biggest side effect is vaginal discharge, which should be expected with all hormonal products as they increase vaginal lactobacilli. Prasterone has never been compared in studies directly against vaginal estrogen, so making statements about which product is better is not possible.

Are "Bioidentical Hormones" Safer?

Bioidentical is a marketing term—medically, it has no meaning. Some people use it to describe hormones that are chemically identical to what the body makes; however, some people use it to for hormones derived from a plant source.

One of the big myths about "bioidentical hormones" is that they are ground-up yam or soy products that have been encapsulated. The chemical formula of estradiol is $C_{18}H_{24}O_2$, and it is the same if synthesized in the ovary or in a lab. The ovary makes estradiol from cholesterol and in a lab the process is the same: cholesterol (or another steroid) is chemically converted into estradiol. The raw hormone is a powder, and either a pharmaceutical company or a compounding pharmacy uses it to make a medication. There are only a few manufacturers of the raw hormone. A big pharmaceutical company and a small compounding pharmacy could be getting their raw hormone from the same source.

So-called "bioidentical hormones" are not safer. They may even have higher risks, as some data shows they can have up to 30 percent more estrogen than advertised. This could put you at risk for endometrial cancer (cancer of the lining of the uterus). In addition, women who start their periods early are at a higher risk of breast cancer, specifically because they have had a longer exposure to the natural hormones made by their ovaries.

What matters is if a medication is safe and effective. Unpredictable dosing is not a safety feature. A more accurate term for "bioidentical hormones" is non-pharmaceutical-grade hormones.

Some practitioners and compounding pharmacists make a big deal about offering concoctions with the three types of estrogen made in the body: estradiol, estriol, and estrone. Any estradiol that you take will be converted into estriol and estrone as needed. No studies suggest offering a compounded version adds anything but expense.

The only time I suggest compounded hormones (and this is estradiol only, not one of the customized concoctions) is when pharmaceutical grade is simply too expensive. In the United States, the pricing is currently (as of 2019) outrageous—a 42.5 g tube of generic estradiol cream is approximately $325. Many compounding pharmacies can make vaginal estradiol under $100. If the alternative is to go without, then compounded estradiol may be considered if there is informed consent about the possibility of inaccurate dosing.

Do I Need Testosterone?

No one has demonstrated that vaginal testosterone is beneficial. It can cause significant clitoral enlargement and can be absorbed into the bloodstream, causing other negative effects.

Nonhormonal Medications

Ospemifene (Osphena) is an oral medication in the class of drugs called selective estrogen receptor modulators (SERMs), meaning it acts like an estrogen on some tissues and like an antiestrogen on others. On vaginal tissues, it acts like an estrogen. It is FDA approved to treat vaginal symptoms of GSM.

For women who dislike vaginal application or who find vaginal application painful, 60 mg of oral ospemifene a day is an option. As it acts like estrogen on the uterus, women who have not had a complete hysterectomy (meaning uterus and cervix removed) will also need to take the hormone progesterone (or a similar drug) to protect against endometrial cancer. A levonorgestrel (hormonal) IUD may also offer this protection. Some women dislike the idea of two medications for a vaginal concern, and others are happy to have an oral option.

Ospemifene has not been studied head-to-head with vaginal estrogen, which we know helps 90 percent of women. In studies, ospemifene showed a statistical difference from placebo for decreasing pain with sex, but it is not clear if the changes were clinically significant—meaning whether it helped enough women in a meaningful way. In one large study, only 30 percent of women taking ospemifene reported no pain with sex. That does not mean it will not help you, but a 30 percent success rate seems low.

Other issues with ospemifene include the following:

- an increased risk of blood clots
- an increase in hot flashes
- drug interactions

What about botanicals and "natural" therapies?

Approximately 10 percent of women with GSM try herbal and other alternative therapies such as black cohosh, red clover, motherwort, and topical vitamin E. There is no data to support using these products. One small study suggests that vitamin D improves the appearance of cells for menopausal women, but there was no difference in pain or irritation among women who took vitamin D versus those who did not.

Women with breast cancer

All women with breast cancer should try moisturizers and lubricants first. If those fail, then the newest guidelines tell us the dose of vaginal estrogen in the ring and the 10 mcg tablets is safe for most women with a history of breast cancer, as they are not absorbed into the bloodstream. We have no data on the safety of vaginal DHEA, although studies tell us it does not seem to raise blood levels of estradiol or testosterone.

While hormonal monitoring is not recommended with vaginal estrogen, many women with a history of breast cancer are understandably apprehensive. Some find it reassuring to check blood levels of estradiol before starting vaginal estradiol, and again after therapy is initiated to make sure there has been no absorption.

The exception is women with breast cancer taking a class of medication called aromatase inhibitors. Those medications are meant to take away every molecule of estrogen for women with hormonally responsive cancer. In this situation any estrogen, even a tiny bit, is too much.

For women who are taking an aromatase inhibitor and have tried two different types of moisturizers (I usually recommend one product have a hyaluronic acid base), there are few options for pain with vaginal sex. Some women find lidocaine (a topical numbing medication at the vaginal opening) helpful. Another option is anal sex, as those tissues are not affected by an aromatase inhibitor, but that is not acceptable for all women.

The Mona Lisa and similar lasers (chapter 23) have been proposed for this situation. Given they are currently understudied, it is hard to make a safe, evidence-based recommendation, although more studies will be published soon and hopefully we will be better able to guide women about these products. However, a woman who is looking at a lifetime of aromatase inhibitors and who is unable to have vaginal intercourse may feel that the risk-benefit ratio, where the long-term risks are largely unknown, is acceptable to her if intercourse is otherwise impossible due to pain and there is no prospect of safely stopping aromatase inhibitors.

BOTTOM LINE

- Pay attention to vulvar care so you are not contributing to moisture loss.
- Moisturizers are most helpful when there is only one bothersome symptom.
- Vaginal estradiol has been studied the most. Doses of 20 mcg a week or less may not be effective for pain with sex
- There are newer options to consider: vaginal DHEA and an oral selective estrogen receptor modulator (SERM).
- Many women with breast cancer can safely use the lower doses of estrogen vaginally.

Medications and Interventions

CHAPTER 20

Cannabis

WITH THE INCREASING LEGALIZATION OF CANNABIS, it should come as no surprise that it has found its way into the vagina. Some women report that cannabis improves their sexual experience—specifically, that it increases desire, orgasm, and satisfaction. Others wonder if vaginal application of cannabis might be helpful for pain conditions, such as painful periods (dysmenorrhea) or pelvic floor muscle spasm (chapter 33).

Like a lot of "next great ideas," there is some basic biologic plausibility, little hard science, and a lot of hype. I have no issue with legalized cannabis, but I am no fan of unfounded claims and undertested products, as neither of those help me inform women.

The Basics

Cannabis is the plant *Cannabis sativa*, and it contains many pharmacologically active compounds known collectively as cannabinoids. The main psychoactive ingredient (i.e., what gives you the high) is tetrahydrocannabinol, or THC, and the other well-known cannabinoid is cannabidiol or CBD, which does not get you high. Including THC and CBD, there are at least sixty different types of cannabinoids. Many believe that CBD may have value for pain, although the data is still sparse. With legalization, we can hopefully expect more studies on the use of the different cannabinoids for pain.

The main cannabinoid receptors are CB1 and CB2. We have receptors for cannabinoids not because we evolved to consume cannabis, but rather because our bodies make our own (or endogenous) cannabinoids called endocannabinoids. The first endocannabinoid identified, in 1992, was named anandamide, which is from *ananda*, the Sanskrit for "bliss" or "joy." We don't make endocannabinoids and store them, they are made on demand.

A medical motto that governs much of what I do, especially when something is understudied, is "we don't know what we don't know." With cannabis, the fact that it was illegal for so long has hampered research. Another complicating factor is the endocannabinoid system, meaning what our naturally occurring endocannabinoids do, and how they do it, is complex and not fully understood. There are endocannabinoid receptors in the uterus, ovaries, and fallopian tubes, hair-bearing skin (like the vulva), and muscles, although we don't yet know if there are endocannabinoid receptors in the vagina. From an OB/GYN standpoint, we believe the endocannabinoid system is important in fertilization and pregnancy, but it may well have a role in other functions.

How Might Cannabis Impact Sex?

Some women report that cannabis enhances their sexual experience. The mechanism is not understood. Some hypotheses include increased blood flow to the vagina, improved nerve signaling either in the vagina or brain (i.e., cranking up the chemicals that tell you that you are feeling good), or a reduction in anxiety and inhibitions helping women let go sexually. The tachycardia (increased heart rate) that can come with cannabis may make some women feel as if they are aroused. There is also the possibility of placebo—if you think something is going to help get you turned on, you may approach that sexual encounter differently.

If cannabis truly impacts sexual function, then how it works matters, because if the impact is on the brain, it makes no sense to use it vaginally.

To help us understand more about the potential impact of cannabis on sexual function for women, a team of researchers studied whether our natural endocannabinoids are linked with the feeling of being aroused as well as the physical signs of arousal. In the study, a vaginal device was inserted that measured changes in vaginal engorgement (a proxy for blood flow) as the women watched a neutral video (either on shallow seas or birds—no shade to birders) and then an erotic video. The blood levels of two natural endocannabinoids were measured. The researchers thought they would go up, but levels of natural endocannabinoids actually went down with the feeling of being aroused and the physical vaginal changes of arousal.

This study is exciting because it does link the endocannabinoid system with physical arousal, just not in a positive way. The study authors point out that the experience of feeling more sexually aroused while sexual performance is actually physically reduced by a substance is a well-known phenomenon—the most notable example is alcohol.

Based on the limited data that we currently have, if women feel that smoking or ingesting cannabis is helping them sexually it may not be due to physically influencing arousal in the vagina or vulva.

What about cannabis lubes?

There are sexual lubricants that claim to enhance sexual functioning, the theory being that topically applied THC/CBD will dilate blood vessels, increasing blood flow, or improve nerve signaling. To make these kinds of claims requires studies, and there are none. The only thing we know is from one 2018 study (the one we just referenced), which suggests natural endocannabinoids go down with physical arousal. We also know that the impact of endocannabinoids on blood vessels varies throughout the body significantly—in some situations they can increase blood flow, and at other times reduce it. And as of 2019, we don't know anything about cannabinoid receptors in the vagina.

The lack of information doesn't stop wild claims. One company claims their product is "proven effective at delivering longer, stronger orgasms in 8 out of 10 women." If your data has not been published in a peer-reviewed medical journal for everyone to read, it has not been proven effective. I guess an advertisement along the lines of, "Lots of people are curious about topical cannabis. If you are one of them, here are our ingredients and the dose" just wouldn't sell. If a product is as effective as a company claims—and in medicine, an 80 percent success rate is truly amazing—then why don't you prove it? I guess there is a reason I am in medicine and not advertising or marketing.

CAN YOU GET HIGH FROM A CANNABIS LUBE? While there are no studies, we know THC could be absorbed from the vagina, as rectal THC is absorbed quite efficiently (for many drugs rectal and vaginal absorption is similar). Rectal doses of 2.5–5 mg of THC can produce blood levels of 1.1–4.1 ng/ml. Other ingredients in the lube could potentially affect absorption, so each lubricant would have to be studied independently to have a real answer.

What do these blood levels mean? For reference, at a blood level of 5–10 ng/ml of THC, approximately 75–90 percent of people exhibit impairment on performance skills related to driving.

How cannabis affects people varies greatly. People who use it regularly will have higher blood levels after using the same amount as someone who has never used. This is because THC is stored in the fat, and so the blood levels include what is being ingested or inhaled as well as what is being released from fat.

One cannabis-based lube claims it has 1.5 mg of THC and 0.5 mg of CBD per pump and advertises a typical use of 5–10 pumps, or 7.5–15 mg of THC. That could theoretically produce significant blood levels. If that is actually the dose needed for an effect, it seems likely the method of action involves getting high—meaning it has an impact on the brain.

If you want to use a cannabis lube and want only a local effect (meaning no high), then sticking with an application that involves less than 5 mg of THC is the best guess I can offer—this is all assuming the dose advertised is what is in the bottle and the product is pharmaceutical grade, meaning each pump delivers the same dose.

Giving recommendations about cannabis lube is like predicting the final image of a ten-piece puzzle based on two pieces. While it's better than zero pieces, it's not a lot to go on. Ultimately, whether you want to put something in your vagina with so little data is up to you.

What About Vaginal Medicinal Cannabis?

Some companies sell cannabis suppositories meant to treat painful periods or pelvic pain. Like cannabis-based lubricants, these products are unstudied. We do know that one drug (not cannabis related) used to stimulate uterine contractions works a little better when given vaginally versus orally, so it is not impossible that a vaginal route of a medication meant for period cramps could potentially have a greater effect with vaginal administration. However, we have no idea what dose of THC or CBD can impact the uterus, if only one or both are needed, or how the endocannabinoid system is even involved in menstrual cramps.

The vaginal suppositories can have significant amounts of THC—one product has 60 mg of THC and 10 mg of CBD, so a 6:1 ratio. For comparison, one cannabis-based drug approved in Canada and the U.K. for muscle pain called nabiximols (trade name Sativex) has THC and CBD in a 1:1 ratio. As we believe CBD is better for pain (whether it is or not is understudied, that is simply the current hypothesis), it seems an unusual medicinal choice to have so much THC versus CBD. As a rectal dose of 2.5–5 mg of THC can produce blood levels just under the level of impairment for driving, there is concern that 60 mg of vaginal THC could produce significant blood levels. We also have no idea if vaginal administration offers something unique for the uterus that smoking or oral use does not.

Hopefully, we will start to see some published research in the area soon so we can offer more guidance.

Are There Risks?

Cannabis has never been tested vaginally.

High doses given regularly to gerbils and rats had a negative impact on the storage sugar glycogen in the uterus—we don't know if it could do the same in the vagina (see chapter 2 for more on glycogen and its importance in feeding good bacteria). Constant administration of cannabis also reduced estrogen levels in that study.

The pH and osmolality of the lubricants has not been tested, so their impact from a safety standpoint is unknown. A high pH or osmolality could potentially damage tissues, causing irritation or increasing the risk of transmission of HIV if exposed.

One study that evaluated risk factors for yeast tells us that women who used cannabis (smoking or eating) in the previous four months were approximately 30 percent more likely to have yeast in their vaginal ecosystem as compared with women who did not. It was a good study where they cultured women for yeast on a regular basis over the course of a year. Studies looking at oral health tell us that cannabis use is associated with increased yeast in the mouth, and chronic cannabis use appears to negatively affect the immune system's response to yeast.

Other potential concerns are the fact that cannabis is an endocrine disruptor, meaning a substance that isn't an estrogen but acts like one, just like BPA in plastics. As vaginal application is untested, we don't know if there is any long-term impact from using an endocrine disruptor in the vagina, which is filled with estrogen receptors.

From a fertility and pregnancy standpoint, we know endocannabinoid signaling is very important in fertilization and early pregnancy, and it is unknown what the impact of a vaginal product could have on getting pregnant or on an early pregnancy.

BOTTOM LINE

- The impact of cannabis on the vagina is poorly tested. The scant data we have strongly suggests a link with yeast and a negative impact on hormones.
- Vaginal cannabis products are untested medically speaking—this is very much a "buyer beware" situation.
- If you want to explore a lubricant sexually and wish to avoid significant absorption (so no high), the best guess I can give is staying at doses of 5 mg or less of THC.
- As the pH and osmolality of cannabis-based lubricants and their impact on lactobacilli is unknown, avoid using them when there is an increased risk of HIV transmission.
- CBD is believed to be more important for pain than THC, and so products with more THC than CBD do not appear to be designed for pain control.

CHAPTER 21

Contraception

CONTRACEPTION METHODS CAN HAVE AN IMPACT on the vaginal ecosystem, although vaginal considerations should probably not be the number one reason you choose a method of birth control. It doesn't matter how awesome an estrogen-containing birth control pill might be for your lactobacilli if you are not the type who can remember to take a pill every day. The method of contraception that you choose has to actually work for you. However, if you are having symptoms, then this chapter may help you figure out if your contraception might be a cause, and if so, whether there is anything that can be done about it. If you have had a lot of vaginal symptoms and are contemplating starting contraception or switching your method, this information may help you make a more informed choice.

Condoms

We're going to start here, because if you partner with either men or women, condoms are the very best thing that you can do for your vagina. Multiple studies show sexual activity can be harmful for the good bacteria. Women who have never partnered with men don't get bacterial vaginosis. Women who partner with women and share vaginal secretions can colonize each other with less robust strains of lactobacilli. Condoms also reduce the risk of sexually transmitted infections (STIs) that can harm the vaginal ecosystem and/or lead to precancer and cancers.

Condoms are the clear winner in the contraception as vagina-defender category.

Multiple studies show women who partner with men who consistently use condoms have healthier vaginal bacteria. This is especially important for women with multiple partners, as the effect on the good bacteria increases with additional partners. If you only have one male partner and he has multiple female partners, that also increases the risk to your ecosystem. Having healthy vaginal bacteria is also the first line of defense against STIs; women who have low or no levels of good bacteria are four times more likely to catch gonorrhea or HIV if exposed.

Don't use condoms with spermicide (typically nonoxynol-9, or N-9). I know that seems counterintuitive, as extra protection sounds better. However, spermicide shortens the shelf life of the condom (without spermicide, most condoms have a five-year expiration date; with spermicide, because it degrades the latex, it's about two years), increases the cost, increases the risk of urinary tract infectious for women, and the spermicide damages the good vaginal bacteria. Spermicide, whether it has N-9 or not, is not effective at preventing infection from any STI.

If you find condoms irritating, make sure they are spermicide-free and lubricant-free and use your own lubricant. If that doesn't work, try a different brand or switch from latex to polyurethane. If that still doesn't work, see your doctor.

Estrogen-Containing Birth Control and Your Vagina

Estrogen-containing oral contraceptives have a beneficial effect on lactobacilli. This is likely because estrogen causes glycogen deposition in the vaginal epithelium—basically, it provides the fertilizer for vaginal bacteria. Studies show there is no negative effect on vaginal pH, although there can be an increase in the normal amount of discharge. Approximately 10 percent of the vaginal contraceptive ring users will report a definite increase in discharge.

Several studies have shown that an estrogen-containing birth control pill is protective against bacterial vaginosis, likely due to the increase in good bacteria. There is also data linking estrogen-containing birth control pills with an increased risk of yeast. Whether it causes yeast to grow faster than the healthy lactobacilli can contain, an impact on the vaginal immune system, or another mechanism is unknown. This doesn't mean that birth control pills will give you yeast; however, it is something to consider if you are struggling with recurrent yeast infections.

Bacteria and Biofilms

Biofilms are protective coatings that bacteria and yeast can make that allow them to avoid detection from the immune system and escape antibiotics or antifungals (yeast medication). Think of biofilm as an invisibility cloak. After treatment is completed, the microorganisms can reemerge, quickly reestablishing an infection.

Some foreign objects makemore likely for biofilm formation, and some organisms have a greater propensity for forming biofilms, like the yeast *Candida krusei*. Biofilms have been identified with both copper and levonorgestrel (hormonal IUDs) as well as the hormonal contraception vaginal ring. The longer an IUD is in place, the more likely it could develop a biofilm. Unfortunately, there are no commercially available tests for vaginal biofilms.

What does this mean? If you have no symptoms, then nothing. However, if you have a problem with recurrent infections, either bacterial vaginosis or yeast, you might want to discard your contraceptive ring (or your estrogen ring, if you are menopausal) before starting therapy and insert a new one after you have finished therapy. Obviously, backup contraception if appropriate should be considered, along with the expense. In the United States, one NuvaRing without insurance is easily over $100.

If you have an IUD and truly have a recurrent infection, yeast or bacterial vaginosis, you may wish to ask your provider about strategies to disrupt the biofilm (more on that in the chapters on yeast and bacterial vaginosis). Obviously, IUD removal is a consideration. In one study when biofilms were present, women with yeast and BV were more likely to have resolution when their IUD was removed. A firm diagnosis should be established first, as 70 percent of women who think they have a vaginal infection are misdiagnosed, and seeing a provider who understands about biofilms would also be helpful.

Does the hormonal IUD have other effects on vaginal bacteria?

While the initial studies suggest there is no impact, this is short-term data for twelve weeks. The method of action of the hormonal (progestin) IUD is changing cervical mucus, and the mucus is a part of the vaginal ecosystem, so it is hard to believe there is no effect when the very mechanism of action involves a change in one of the components of vaginal discharge!

Some data suggests there may be an increased risk of colonization with BV-associated bacteria with the hormonal IUD, but the connection is not definitive. Overall, the risk of bacterial vaginosis for IUD users, especially hormonal IUD users, may be slightly increased, but whether this is due to changes in bacteria or ongoing spotting (this can change pH and affect lactobacilli levels) is not known.

About 7 percent of women who use IUDs will have a bacteria called *Actinomyces* identified on Pap smear, possibly related to biofilms on the string. While this organism is implicated in pelvic infections, in this situation—when identified by chance on a Pap smear and there are no symptoms—it is considered an incidental finding and can be ignored, meaning no antibiotics are needed and the IUD does not need to be removed.

Hormonal contraception and HIV transmission with vaginal-penile sex

How might hormonal contraception possibly impact HIV transmission? Theories include impacts on lactobacilli, mucus, the vaginal epithelium or immune system, and lubrication, which decreases microtrauma with vaginal penetration. Some early data suggested a possible link, so there has been a lot of work trying to figure out if there truly is a connection or not. Women who are using hormonal contraception may be having more sex or different sex, and so a link may simply imply correlation (today it is sunny, and I read the newspaper—two events that happened on the same day, but no cause and effect) versus causation (it is sunny so I am wearing sunglasses—direct cause and effect).

The WHO has looked extensively at the risks of HIV transmission and different methods of hormonal birth control, and their conclusions are as follows:

- Estrogen-containing birth control pills: No link.
- Progestin-only birth control pills (no estrogen): No link (although the data is slightly less robust).
- Lenonorgestrel IUD: No link.
- Etonogestrel implant: No link.
- Injectable progestins (such as Depo-Provera): Despite multiple studies, there are still some unknowns and uncertainty whether there is a true link or not. The WHO still states the benefits are likely to outweigh the risks, but this is information women who are at high risk for HIV may wish to consider.

Progestin-Only Contraception and Vaginal Irritation, Discharge, and Pain with Sex

Anecdotally, some women who have been using a progestin-only method of contraception report vaginal irritation or dryness with sex. On exam, some have changes that look similar to the changes seen with menopause or low estrogen, including microscopic inflammation, although not as severe. Progesterone can block the effect of estrogen on some tissues, and the cells in the vagina are hormonally sensitive, so the hypothesis is plausible. One study has looked at whether progestin-only contraception can thin the lining of the vagina and found no effect; however, they only evaluated twenty-three women. (I imagine it is not easy to recruit women for a study that involves a vaginal biopsy.) Another study found a change in glycogen (the storage sugar that feeds the healthy bacteria) in the vagina, so this could be a mechanism.

BOTTOM LINE

- Condoms are highly protective for vaginal bacteria.
- The estrogen-containing birth control pill and the contraceptive ring may increase vaginal discharge.
- The estrogen-containing birth control pill increases healthy vaginal bacteria, but it may be associated with a small increased risk of yeast.
- Most women will have no vaginal issues from IUDs, but with recurrent yeast and BV the possibility of a biofilm should be considered.
- Hormonal birth control does not appear to be associated with an increased risk of transmission of HIV, with the exception of injectable medroxyprogesterone acetate (Depo-Provera)—whether there is a true link or not is not clear.

CHAPTER 22

Antibiotics and Probiotics

THERE ARE A LOT OF MYTHS about the impact of antibiotics and probiotics on the vaginal ecosystem. I've heard statements from self-described "wellness" gurus that "antibiotics are napalm" or that some food or plant, for example garlic or echinacea, can take the place of antibiotics.

These claims are false and harmful.

If you need antibiotics, you need them. If you don't, you don't. However, many people worry about the impact of their antibiotics, often because of this destructive kind of messaging, and this can lead to people stopping their antibiotic prematurely with the idea that fewer doses will reduce harm to their vaginal ecosystem. If you don't take the entire course of antibiotics—43 percent of people do this, for a variety of reasons—you risk not only getting sicker when your partially treated infection returns, but you also paradoxically contribute to the development of resistant organisms that could harm you and other people.

It is true that millions of antibiotic prescriptions in the United States (47 million, or about 30 percent) are unnecessary. Unnecessary antibiotic exposure not only contributes to yeast infections, but also the growing and very serious problem of antibiotic resistance as well as antibiotic-related diarrhea. So there is reason to be concerned about the impact of overprescribing antibiotics.

Medically, the most appropriate course of action is to make sure you really need those antibiotics to begin with (this is called antibiotic stewardship). For example, one third of people erroneously believe antibiotics can help colds, but a cold is due to a virus, so no antibiotics are needed. Have a sore throat? Only 5–10 percent are due to bacteria that require antibiotics. Have a cough with dark yellow or green sputum? It's a myth that colored sputum means you have a bacterial infection, and antibiotics are not recommended for acute bronchitis. If you think you have a bladder infection—well, hang on, because there is a whole chapter (chapter 36) that can help you decide if you should get antibiotics over the phone or if you should get tested and wait.

If I Take an Antibiotic, Will I Get a Yeast Infection?

Two studies have shown that 23 percent of women develop a symptomatic yeast infection after antibiotics. The fact that two studies—done in different ways by different researchers in different countries—show this suggests it is reliable data. In one of these studies, women with a history of antibiotic-induced yeast infections were at higher risk of a post-antibiotic yeast infection. The chance of being colonized with yeast (meaning yeast is present but does not cause symptoms) also increases with a course of antibiotics.

The prevailing belief is that antibiotics lead to yeast infections by killing the lactobacilli (good bacteria) in the vagina, as well as killing the pathogenic (harmful) bacteria that they were prescribed to treat. The temporary drop in lactobacilli allows yeast, which is often normally present, to overgrow. Antibiotics that do not kill lactobacilli are not associated with yeast infections, supporting this theory.

It is hard to recommend a strategy of taking yeast medication for every woman appropriately given antibiotics—this would expose 77 percent of women to medications they don't need, and inappropriate use of yeast medications is increasing problems with resistance. If you regularly get yeast infections after antibiotics, it may be a reasonable strategy to co-treat, meaning starting yeast treatment when you start antibiotics, or 2–3 days into your antibiotics, although this strategy has not been tested. It is best to make sure that at least one of your previous antibiotic-induced yeast infections has been confirmed by a culture (see chapter 31 for more on that point because it is important).

Is there an antibiotic least likely to cause a yeast infection?

Medically you always want the most appropriate antibiotic—the one that can best treat your infection and has the lowest potential to cause collateral damage, meaning least likely to contribute to the growing problem of antibiotic resistance and the lowest risk of causing antibiotic-associated to diarrhea.

Antibiotics can be broad spectrum, killing many different kinds of bacteria, or they can be narrow spectrum and kill a very specific type of bacteria. There are definitely times where broad-spectrum antibiotics are indicated—a serious infection with an unknown cause is one example. However, in many situations guidelines call for narrow-spectrum antibiotics, and so medically they are preferred when possible. When getting an antibiotic, ask if this is the narrowest-spectrum antibiotic you can have for this infection. Most doctors I know would be thrilled to be asked! Antibiotic stewardship, or choosing the right antibiotic for the right infection, benefits everyone, and so we doctors need to enlist everyone in this cause.

Understanding there are no good studies that suggest which antibiotics are the worst for the vaginal ecosystem, I have some considerations for the least vaginal fallout, assuming these antibiotics are in the acceptable-for-your-infection category:

- **NITROFURANTOIN:** This antibiotic can only be used for bladder infections. It doesn't penetrate into tissues, and in a recent study for bladder infections only 1 percent of women reported vaginal symptoms (this is likely a nocebo, or negative placebo, effect). This is also the first-line drug recommended for uncomplicated bladder infections.
- **FOSFOMYCIN:** Also for bladder infections, here the risk of vaginal discharge and irritation in a recent study for bladder infections was reported as < 1 percent. Cultures for yeast were not done, so the cause of the symptoms is not known.

- **TRIMETHOPRIM-SULFAMETHOXAZOLE, METRONIDAZOLE, AND NOR-FLOXACIN:** Lactobacilli are naturally resistant to these antibiotics. One study specifically looked at norfloxacin and found no increased risk of yeast colonization. Metronidazole is used for bacterial vaginosis and trichomoniasis, so prescribing a medication for yeast at the same time is not indicated. Trimethoprim-sulfamethoxazole can be used for urinary tract infections and for skin infections (among other things).

Obviously there may be other reasons these antibiotics are not appropriate for you, and the fact they are least likely to damage the lactobacilli is only one factor to consider in their use.

What about vaginal antibiotics?

The two antibiotics used most commonly in the vagina are metronidazole gel and clindamycin cream. Clindamycin cream and suppositories have mineral oil, so they are not compatible with latex condoms—if you rely on condoms for disease protection or birth control, you should not have sex while using clindamycin or for seventy-two hours afterwards. No one has actually studied how long it takes for product to clear the vagina, so the seventy-two hours is a best guess. I can see tiny globules of most products under the microscope for the first forty-eight hours after the last use, but by seventy-two hours microscopically it seems to mostly have cleared.

Unlike most oral antibiotics, we have good data on the risk of yeast infections as these formulations are relatively new, and when the brand-name drugs were submitted to the FDA for approval, they included the risk of yeast infections in the studies. The chance of developing a yeast infection from these products is as follows:

- **VAGINAL METRONIDAZOLE:** 1 percent (This was lower than the risk with the placebo gel!)
- **VAGINAL CLINDAMYCIN 7-DAY CREAM:** 10 percent
- **VAGINAL CLINDAMYCIN 3-DAY CREAM:** 8 percent
- **VAGINAL CLINDAMYCIN 3-DAY OVULES:** 3 percent (Why there is a difference between the cream and ovules is not known.)

What About Probiotics?

According to the Food and Agriculture Organization of the United Nations and the World Health Organization, probiotics are live microorganisms that, when administered in adequate amounts, confer a health benefit on the host. Worldwide, probiotics are big business, and interest in them continues to grow. In 2012, 1.6 percent of Americans were using probiotics, four times more than were taking them in 2007.

In the U.S. alone, millions and millions of dollars are spent every year on probiotics. Despite all of that money, there is very little quality research. It is very discouraging to see so many people spend so much money and to be able to offer so little useful information for guidance. If everyone gave the money they were going to give to a probiotic company to a research fund, I wonder how long it would take us to figure out how probiotics could help and for what medical conditions?

Probiotics for otherwise healthy people

If you are feeling well and have no symptoms, probiotics are unlikely to enhance or improve your gut bacteria. There is data to suggest taking a probiotic with antibiotics can help reduce antibiotic-associated diarrhea, which is a good thing. However, a recent small study found probiotics after antibiotics actually delayed repopulation of good bacteria in the gastrointestinal tract. So it is fair to say that there are many things about probiotics and gut bacteria that we do not fully understand.

Probiotics for vulvovaginal conditions

The three gynecologic indications for which probiotics are promoted are recurrent bacterial vaginosis, recurrent yeast infections, and recurrent bladder infections. Deficient or low levels of lactobacilli are associated with bacterial vaginosis and may have a role in yeast infections and urinary tract infections, so the hypothesis is sound. If the bowel could be populated with healthy bacteria, might some find its way into the vagina?

There have been a few studies, and when probiotics are analyzed rigorously there is no proof they benefit any of these three conditions. The data is lower quality, and none of the studies addressed whether or not the probiotics increased vaginal lactobacilli.

Other reasons why the data on probiotics has been discouraging include studying the wrong strains (the strains that we believe to be most important for vaginal health are difficult to grow outside the vagina) and that women may need strains individualized for their own flora or specific medical condition. It is also possible that the tested brands were mislabeled, and so there is no way to know what was actually tested.

Anecdotally, I have seen no benefit. I admit it is not a study, but fifteen years ago I recommended probiotics enthusiastically, and over the years it seems that they have not helped many women. Many women are frustrated that they have been taking these expensive products, sometimes for years, and yet they are still symptomatic.

Do probiotics have risks?

The biggest issue is they may not help and you have wasted money in addition to the frustration of committing to a regimen. Whether it is changing laundry detergent, wearing cotton underwear, or giving up bubble baths, the frustration of the unscientific "well, it won't hurt!" recommendations given to women about their bodies add up. It makes women feel like they are doing so many things for their health, and they are—it's just none of them have been proven to help. There are only so many hoops one can jump through and retain one's sanity.

I call this phenomenon the burden of "well, it can't hurt." Women only get frustrated with therapies and recommendations that are based on little more than a hypothesis, and when they don't get better it can make some feel as if they can never get better (they have tried all of these interventions in good faith, so when they don't work they feel that they are untreatable, but it's just that ineffective therapies don't work). This can lead some women to try other ineffective and potentially harmful alternative therapies or to give up on care altogether.

The most concerning health risk with probiotics is that bacteria might inadvertently get into the bloodstream, causing a serious infection. There are reports of this happening in situations with a compromised immune system, severe bowel inflammation, or reduced blood flow to the bowel (these latter two situations may make it easier for the probiotic bacteria to cross the bowel into the bloodstream). If you have any significant immune-system problems or are taking medications that suppress your immune system, you should check with your doctor before starting probiotics. Similarly, if you have bowel inflammation or a significant heart condition, you should also check in before starting.

Some probiotics formulated for the bowel contain the yeast *Saccharomyces cerevisiae*. If you have an issue with chronic yeast infections and are the rare person for whom *S. cerevisiae* is the culprit, then it's probably best to not use a probiotic that contains the same yeast. Whether probiotics with *S. cerevisiae* can actually cause vaginal yeast infections is unknown, but I think if you are trying to prevent yeast it is probably a good commonsense idea to not take a probiotic with a yeast.

Finally, you simply don't know what you are taking. A recent study found that 33 percent of probiotics contain fewer colonies than indicated on the label, and 42 percent were incorrectly labeled, with either mislabeled species, missing species, or species not included on the label. Mislabeling and unknown ingredients are unfortunately common in the supplement industry. The New York Attorney General commissioned an investigation in 2015 that revealed only 21 percent of the dietary supplements tested (not probiotics, but regulated the same way) contained the ingredients that were on the label. Unlisted contaminants were often the only ingredients. Another 2013 study also found contamination and substitution were common with herbal supplements. As the ingredients, purity, and doses for supplements—including probiotics—in the United States are on the honor system, it is very much buyer beware.

I want to try probiotics—can you make recommendations?

It is not possible to make a strong recommendation for probiotics based on the data, but if you don't have any contraindications, choosing a product that claims to contain *Lactobacillus rhamnosus*, *Lactobacillus reuteri*, and *Lactobacillus gasseri* is the most evidence-based (such as it is) recommendation I can give, as these strains are considered important in the vaginal ecosystem. If after 2–3 months you have not seen any impact, then any further use is probably a waste of money.

I don't recommend vaginal probiotics, as one well-known investigator told me she had to halt a vaginal probiotic study because the food source in the capsules meant to keep the probiotics alive also fed the bad bacteria, and women who used them developed more infections than anticipated. Basically, the weeds grew faster with the enhanced food source than the flowers. This anecdote also shows all the information we miss because negative studies are less likely to get published. Everyone wants to find a cure, not show that something is ineffective, even though they are both very important information.

Before buying probiotics, as they are expensive, I recommend every woman look at her diet to make sure it is healthy. Some basics are 1–2 servings of fish a week, no trans fats, no fast food, and 25 g of fiber a day. There will likely be far more benefit from eating a healthy, balanced diet than from taking probiotics. If you have an extra $40 or more a month for probiotics and your diet could use some help, it is probably a better idea to spend that extra money on dietary changes.

Should I Use Boric Acid Weekly to Help My Vaginal pH?

No!

Boric acid does not work by acidifying the vagina. It works because it is toxic to cells. It appears to be more toxic to yeast cells and biofilms (colonies of bacteria) than vaginal tissue, although it is still harmful to vaginal tissue. After 2–3 weeks of use, there is visible redness and inflammation in the vagina.

Antibiotics and antifungals do not typically affect human cells at all— they target enzymes or structures seen only in bacteria or yeast cells. Boric acid pretty much kills everything in its path.

We do not have information on how boric acid impacts the vaginal ecosystem, but looking under the microscope after 2–3 weeks of boric acid my experience is there is very little lactobacilli. Vaginal pH is not affected for more than 1–2 hours by a vaginal application of an acid; to maintain a pH less than 4.5 requires lactic acid–producing bacteria.

There are currently two indications for vaginal boric acid:

- For yeast that is known to be resistant to the regular prescription and over-the-counter medications
- As part of a regimen for recurrent bacterial vaginosis to disrupt a suspected biofilm
- Boric acid should only be used when medically there are no other alternatives.

BOTTOM LINE

- Practice antibiotic stewardship and ask your doctor if you are on the narrowest-spectrum antibiotic that is appropriate for your condition.
- Approximately 23 percent of women will develop a yeast infection after antibiotics.
- Some antibiotics have a very low/no risk of causing vaginal yeast infections. Some names to remember are nitrofurantoin, fosfomycin, metronidazole, and trimethoprim-sulfamethoxazole.
- Studies on probiotics for vaginal health or preventing bladder infections are very low quality, and so we have no good evidence to say they help or don't help.
- Boric acid does not work by acidifying the vagina; it is cytotoxic (kills cells).

CHAPTER 23

Cosmetic Procedures, Injections, and "Rejuvenation"

THERE IS AN EVER-GROWING MARKET for cosmetic procedures and "enhancements" for the vulva. Many of these products and procedures are undertested or completely untested. Some are offered with predatory marketing, amazing promises that capitalize on genital shame and fear of aging inflicted upon women by the patriarchy. I hear from women that while they are sitting half-dressed or completely naked at their doctor's office, they see posters for vulvar cosmetic surgery and vaginal "rejuvenation," which in that most vulnerable state leaves them feeling, "Maybe there is something wrong with me?" I also hear from women having surgery for incontinence about getting a hard sell regarding add-on "cosmetic" procedures.

When it comes to procedures, words like "rejuvenation" and "renewal" are medically meaningless. I would steer clear of any procedure marketed with that terminology. If they are using made-up terminology, whether they don't know or don't care doesn't matter—what else is made up?

I personally believe that cosmetic procedures and surgery for a health indication should not be done by the same surgeon at the same time. It's one thing to plan a hysterectomy for your patient, have her seek out a cosmetic surgeon and inquire about an abdominoplasty (tummy tuck) at the same time, and then have her plastic surgeon call you to arrange the details. The plastic surgery could not have affected my surgical decision to recommend a hysterectomy. However, what if I also performed abdominoplasties? They reimburse a surgeon more than a hysterectomy. Would I be tempted to offer more hysterectomies, and then suggest to my patients that they could also get abdominoplasties? It gets very complicated, and it is hard for us to be aware of all our biases.

Labiaplasty

This surgery for reducing and/or reshaping the size of the labia minora is on the rise. Between 2015 and 2016, there was a 39 percent increase in these procedures—97 percent of primary care doctors in Australia report they have cared for a woman who has expressed anxiety about her labia.

While there are no studies, my experience and that of several other OB/GYNs with whom I have discussed this issue suggest that seeking surgery for reducing the labia minora used to be confined to women with a significant size discrepancy, typically relating to a previous vaginal delivery or significant weight loss, where one labia minora is significantly larger in width (meaning 3–4 cm larger) than the other. I have heard women tell me they have to roll one labia minora up and tuck it into their underwear like a Dumbo ear and stories of one long labia being dragged into the vagina during sex. I can appreciate being bothered by these situations and wanting to restore anatomy to how it was before—symmetrical.

We know there is no "normal" size for labia minora. Among women without symptoms, the labia minora are 2–10 cm in length and 0.7–5 cm in width. We also know that larger labia minora do not cause itching and irritation; however, chronic scratching and pulling and tugging can cause the labia to get larger. There is an African culture where women practice labial elongation, as it is a desired sexual characteristic with no associated negative symptoms or sexual difficulties.

While occasionally women who seek reduction surgery have labia minora at the larger end of the width scale and report issues with their underwear or catching during sex, the majority of women seeking this surgery have labia well within the typical range. A study of women in the United Kingdom presenting for labial reduction found that every woman had labia minora of 5 cm or less in width, and the average width was 2.7 cm on the left and 2.5 cm on the right.

We know that 50 percent of women have labia minora that protrude beyond the labia majora, and yet 75 percent of women who are built this way think it is abnormal. Perhaps women are more aware of their protruding labia due to pubic hair removal, or maybe the naked and nearly naked images of women online and in porn have an impact, as they appear to favor smaller labia. We know that viewing modified genitalia alters the perception of normality among women ages 18–30, so seeing images of surgically or naturally smaller labia minora in pornography can alter women's perception of what is typical. Research also tells us that approximately one third of women who seek labiaplasty recall specific negative comments about their labia versus 3 percent of women who don't seek surgery.

I hear that some mothers are concerned about the size of their teen's labia minora. My advice is stop looking at your daughter's labia minora. Right now. If you have caught a glimpse of something you feel seems atypical, do not make a big deal about it. If your daughter is not bothered by symptoms, it is almost always going to be completely normal. However, if you need reassurance, call her pediatrician or gynecologist. It is important not to discuss this over and over again, as it is very easy for young girls to develop body image disorders. If a doctor reassures you that your daughter's labia are normal, believe it. Labial reduction for women under the age of eighteen, except in extreme circumstances, is rightfully considered female genital mutilation in the United States and is a crime.

Before considering labial reduction surgery, it is important to remember that the labia minora are sexually responsive structures. They have erectile tissue, have specialized nerve endings, they engorge, and they are attached at the top to the clitoral hood, and so traction may enhance clitoral stimulation. The labia minora also have an important role, as they protect the vestibule (vaginal opening). Surgically reducing the labia should be considered the exact same thing as surgically reducing the size of the penis.

Women who choose labiaplasty for cosmetic reasons are generally happy with the outcome, although there are reports of some women feeling that their clitoral hood looks large by comparison after the surgery and are displeased with that outcome. It also cannot be emphasized enough that the long-term medical implications of labial reduction are unknown. The impact of labial reduction on sensation or sexual function has not been adequately studied. We do know that labia minora shrink a little with age, and whether or not a surgically reduced labia combined with age-related changes will lead to symptoms is unknown.

I have read about plastic surgeons who do labiaplasty so women can look "sleeker in so-called athleisure wear." I know some people call this look "camel toe," but I prefer "labial cleavage," and the answer is not surgery—it is better-fitting athletic wear. I've stared at more male butt cracks (gluteal clefts) than I care to remember, whether it was just some guy bending over or gravity-defying pants that appear to hover like magic just above the anus without a belt. What I never hear is that men should seek out plastic surgeons to get their gluteal clefts sewn shut. I also can't imagine a similar industry for men that profits from surgically trimming penises so they look better in tight jeans.

Perhaps gyms and stores that sell yoga pants could put up signs, "Love Your Labial Cleavage."

The gender and specialty of the doctor a woman sees for consideration of labial surgery make a difference in whether the surgery is recommended. Plastic surgeons are more likely to agree to labial reduction than gynecologists, and men more likely than women. Some plastic surgery literature suggests labiaplasty could be offered when the labia minora are 3 cm in width or greater—which would apply to almost 50 percent of women! I can't imagine anyone suggesting 50 percent of men are eligible for penile reducing surgery.

The best guidance that I can give is that if you have symptoms of itch or irritation, see a gynecologist or even a vulvar specialist. Labia don't cause these symptoms. Remember, 50 percent of the population has a penis hanging between their legs—larger than any labia—and are able to avoid catching their penises in their underwear, ride a bike, and sit comfortably.

If you are concerned about size discrepancy, understand that the labia are part of the sexual response, and if, with this knowledge, you wish to go ahead, opt for the smallest reduction that will make you close to symmetrical (it is rare to have perfect symmetry—remember: sisters, not twins). If your labia are greater than 5 cm in width or you have smaller labia but are adamant the surgery is for you, seek two opinions before getting the surgery—I recommend that at least one be from a female gynecologist.

The best surgical technique for labiaplasty is a wedge resection. This involves removing a wedge of tissue at the bottom and leaves the delicate connections with the clitoral complex alone. The other surgery essentially involves trimming the edge. While this sounds simpler, it removes the specialized nerve endings and can compromise the area where the top of the labia, the frenulum, meets the clitoral hood. It also can present some challenging cosmetics closer to the clitoral hood.

The "G-Shot"

This involves injecting collagen into the anterior vaginal wall, where some doctors apparently erroneously believe the "G-spot" exists. If you read chapters 2 and 4, you know there is no specific G-spot. The sensitive area on the anterior vaginal wall is the extension of the clitoral complex. What feels stimulating in that area may also change depending on how engorged and excited you are, so it is not as if most (any?) women can point to a spot in a clinical setting and say, "Right here, this is the money shot." For some women that area feels great, and for others less so. It's all cool, and we are all built just a little differently.

Fillers like collagen and hyaluronic acid plump up tissue by filling spaces around cells and collagen fibers—basically, a G-shot is like blowing in insulation. The idea that this could enhance sexual pleasure is biologically preposterous.

The "O-Shot"

This is a procedure where platelet-rich plasma (basically your own blood minus the red blood cells and white blood cells) is taken out of your body and then injected into your clitoris. The idea is that this is supposed to enhance sexual pleasure, and it is so many layers of horrific, it's hard to know where to begin.

The only study is of such poor quality that it is only fit to line a birdcage—the medical condition that was supposedly treated in the paper is even misspelled repeatedly. We have no idea what this injection could do to the clitoris or vaginal mucosa, and we don't know if it could reactivate a dormant HPV infection. There is also no data to tell us what this does to vaginal or vulvar tissue.

The O-shot is a no shot.

Stem Cells

Stem cells are cells with the ability to differentiate or turn into other cells. Stem cells can be harvested from several sources, such as the umbilical cord, the bone marrow, and even fat (adipose tissue).

Despite the lack of research for vulvar and vaginal applications, women are being offered stem-cell injections for vaginal dryness, incontinence, difficulties achieving orgasm, and skin conditions such as lichen sclerosus. In the United States, the technique that women are offered is injection with stem cells harvested from their own fat, so there is a liposuction component that increases the appeal. The stem cells are typically injected into the vulva.

Who doesn't want to renew your vulva and lose fat? If something sounds too good to be true—for example, a brand-new, youthful vulva and less fat—it typically is.

One study of five patients (some were men who had penile injections; the injections were lumped together as "genital," as if the penis and scrotum and the vulva are the same thing) had uninterpretable results. The scant studies that exist are very low quality, and this is a serious concern.

The biggest reason to be worried by stem-cell injections is that they can cause unregulated growth—there is data emerging of people who have had injections in various body parts developing horrific tumors and other serious complications.

Vaginal Rejuvenation

It is hard to explain a procedure that is not defined, but it seems two surgeries are offered under this vague umbrella: a perineoplasty, which is cutting the muscles at the vaginal opening and sewing them up tighter, and laser to the vaginal tissues to make the tissues more "elastic" but also sometimes advertised as making them "tighter" (elastic and tighter are not the same thing!).

A perineoplasty is a valid procedure. Occasionally when a vaginal delivery has resulted in a tear and there is poor healing because the muscles have healed too far apart, this procedure will be offered to restore anatomy. It is also sometimes done as part of prolapse surgery. What a perineoplasty won't do is give you better sex. It can treat prolapse, but if it is done too aggressively it will create a smaller vaginal opening, and often this can cause pain with penile insertion. The surgery can also trigger painful muscle spasms.

If you feel that your vagina is looser after delivery, the answer is usually Kegel exercises and physical therapy, not surgery.

The laser procedures are more problematic. The technology claims to cause a superficial injury and then the healing process increases blood flow that stimulates the growth of collagen and somehow leads to glycogen deposition, which then improves the bacterial colonization with lactobacilli. As the vaginal mucosa (skin cells) repopulate every ninety-six hours, it is hard to see how these changes could be long lasting, although it is claimed that some of the procedures last six months or more.

The manufacturers of these lasers have advertised that they treat GSM (symptoms of low estrogen) and incontinence. The marketing is intense, and a celebrity has gone public saying this left her vagina brand new, "like a peach."

It's a vagina, not fruit.

These lasers were not FDA approved for GSM or incontinence, and so it is not legal for the company to make these claims. They were cleared for other uses. In addition, in the case of the Mona Lisa device, the handpiece that goes into the vagina was modified after it was cleared for use but the FDA was not notified.

The FDA has received several reports of vaginal injuries, and I have personally heard from OB/GYNs across the country about a few. I've also heard the device is not intuitive to use, and it could be easy to use the wrong settings and cause an injury. Whether injuries have resulted from improper use, meaning the device is fine; improper patient selection (woman with that vulvar and vaginal skin conditions that could possibly be made worse by the trauma); or whether the injuries are true consequences of the device being used perfectly is not known.

The American College of Obstetricians and Gynecologists (ACOG) advises caution with these devices, noting that they are understudied (as of early 2019), and does not recommend their use outside of research protocols. If you haven't already guessed, I hate expensive flashy devices that are rolled out with huge promises and limited data. Women deserve better than inadequately tested devices, especially when they are paying thousands of dollars per treatment session.

If the device is so revolutionary, then the companies should step up and fund a multicenter randomized, double-blinded placebo-controlled trial comparing the device with appropriate doses of vaginal estrogen. Currently, the only study comparing the device with estrogen used a dose of estrogen that has been proven to be ineffective. The device was as good as the ineffective dose of estrogen.

There is a new study going to press that is apparently of much higher quality, so hopefully we will get some data soon to see how these therapies fit in for women with vaginal symptoms of menopause and incontinence.

BOTTOM LINE

- Labial reduction surgery is best reserved for women who have labia greater than 5 cm in width or a size discrepancy of greater than 3 cm between sides who are bothered by this appearance or have symptoms related to trapping of the labia.
- All women getting labial reduction surgery should be counseled that the labia are part of the sexual response, and we do not know how labial reduction impacts sexual functioning.
- Female surgeons are less likely to recommend labial reduction than male surgeons.
- Under no circumstances can I recommend the G-shot, the O-shot, or stem-cell injections.
- Laser to treat GSM and incontinence is understudied, and there is no data about using these devices to "tighten" the vagina.

Sexually Transmitted Infections (STIs)

CHAPTER 24

General STI Information

APPROXIMATELY 80 PERCENT OF WOMEN who have ever been sexually active with a man will have had at least one sexually transmitted infection (STI). Numbers for LGBTQ+ women are harder to come by as lesbian, bi, and trans women and trans men who have a vagina have largely been ignored by research, partly due to marginalization by the medical community but also due to preconceived and mistaken ideas about risk.

Many STIs have important health consequences, ranging from annoying (think genital warts) to very serious (think infertility or cancer). The other rarely discussed but very important consequence is that almost all STIs increase the risk of acquiring HIV (human immunodeficiency virus) if exposed, so reducing STIs is an important weapon in the global fight against new HIV infections.

Am I at Risk for an STI?

Are you having sex or have you ever had penetrative vaginal, anal sex, or oral sex with anyone? If so, then the answer is yes. Some STIs can even be transmitted by non-penetrative sexual activities, like genital rubbing.

While it is true that it just takes one encounter with a person who has an STI to be at risk for an infection, there are some factors that increase your risk, including the following:

- **BEING UNDER THE AGE OF TWENTY-FIVE:** Certain STIs are more common in this age-group, and the cervix may be more vulnerable to infection in younger women.
- **MULTIPLE PARTNERS.**
- **A RECENT CHANGE IN PARTNER.**
- **NOT USING BARRIER PROTECTION.**
- **BACTERIAL VAGINOSIS (BV):** This indicates low levels of protective bacteria. A woman with BV is four times more likely to get gonorrhea or HIV if exposed.
- **RECEPTIVE ANAL SEX:** There is more microtrauma, making it easier for bacteria or viruses to establish an infection. The lining of the anal canal is also more susceptible to infection.
- **PARTNERING WITH A MAN WHO IS BISEXUAL:** Men who have sex with men have a higher rate of some STIs.
- **TRANS MEN WITH A VAGINA WHO ARE TAKING TESTOSTERONE AND PRACTICE PENILE-VAGINAL SEX:** The testosterone-related changes can facilitate transmission of STIs if exposed.

Many studies tell us that race can be a risk factor for some women. While this is almost always due to socioeconomic factors that affect access to affordable health care, as we learn more about the different microbial communities in the vagina we may find other reasons.

Knowing your risk factors can help you decide if you should advocate for more testing. For example, national guidelines suggest we should only screen women under sixty-four years of age for HIV. On a population level this seems cost-effective, as on average a sixty-five-year-old woman likely has fewer sex partners than a twenty-six-year-old. However, when this book is published I'll be fifty-three (writing that down makes me feel in a little way that I will forever be fifty-three, which honestly isn't too bad), and if I find myself single when I am sixty-five years old, I will be looking for a new partner (my goal is to be sexually active as long as possible), and I may want to be screened for HIV.

Many STIs Are on the Rise

It's hard to pin down a specific reason, but it is likely a combination of some or all of the following:

- **LACK OF FUNDING FOR PUBLIC HEALTH DEPARTMENTS:** County health departments provide low-cost or no-cost screening, assist with partner notification, and provide treatment for reportable infections. With fewer staff and with many closing down, fewer people get screened and treated.
- **DATING APPS:** Not everyone uses their real name, and if you only ever hooked up via messaging on the app and don't have someone's phone number it is hard to pass along their contact information to the health department. Also, if you get ghosted afterwards, you may not feel inclined to go to great lengths to track someone down. There may also be other ways that apps change how people engage sexually, like condom use at the first sexual encounter—exchanging messages may provide an illusion that you know someone so the first time you meet it feels as if you've already had ten dates.
- **CONDOM USE IS DROPPING:** Reasons are complex and may differ from woman to woman. Alcohol use and not being at risk for pregnancy because of highly reliable contraception, like the IUD or birth control implant, may affect condom use.
- **OVERRELIANCE ON CONDOMS:** Condoms are not a "Get out of Jail Free" card. They reduce STIs in the same way that seat belts reduce death in car accidents. Condoms reduce transmission, but they are not 100 percent protective.
- **PUBIC HAIR REMOVAL:** The microtrauma of pubic hair removal may increase the transmission of some STIs, although removal is associated with a reduction in pubic lice.
- **EARLY ACCESS TO PORN:** Male condoms are used about 3 percent of the time in heterosexual porn, and dental dams are almost never used. Some data suggests that people with less sexual experience may be less inclined to use condoms after viewing porn as compared with those who are not condom naive or who have already received quality sex education.

Incidence and Prevalence

You will hear these two terms mentioned a lot when discussing STIs. Incidence is the number of new cases and prevalence is the number of total cases. Think of a tub being filled with water: the water in the tub is the prevalence, and the water coming out of the tap is the incidence. Some water is always leaking out of the tub via the drain (for example, people getting treated or developing immunity and clearing the infection); that is why the prevalence never gets to 100 percent.

What STI Tests Do I Need?

There isn't really a standard STI screening panel—what you are offered may vary based on your age, where you live (there are regional variations in STIs), if you are pregnant, and what your provider believes is appropriate testing. STI screening can include testing for chlamydia, gonorrhea, syphilis, trichomoniasis, human immunodeficiency virus (HIV), hepatitis B (HBV), and herpes. Chlamydia, gonorrhea, trichomoniasis, and herpes each have their own chapter, and you can read through those for testing recommendations. Syphilis screening for nonpregnant women is based on risk. Your state health department is a good place to check for local syphilis testing recommendations. Testing for HIV for sexually active individuals is recommended annually until you are sixty-five years of age.

While you should be tested if you have concerns about exposure, STI testing is recommended for women if they have had more than one partner or a new partner in the previous year or if their partner has had other partners.

There are several ways to test for STIs. Sometimes we look for the organism itself, and other times it is the body's response to the organism. Here are some basics:

- **NUCLEIC ACID TESTS:** A fragment of genetic material from the infection is identified. Think of looking for a needle in a haystack. This test attaches a magnet to the needle, making it easier to see, and then replicates the magnet-needle combination millions of times so it is easy to find. Nucleic acid testing is very accurate.

- **CULTURE:** Growing the bacteria or virus in a lab. If it grows, the test is 100 percent accurate, but if it does not it does not always mean the test is negative. Some bacteria and viruses grow easily in the vagina and yet are very hard to grow in a lab.
- **MICROSCOPY:** Taking a swab from the skin, cervix, or vagina and looking under the microscope for the infection or signs suggestive of an infection. This is typically only used for trichomoniasis (chapter 29).
- **ANTIGEN:** Identifies a protein on the surface of a bacteria or virus. These tests are done on blood or on a swab from the area of infection depending on the infection. The blood tests are very accurate, but tests on swabs from the site of the infection are rarely used, because nucleic acid tests are more reliable.
- **ANTIBODY:** A blood test that identifies the immune response to a virus or bacteria. It can take 1–6 months for an antibody test to turn positive, depending on the infection.

Is the Test FDA Approved?

FDA approval means the Food and Drug Administration has looked at data sent by the company and evaluated it for accuracy. A test does not have to be FDA approved to be used in the United States. A test that is not FDA approved might be fine, but it may also be inaccurate, and so how the results are interpreted may vary.

Where Can I Get Tested?

Testing for STIs can happen at your provider's office, an STI clinic, your local health department, and even at home. Urine and blood specimens can be used to screen for many STIs, so you may be able to skip an appointment and just go to a lab. If you don't know where to get tested in the United States or want someone other than your own provider, the best resource to find testing is through the CDC: gettested.cdc.gov.

There are a variety of home testing kits that you take to a lab or mail back self-collected specimens. There is also a home HIV test. Testing outside of the medical office can identify a lot of STIs that would other-wise have gone undetected. A project in Baltimore that mailed free testing kits found 10 percent were positive for chlamydia and 1 percent for gon-orrhea, and 86 percent of women who returned the kits said they would use them again. Not everyone is comfortable with public-sector services, especially if they have had negative interactions with providers or the gov-ernment. Home testing for STIs is used routinely in many countries, such as Sweden, Denmark, the United Kingdom, and the Netherlands. If you buy a self-testing kit in the United States, your credit card is typically charged with a generic-sounding product, but if that matters to you, it is wise to ask or read the fine print before ordering.

Home testing can be expensive. Each individual test can be $60–170, and the sites often try to sell you tests you may not need, the most com-mon being blood tests for herpes and hepatitis C (which is no longer considered an STI in the United States). A full home panel with many of these tests can be $800. You can be tested for most STIs free or for very low cost at a health department. Planned Parenthood and a variety of community clinics also have low-cost or sliding-scale options.

I'm Under Eighteen; Can I Get Tested and Treated Without My Parents' Knowledge?

Most states allow testing without parental consent at 12–14 years of age, but some states allow providers to inform parents without the permission of the patient if a minor is seeking or receiving STI services. This is obvi-ously concerning, as many young people do not want their parents to know. Minors who get tested and treated for STIs without their parents getting involved do not have worse outcomes. Forced parental involve-ment or the fear of parental involvement just prevents some kids from getting tested.

The states that allow parental notification (as of 2019) include the fol-lowing: Alabama, Arkansas, Delaware, Georgia, Hawaii, Illinois, Kansas, Kentucky, Louisiana, Maine, Maryland, Michigan, Minnesota, Missouri, Montana, New Jersey, Oklahoma, and Texas. Laws change, so if this mat-ters to you, get the latest information at guttmacher.org, which provides a wealth of information about reproductive health care laws.

What Do You Mean by a Reportable STI?

The positive results go to the state health department and the Centers for Disease Control and Prevention (CDC). It's not just STIs; many infections and health conditions that have nothing to do with sex, like tuberculosis and elevated lead levels in children, are reportable. This is for tracking trends and hopefully preventing or curtailing outbreaks. It's also a good way to know if efforts to control an infection or health condition are working. The STIs that are currently reportable in the U.S. include the following:

- Chancroid (from 2012 to 2016 there have only been 6–15 cases per year in all of the U.S., and they were all in men, so that's all I am going to say about chancroid).
- Chlamydia
- Gonorrhea
- Hepatitis B
- HIV
- Syphilis

If you test positive for one of these STIs, the lab will automatically notify your state health department and the CDC. Typically, a health official will contact you to try to ensure you received your results and, in the case of gonorrhea, chlamydia, or syphilis, that you received treatment. They will also ask about partners and notify them of their exposure. Partner-notification is confidential, so your name will not be revealed. The health department may also give you the option of notifying your partners yourself. If you used a home kit, the CDC will be notified of a positive result for tracking, but they will not know who you are, so you will not be contacted.

I tested positive for an STI that is not reportable or I used a home test—I want to notify my partner, but I'm too scared

You can call your local health department and ask for help. They may be willing to call for you or give you a script to use to help get you started. If you are concerned about your safety, that comes first, although your local health department still may be able to help you in an anonymous way. There are services that will anonymously notify your sex partner for you, such as inspot.com and STDcheck.com. You enter a phone number or email and send a standard message about exposure. These sites typically sell STI testing, so be mindful of the advertisements.

If I had an STI conundrum I couldn't work out, I would personally start at a county STI clinic. I spent a lot of time working at the Wyandotte County STI clinic in Kansas City, and while that is only one clinic, it seemed they had seen it all and knew how to help a lot of people in very creative ways. I've also spoken to many county STI clinic workers at conferences, and they have all seemed like incredibly passionate and dedicated people.

BOTTOM LINE

- Anyone who has ever had sex of any kind is at risk for STIs, but women twenty-four years and younger, with multiple partners, a recent change in partner, or not using barrier contraception are at greatest risk.
- Bacterial vaginosis, a bacterial imbalance of the vagina, increases your risk for STIs if exposed.
- There are many places you can get screened: at a provider, the health department, and even at home.
- Local health departments and home tests are an option for those who are really worried about privacy.
- In the United States, you do not have to be eighteen to consent to testing, but in some states the provider can legally contact your parent or guardian if they choose to.

CHAPTER 25

STI Prevention

MANY THINK ONLY OF ABSTINENCE OR CONDOMS regarding prevention of sexually transmitted infections (STIs). This is unfortunately a narrow view. Abstinence is not a desired strategy for many women, and while condoms are definitely helpful, there are other complementary approaches that are underused.

Many women do not learn about all the options, as the quality of sex education varies greatly depending on where you live and where you go to school. Some schools still teach an abstinence-only policy, which is ineffective. Compounding this issue is the fact that women are often hesitant to discuss their sex lives with medical professionals, as they have been inappropriately judged previously or previous efforts to ask questions were ignored. Some health care providers may not know all of these options or may not be comfortable discussing them. Many women do not understand the extent of their risk. Not everyone knows if their partner has other sexual contacts or if their partner has an STI.

STIs: There's a Vaccine for That!

There are highly effective vaccines for two STIs: hepatitis B (HBV) and human papilloma virus (HPV). You can think of these as anticancer vaccines, because HPV is the cause of cervical cancer and many cancers of the vagina, vulva, and anus, and HBV causes liver cancer. You hear lots of talk about a cancer moon shot, but we already have two with these vaccines. That is pretty cool. The unfortunate part is not every woman has received this protection.

Tell me more about the hepatitis B vaccine

HBV is a sexually transmitted virus that causes liver disease. I'm not going to go into detail about HBV infection because it does not directly impact the vagina, vulva, or rectum. What you need to know GYN-wise is that the genital tract is a portal of entry (you can also acquire HBV by sharing needles). HBV can cause acute hepatitis, which is fatal 1.5 percent of the time. If you get HBV as a teen or an adult, the risk of developing a chronic infection that can damage the liver, potentially causing liver cancer, is approximately 10–12 percent.

HBV can remain infectious on surfaces for seven days and it is highly infectious—even microscopic blood on a shared toothbrush can potentially transmit the infection. While people with multiple sexual partners and those who use IV drugs are at the highest risk, about 50 percent of adults who get hepatitis B have no identifiable major risk factor. A vaccine protects you no matter how you might be exposed.

The CDC recommends universal vaccination against HBV at birth, but many people miss out, as some parents balk at a vaccine against an STI at birth, thinking their child can get vaccinated later on. We want people vaccinated before they are sexually active, so waiting potentially exposes a lot of people unnecessarily. For example, in California approximately 10 percent of kids ages thirteen to seventeen are unvaccinated against HBV, yet by the 12th grade, 39 percent of teens have been sexually active, 19 percent of high school students have had sex with four or more partners, and 4 percent of kids have already had sexual intercourse before the age of thirteen. Yes, before.

If you don't know if you have been vaccinated, ask your doctor for a blood test for antibodies to HBV. If it is negative, get the vaccine. It is very safe and highly effective.

Human papilloma virus vaccine

We are going to get into HPV in depth in the next chapter, but as a primer you need to know that this is the cause of cervical cancer as well as many vaginal, vulvar, and anal cancers for women. The HPV vaccines are approved in the United States up to the age of forty-five. This has nothing to do with safety; the studies submitted to the Food and Drug Administration (FDA) involved this age range.

There are three HPV vaccines on the market:

- **GARDASIL 9:** Vaccinates against seven cancer-causing types of HPV (16, 18, 31, 33, 45, 52, and 58) and two that cause genital warts (6 and 11).
- **GARDASIL 4:** Vaccinates against 16 and 18 (cancer causing) and 6 and 11 (genital warts).
- **CERVARIX:** Vaccinates against 16 and 18.

Ideally the vaccine is given between the ages of nine and twelve, as before the HPV vaccine was introduced, 33 percent of girls were already exposed to one type of HPV by the age of nineteen. The vaccine will not protect you once you have been exposed and developed antibodies. The other benefit of vaccinating early is there is a stronger immune response. Before the age of fifteen only two doses are enough, but once you turn fifteen you need three doses.

These vaccines are highly effective. They protect against cervical cancer, precancer of the cervix, and precancer of the anus. The vaccines that include types 6 and 11 also are very effective against genital warts. With time, we expect they will be shown to reduce the vulvar and vaginal cancers that are HPV-related. While the benefit of preventing cancer is clear to most people, many do not realize the burden of precancerous changes, including the stress of abnormal results and the physical and emotional pain of biopsies and procedures to remove precancerous changes. It can take years of repeat testing for many women. Never having that worry and pain is a hard thing to quantify.

The HPV vaccine is very safe. More than 200 million doses have been given worldwide, many with fifteen years of follow-up. The illnesses attributed to the vaccine that you may read about online, often in stories about the "Gardasil girls," have never appeared in the long-term studies. This does not mean these girls do not have symptoms; it means their medical conditions are not the result of the vaccine. Studies have proven there are no links between the HPV vaccine and autoimmune conditions or premature ovarian failure.

Another online myth about the HPV vaccine is that it does not protect African American women, but that is not the case. If you look at the seven types of cancer-causing HPV types that Gardasil 9 protects against, they cause 79 percent of cervical cancers for white women, 82 percent of cervical cancers for African American women, and 81 percent of cancers for Hispanic women. The vaccine offers equal cancer protection for all women.

In the United States, the HPV vaccine is underutilized—only 57 percent of thirteen- through seventeen-year-old girls have received one dose, and only about one third are fully vaccinated. Vaccinating kids does not make them more likely to have risky sex. This has been proven by studies. (Also, no one worries that teaching kids to buckle up produces unsafe drivers.)

I'm worried about vaccines

There are so many internet myths about vaccines that people have written entire books on them (a great one is *The Panic Virus* by Seth Mnookin). Here is a short list of vaccine concerns and how they relate to the HBV and HPV vaccines:

- **VACCINES CONTAIN FORMALDEHYDE:** Formaldehyde is used in the manufacturing of some vaccines, and in high doses it can cause cancer. Almost every substance is dangerous at some level and safe at others. Too much oxygen can make you go blind and damage your lungs, but we breathe air, which is about 20 percent oxygen, without any issue. This is the same for formaldehyde. We all have microscopic amounts that help us make DNA and amino acids, the building blocks of protein. A 50 kg (110 lb) women has approximately 8.75 mg of formaldehyde circulating in her body, and the teen/adult dose of the HBV vaccine has less than 0.015 mg of formaldehyde, or less than 0.002 percent of what is naturally in a 50 kg body. Formaldehyde is also found naturally in many foods. An average apple has 0.945 mg of formaldehyde, or sixty-three times the amount in the HBV vaccine.

- **MERCURY:** Some vaccines contain ethylmercury, which is not the same as methylmercury, the chemical that can cause mercury poisoning. They sound the same, but chemically they are very different. Ethylmercury has been proven to be safe, but we don't even need to discuss it further because it is not in either the HBV or the HPV vaccines.
- **ALUMINUM:** This is an adjuvant, meaning it boosts the vaccine and helps your body make more protective antibodies. Both the HBV and HPV vaccines have aluminum. It has been studied extensively for almost one hundred years, and the dose in vaccines is known to be safe. Aluminum is not essential for our body, but it is in almost everything we eat because it is in the soil. The dose of aluminum in HBV and HPV vaccines is approximately 0.5 mg. To put that in perspective, after two days of taking aluminum-containing antacids at the recommended dose, you will have absorbed the same amount of aluminum into your bloodstream.
- **VACCINES ARE TOO HARD ON THE IMMUNE SYSTEM:** Vaccines stimulate an immune response. They do this via an antigen (a protein or a carbohydrate) that the immune system confuses for the infection, which triggers the production of protective antibodies. The smallpox vaccine I received at birth in 1966 had approximately two hundred antigens. The HBV vaccine has one antigen, Cervarix has two antigens, Gardasil 4 has four, and Gardasil 9 has nine. A cold exposes you to 4–10 antigens and strep throat to 25–50.

Barrier Protection

Many women and a lot of men get little to no information on the appropriate use of condoms, either in sex education, at home, or from a health care provider. They also almost never appear in movies or television and are nearly absent in porn, so it is easy to see how culturally they are erroneously assigned little to no value.

It is also important to remember not all women have a choice with condoms. Many can't ask their male partner out of perceived risk of sexual or physical violence. If this is you, please tell your medical provider or call the National Domestic Violence Hotline at 1-800-799-SAFE (7233). If chatting online is better, go to thehotline.org.

Finally, I am just going to say consistent condom use is hard, even for the most dedicated condom user. I understand that, but they are an important safety strategy. Keeping them on hand so you are not dependent on a partner is a good way to help with consistent use.

Male (external) condoms

Male condoms can be used on a penis or on sex toys, and are made of latex, polyurethane, or sheep intestine, usually called sheepskin. Sheepskin condoms are not effective for STI prevention, as the pores in the material are large enough that viruses can pass through. Latex condoms are slightly better than polyurethane for STI prevention, probably because they have more stretch and result in a better fit. If you have irritation, feel you are getting infections from condoms, or want to know more about how condoms benefit the vagina, head back to chapter 21 for a refresher.

Getting precise statistics on condom effectiveness in preventing infections is difficult. It is unethical to tell one group in a study not to use condoms to see who develops an infection and who does not. In addition, the infection status of the partner(s) isn't always known, so researchers do not always know who is being exposed to an STI and who is not.

What we do know is that if you are exposed to gonorrhea or chlamydia and you use condoms consistently, they reduce transmission by approximately 90 percent. Trichomoniasis has not been studied, but it is probably in the same range. For HIV, condoms reduce the risk of transmission by about 85 percent, and for herpes and human papilloma virus (HPV) the reduction is between 70 and 80 percent. Herpes and HPV don't just infect the shaft of the penis, so there will be rubbing on the exposed vulva or scrotum during sex. There is no data on syphilis (probably because the number of cases in women is much lower than men), hepatitis B, or mycoplasma. Condoms will not prevent transmission of pubic lice.

DO I NEED ORGANIC LATEX CONDOMS? Sites that sell so-called "organic" or "natural" condoms have been promoting them as "safer." You do not need to know your latex farmer.

The concern promoted by people who profit by scaring the public about condoms (usually people selling supposedly safer but more expensive condoms or certain religious groups) is the group of chemicals called nitrosamines. They can be formed during the processing of rubber into latex. While nitrosamines can be found in latex condoms, they are also in beer, some cheeses, deli meats, and a lot of cosmetics. A single 1 g dose of nitrosamines is believed to be cancer causing—but during intercourse, about 0.6 ng of nitrosamines may migrate from the condom to the vagina. Using about one condom a week for thirty years would result in about 0.9 micrograms of absorbed nitrosamines, which is one millionth of that single carcinogenic dose.

If knowing there are no nitrosamines in a condom matters to you, you do not need artisanal condoms. A study from 2014 showed the following condoms had no detectable nitrosamines:

- Durex Extra Sensitive
- LifeStyles Skyn
- Trojan BareSkin

HOW TO USE A MALE CONDOM. When used perfectly, the condom breakage rate is only 2 percent, yet in the real world up to 29 percent break and 13 percent of them slip. It's easy to see, given the number of steps and in the heat of the anticipated moment, how correct use can be a challenge. I've been in that "for the love of all that is good, just get on with it" moment. If you become proficient and always bring your own condom and lubricant, then you control many of the user variables. A confident women putting a condom on her male partner to protect both of them should be in the dating plus category. There are also female condoms (keep reading for more on those).

If you don't have a penis to practice on, use a cucumber or banana, because figuring it out the first time when the pressure is on is hard. But even proficient users make mistakes. I was a very proficient condom user in my twenties and early thirties. When I started dating after divorce, the first time I put a condom on a partner I put it on inside out. Just saying.

Here is the definitive "how to put a condom on a penis" checklist:

1. Keep one in a wallet or purse less than a month.
2. Make sure it's not expired.

3. Open the package with your hands—not your teeth, as you could tear the condom.

4. Check for visual damage.

5. Put it on the right way, meaning not inside out: if you pinch the tip immediately after opening the package, then you are holding the outside.

6. Hold the tip to leave space for the ejaculate as you roll on the condom.

7. Put the condom on before starting sex: 43 percent of men report they have often put their condoms on after some penetration.

8. Make sure the condom is unrolled completely on the penis: not doing this is in the list of top ten condom errors.

9. Use lubricant: this reduces breakage and makes sex more comfortable for the female partner. Water-based and silicone lubricants are fine for latex, but any oil product, like mineral oil, baby oil, or coconut oil, could degrade the latex. You can use any lube with a polyurethane condom.

10. Make sure the condom is not removed during sex: this is called "stealthing." It is condom sabotage, and up to 9 percent of men have admitted to doing it. Be explicit beforehand if this is not acceptable to you.

11. Grasp the base of the condom during withdrawal so it doesn't slip off.

12. Don't assume your male partner knows all these steps.

Female (internal) condoms

These condoms are inserted vaginally before sex. Partner participation is not required, giving you more control, and they do not require a full erection for application. Erectile dysfunction (ED) prevents many men from using condoms. The incidence of ED climbs with age, so if your partner is over forty years old and you need protection, keep some female condoms in stock. These condoms can also be used for women who partner with women and wish to share sex toys. They can also be used for anal sex.

A female condom is a polyurethane sheath with a ring at either end. Any kind of lube is fine, and there is no worry about latex allergy. They are more expensive than a male condom (up to 2–3 times the cost). Some family planning clinics offer them for free or for a low cost. Don't double up using a male and female condom. This causes more friction and can lead to condom failure.

A female condom takes practice, but the user failure rate is pretty low once you have your lady condom skills. It requires slightly more dexterity than inserting a tampon, but less than removing a menstrual cup filled with blood. The failure rate (meaning leakage or slipping enough that there is fluid transmission) with first time use is 7–8 percent, the second time it is 3.2 percent, and by the fourth use it is 1.2 percent. By the twentieth use, the failure rate is 0.5 percent.

There are great videos online that can show you the mechanics. Given it takes a few tries to get the technique down, I recommend trying it at home by yourself a few times without the pressure of an eager partner.

Dental dams

There is barely enough information about dental dams, a barrier to offer protection while performing oral sex, or anilingus, to even have misinformation.

Dental dams are a square sheet of latex to cover the vulva or anus before oral sex. They were originally used in dentistry (hence the name). A cut-up latex condom can also be used, but there are no studies looking at effectiveness with either dams or cut-up condoms. Only 10 percent of women have used dental dams, and most do not use them regularly.

Dental dams have to be held in place, although there are harnesses to purchase. The taste of latex can be a little clinical, so there are flavored products. Putting lubricant on the person on the receiving end improves the sensation. They are single use only; do not flip them over to use a second time.

Dental dams are often hard to find in drugstores, but you can get them at most sex shops and, of course, online.

Pre-Exposure Prophylaxis (PrEP) for HIV

PrEP involves taking medications every day to prevent HIV. In many ways it is like a vaccine. With a vaccine, your body's immune system is stimulated to kill the virus or bacteria, and with PrEP there is medication circulating in your body to kill the virus. A vaccine offers the convenience of two or three shots and then you are done, but with PrEP you must take the medication every day. If you forget, the amount in your bloodstream may not be enough to fight off the infection.

PrEP is for HIV-negative individuals at high risk of acquiring HIV. It is well over 90 percent effective at preventing HIV infection if exposed (some newer data suggests when prescribed and taken appropriately it is close to 100% effective). Less than 10 percent of people who are eligible are on the medication, and uptake among heterosexual women has been much lower than among gay men. It has been approved since 2012 in the United States, but many people, doctors included, do not know much (if anything) about it.

PrEP is two anti-HIV medications, tenofovir and emtricitabine, sold under the brand-name Truvada. The most common side effect is nausea, but that usually goes away after a month. A generic has been approved and is available in many countries, but is still not available in the United States because the company that makes Truvada has held up the generic with lawsuits. In the United States, the brand-name Truvada is $2,000 a month (without insurance). What makes this pricing particularly egregious is that much of the research was funded by the government and private foundations, not the drug company. In the United States, most private health insurance policies and Medicaid cover PrEP. In Canada, some health plans cover the generic and others do not. The cost in Canada for the generic is $200 a month. In most other countries around the world, PrEP can be purchased for the equivalent of less than $100 a month, often much less.

To start PrEP, you must be HIV negative and get tested every three months—if you become HIV positive, different medication is needed.

HIV-negative women or teens who weigh at least 35 kg (approximately 77 lbs) who fit into one of these categories should consider PrEP:

- Women who have an HIV-positive partner
- Heterosexual women who do not regularly use condoms during sex with partners of unknown HIV status, especially if they engage in unprotected receptive anal sex, which has the highest risk for HIV transmission

- Women with bisexual male partners
- Trans men who have vaginal sex or anal sex with men who partner with men

---

BOTTOM LINE

- Make sure you are vaccinated against HBV, and ask your sexual partners if they have been vaccinated.
- If you are twenty-six or younger, get the HPV vaccine. If you are 27–45, there may still be a benefit, and considering Gardasil 9 may not unreasonable depending on your individual risk factors and Pap smear history.
- When used correctly, male condoms reduce the risk of transmission of almost all STIs except pubic lice.
- Do not forget about female condoms and dental dams.
- PrEP is very effective at reducing the risk of HIV transmission.

CHAPTER 26

The Human Papilloma Virus (HPV)

THE HUMAN PAPILLOMA VIRUS (HPV) is the most common sexually transmitted infection (STI) in the world. There are over 200 different types, and
about forty infect the genital tissues. The impact of genital HPV ranges
from a mild, transient infection that you never knew you had that clears
within a year to cancer of the cervix, vulva, vagina, and anus. Genital HPV
can also cause warts and cancer of the mouth and throat.

Genital HPV Infection Is Ubiquitous

If you are going to have sex, you are almost certainly going to be exposed
to HPV. This doesn't make you dirty or bad or promiscuous, it just makes
you human.

Up to 80 percent of American and Canadian women will have at least
one infection with HPV in her lifetime (it is possible to have more than
one). The prevalence of HPV, meaning the number of people currently
infected, varies from country to country. The exact reasons are not well
understood, probably a complex mix of biology (vaginal microbiomes
vary regionally), genetic factors, and male circumcision (may reduce
transmission to female partners, and women with circumcised male partners may be more likely to clear the infection). Social determinants of

health that affect access to condoms, education about safe sex, availability of the HPV vaccine, and the willingness to have the vaccine clearly play a big role.

Studies that look at antibody levels against HPV tell us that the prevalence (total cases) decreases with age. Medicine does not know if antibody levels against some types of HPV drop over time (so women who were positive on blood testing now appear falsely as negative, although antibody levels to HPV 16 don't appear to drop with age), this is due to clearing the virus, or different cumulative sexual practices.

The biggest modifiable risk factor for HPV is the number of sexual partners—three or more lifetime partners increases the risk of having one of the cancer-causing types sixfold. A history of having chlamydia almost doubles the risk of HPV. It's possible the cervical inflammation of chlamydia could make it easier to acquire HPV if exposed.

Understanding HPV Infection

A virus is a tiny organism made of genetic material within a protective membrane that depends on the host for food, energy, and reproduction. It is parasitic, meaning dependent on a host to live, but not a true parasite. A parasite reproduces outside our cells, while a virus lives its entire life cycle inside a cell. Viruses are everywhere in our environment. They infect plants, animals, humans, and bacteria—they can even infect parasites!

HPV has evolved to match the life cycle of skin cells. It infects the basal (bottom) layer of skin cells and then inserts itself into the nucleus, which is the command center of a cell. The basal layer produces new skin cells, so once infected with HPV each new cell now contains HPV in its nucleus.

New skin cells are immature. The DNA is preprogrammed with instructions on how to develop into a mature skin cell. HPV hijacks the cell's DNA to make more HPV and instructs the cell to assemble the DNA into new viral particles. It is like stealing into a house and using the printer and envelopes for your own purpose. When the skin cell dies, it releases these new HPV viral particles, which are ready to infect more cells. HPV types are highly adapted to specific skin cells, which is why plantar warts (also due to HPV) do not grow on the vulva and genital warts do not grow on the feet.

As HPV needs to infect the basal layer of cells, trauma—even microtrauma—is a great facilitator. This is why genital warts are most common at the lowest part of the vestibule (vaginal opening), as this area receives the most microtrauma during sex. This may also be the reason pubic hair removal, which involves microtrauma, is associated with an increased risk of both HPV and precancer of the vulva.

How does an HPV infection cause cancer?

Some HPV types are oncogenic, or cancer causing. HPV 16 and HPV 18 cause about 70 percent of cervical cancers and types 31, 33, 35, 39, 45, 51, 52, 56, 58, 59, 68, 69, and 82 cause the rest. The breakdown of HPV types for cancer of the vulva, vagina, and anus is not as well known, but HPV 16 and 18 are the most likely to trigger precancerous changes. High-risk HPV can also cause cancer of the mouth and throat.

When healthy cells divide, there are normal mix-ups and mutations with DNA, some of which can be cancerous. DNA has a variety of repair mechanisms that work like spell-check and look for and fix these mistakes. When the mistake is not reparable, these safety mechanisms may even kill the cell. Oncogenic HPV types interfere with a specific repair mechanism, so mutations go unchecked and are more likely to become cancer.

An infection with an oncogenic type of HPV does not mean that you will get cancer—it means you are at risk. In most cases, the immune system takes care of the virus—by two years after infection, 90 percent of women have cleared or show no signs of infection. The concern with HPV is when the virus doesn't clear. It is this viral persistence that puts women at risk for cancer.

It takes a long time for an infection with an oncogenic strain to become cancer. The first step is dysplasia, or precancerous changes, which typically appears several years after infection. The immune system may be able to clear early precancerous changes. The time from infection to cancer is typically more than ten years.

HPV 6 and HPV 11 cause most cases of genital warts. The mechanism is the same—hijacked DNA—but instead of affecting tumor suppression, the DNA changes cause the cells to change into warts.

One major modifiable risk for cervical cancer is smoking—cigarette smoking significantly increases the risk that an HPV infection will progress to cancer.

How common are HPV-related cancers?

Cervical cancer is the fourth most frequent cancer among women worldwide and the second most common cancer among women of reproductive age (15–44). Over 500,000 women worldwide are diagnosed with and over 250,000 women die from cervical cancer each year. The bulk of this cancer burden is for women in countries with no access to the HPV vaccine, screening for precancer, or treatment for precancer or cancer. Cancers of the vulva, vagina, and anus are less common than cervical cancer. HPV-related anal cancer appears to be on the rise.

What Is the Screening for HPV?

This is cervical screening, and the goal is to identify oncogenic or cancer-causing viruses or early precancerous changes so they can be monitored and treated if needed to prevent cancer. The methods are the Pap smear, which is a light scraping of cells from the surface of the cervix that a pathologist evaluates under the microscope, a swab that looks for oncogenic strains of HPV with a nucleic acid (DNA) test, or both.

In the United States, cervical screening starts at twenty-one years of age and continues to sixty-five years of age. Vaccination against HPV does not affect your screening. There are several algorithms approved for testing:

- A Pap smear every three years at ages 21–29 years of age. At ages 30–65, women should either receive a Pap test every three years or a Pap test plus HPV test (co-test) every five years; co-testing can be done by either collecting one swab for the Pap test and another for the HPV test or by using the remaining liquid cytology material for the HPV test.

- High-risk HPV testing every three years in women 25 years of age and older. Your provider may be comfortable collecting this without a speculum.

Women with a history of negative tests can stop screening after sixty-five years of age.

There is no need to test for the nononcogenic strains of HPV. We have no treatment or recommendations for women who are positive. There is a good unwritten rule in medicine—if the test is not going to change the plan, don't order it! Testing for high-risk strains under the age of twenty-five is also not recommended, as women are very often positive, and we know this leads to worry and testing that is much more likely to cause harm than help, given the length of time it usually takes for cervical cancer to develop.

Abnormal results (either the Pap smear or the HPV test) require further evaluation. That may be a repeat Pap smear and HPV test or colposcopy, a procedure where your doctor or provider looks at your cervix with a special magnifying lens. They may take one or more biopsies (small samples of tissue) from the cervix. There are a lot of permutations and combinations of results, something beyond the scope of this book. However, low-grade lesions (LSIL) mean a very low risk of developing cancer, and management is often observation and follow-up in a year. High-grade lesions (HSIL) generally require treatment—the risk of progression to cancer is 4 percent in the first twelve months and increases over time.

There are a variety of methods for removing the abnormal cells of high-grade lesions, and several factors need to be considered. As removal can impact the cervix for future pregnancies or a current pregnancy, removal is not recommended for women twenty-one through twenty-four years of age or for pregnant women unless there is a high suspicion of cancer.

If I Had HPV and Now Test Negative, Could the Virus be Hiding?

Latency means the virus is hiding, but could be reawakened at some point. There is no direct evidence proving latent HPV infections occur, but admittedly it is hard to prove, because finding a virus hiding inside a cell is not easy. Some indirect data suggests that it could happen; for example, during pregnancy some women who have never tested positive for HPV can develop an HPV infection. Pregnancy suppresses the immune system, which may allow a latent virus to reactivate.

If you did have an HPV test that was positive and now it has reverted to negative, there is no way of knowing if it could become positive again. What we do know is if the DNA test is negative, there is no active infection and no risk of transmission. There is no test to tell if you have a latent HPV infection, so you just have to let that idea go.

What About Anal Cancer?

Anal cancer is often caused by HPV. While we used to believe that recep-tive anal sex with a male partner was the biggest risk factor, newer studies are emerging that suggest that is not the case. HPV has what we call a field effect, and so HPV deposited on the cervix or the labia can infect any cells in the genital field.

If you have anal symptoms, for example a persistent itch or irritation, then you need a rectal exam. That doesn't mean you have anal HPV—lots of very common conditions cause anal itch and irritation. Women with HIV and women who have certain kinds of precancerous changes of their cervix due to HPV may be candidates for anal Pap smears, but unfortunately as of early 2019 there are no clear guidelines to turn to for advice. Currently, rou-tine screening for anal cancer or anal HSIL is not recommended for healthy women with no known risk factors or anal cancer symptoms.

Can You Transmit HPV During Birth?

This is called perinatal transmission and the short answer is yes, but it is rare.

Transmission of HPV during birth has been documented during vaginal delivery and C-section and can result in warts on the vocal cords for the baby. This is a rare condition (the number of people af-fected is approximately 2–4 per 100,000) and is called juvenile-onset respiratory papillomatosis. It can lead to multiple surgeries. Given how many women have infections with genital HPV and the rarity of juvenile-onset respiratory papillomatosis, it clearly takes more than viral exposure. It is not clear if mother-to-child genital transmission can occur during delivery.

If I Have HPV, What Do I Tell My Sex Partner?

An abnormal Pap smear due to HPV infection or a positive DNA test means you will shed the virus and there is a potential risk of passing the infection on to your sex partner. If you partner with men, as men do not get screened for genital HPV, some women feel at a disadvantage with disclosing. We generally recommend that honesty is the best policy.

If you have been sexually active with this partner, then he or she may already have been exposed, and of course you have no way of knowing if you contracted HPV from this person or from another partner. Female partners should make sure they are up to date on their cervical screening. Condoms can be used as a protection strategy if desired. If your partner has not been vaccinated against HPV, that is another good strategy to consider.

Can I Catch HPV from Sex Toys?

Aside from penetrative sex, rubbing, and oral sex, theoretically HPV can potentially be transmitted by sex toys. In one study, women were given two different kinds of vibrators, one made of a thermoplastic elastomer and another of silicone, as well as a cleaning solution and instructions for cleaning. The women were asked to self-collect vaginal swabs for HPV and swab the vibrators before and after use and also after cleaning.

It's a small study. Only nine women were HPV positive and submitted results for testing. The shaft of the thermoplastic elastomer vibrator (a "rabbit" style) was HPV positive immediately after use for 89 percent of women, 56 percent were HPV positive immediately after cleaning, and 40 percent were still positive twenty-four hours after cleaning. The handle wasn't much different. The silicone vibrator was similarly positive immediately after use and cleaning, but twenty-four hours later none were positive; however, there were only four samples to evaluate.

It is hard to draw conclusions from such a small study, but clearly HPV can be identified on vibrators after use, which is no surprise as it can live for seven days on surfaces. It is clear we need more research into the cleaning of sex toys to help prevent transmission between partners and more research to see if viral persistence is perhaps more limited on silicone surfaces. Until we know that answer, women who are HPV positive may wish to consider shared sex toys potential vehicles for transmitting genital HPBV infections.

What About Genital Warts?

A wart can look flat or raised. Often it looks thickened because the virus triggered additional production of the protein keratin. Genital warts affect approximately 1 percent of people, and they are caused by infection with HPV 6 or 11.

Warts do not become cancer, but a precancer of the vulva or vagina could be misdiagnosed as a wart as they look similar. Women who have acquired a low-risk virus, like HPV 6 or 11, may also have acquired a high-risk, potentially cancer-causing, type of HPV, so genital warts are a risk factor for abnormal Pap smears.

If a wart looks classic and a woman is under the age of forty, it does not need a biopsy. If the wart is pigmented (dark), ulcerated, or otherwise looks atypical, a woman is over forty, or has a compromised immune system (for example, is on immune-suppressive medications for a transplant or arthritis), the wart recurs after treatment, or treatment is ineffective, then a biopsy is needed to rule out precancer or cancer. Warts around the anus (perianal warts) should be evaluated by a provider who can do anoscopy (look inside the anus) to see if you have internal warts that need treatment.

Genital warts may go away on their own, so it is acceptable to adopt a wait-and-see approach. If they have been there for a year or more, spontaneous remission is very unlikely. There are many different therapies, and none have been shown to be superior. The choice of treatment depends on many factors, including number and size of warts, cost, pregnancy risk, and patient preference.

Treatment options are divided into patient-applied (you put the medication on at home) and provider-applied.

Patient-applied therapies include the following:

- **IMIQUIMOD:** Stimulates the immune system to fight the wart. The 5 percent cream is applied three times a week and the 3.75 percent cream daily to the warts for up to sixteen weeks. The treatment is washed off 6–10 hours later. Irritation, redness, and ulcerations can be side effects. It is not a concern if the medication gets on unaffected skin. There is no good safety data for pregnancy, but accidental exposure is probably low risk. Imiquimod is probably the best patient-applied option when there are a lot of warts.
- **PODOPHYLLOTOXIN:** Blocks the ability of HPV DNA to replicate (make more copies). It is caustic, meaning it will irritate surrounding skin, so being precise with the application matters. A solution is applied with a cotton swab or a gel with a finger to the warts twice a day for three days followed by a four-day break. This cycle can be repeated four times. There is a limit to the amount that you can use each day (0.5 ml). It is best if your provider applies the medication the first time so you know exactly what you should be doing and to be sure you can reach all the warts. Should not be used in pregnancy due to a risk of birth defects.
- **SINECATECHINS:** A green tea extract applied three times a day to each wart for up to sixteen weeks. Redness, burning, and ulcerations are side effects. It is not recommended for people with HIV, who are immunocompromised, or who have genital herpes. The safety in pregnancy is unknown.

Provider-administered therapies for genital warts include the following:

- **CRYOTHERAPY:** Liquid nitrogen or a special probe freezes the warts. Cycles of freezing and thawing cause the cells infected with the virus to die. This is usually performed in the office. Local anesthetic (injections) can help reduce the pain if need be, although generally the procedure is well tolerated without. Several treatments may be needed.
- **SURGICAL REMOVAL:** The warts are cut off with a scalpel, scissors, laser, or electrocautery in the doctor's office, a surgical suite, or

an operating room depending on the size and number of warts needing removal. The advantage of surgery is there is a specimen that can go to the pathologist to rule out precancer or cancer. The disadvantage is pain, potential need for anesthesia, bleeding, and scarring if the procedure is not done correctly or if there are complications. Usually the most expensive option.

- **TRICHLORACETIC ACID (TCA) OR BICHLORACETIC ACID (BCA):** Chemically destroys the proteins in the wart. It is very caustic and must only be applied to the warts. A tiny amount is applied, typically with the wooden end of a cotton swab or even a toothpick, and allowed to dry. The tissue will turn white so the provider can see they have only treated the wart. If any gets on the skin, it should be washed off immediately. The advantage is this is very cheap and can be used during pregnancy, the disadvantage is weekly applications are often needed, and if not done correctly, it can cause redness and blistering on the surrounding skin.

BOTTOM LINE

- Failure to clear an oncogenic or cancer-causing strain of HPV is the risk factor for cervical cancer.
- Cervical cancer screening starts at the age of twenty-one.
- Testing for low-risk viruses is not recommended, and testing for high-risk viruses should not be done before the age of twenty-five.
- Optimal screening for anal cancer is not yet known.
- HPV may persist on sex toys, even after cleaning.

CHAPTER 27

Herpes (HSV)

THERE ARE OVER ONE HUNDRED different kinds of herpesviruses, but only eight cause infection in humans. Two are sexually transmitted: herpes simplex virus 1 (HSV-1) and herpes simplex virus 2 (HSV-2).

One of the defining characteristics of a herpesvirus is the ability to establish latency, which means after the initial infection you don't clear the virus; rather, it goes into hiding in cells and can be triggered to reactivate at a later date.

The idea of latency, a virus hibernating in tissues, bothers a lot of people, but this is not unique to HSV-1 or HSV-2. Chicken pox (the varicella-zoster virus) and infectious mononucleosis (Epstein-Barr virus, or EBV) are also herpesviruses that cause infection and can be reactivated later. With chicken pox, the reactivation is the blisteringly painful shingles. Reactivation of EBV doesn't cause symptoms; people simply shed the virus from their mouth and are unaware of that fact. Almost everyone has one or more herpesviruses in their body.

With HSV-1 and HSV-2, the infection starts in the skin. From a genital tract standpoint, this can be the vulva, the vagina, or even the anus. The virus enters through microscopic trauma. Women are more likely to acquire herpes through sexual contact than men because women have more microtrauma during heterosexual sex and the mucosa (skin) of the vagina is more susceptible to infection than the penis.

The HSV virus enters the skin and starts to replicate or reproduce, making more viral copies. Sometimes this leads to a blister or an ulcer, a painful and visible sign of an infection, but more often than not this initial infection causes no symptoms. The virus reproduces itself, and once infection is established it enters a nerve and travels up the nerve to the cell body, which is actually close to the spinal cord, where it lies dormant. This is why both the initial infection and reactivation or herpes are painful, as the nerve is inflamed.

With reactivation, the virus travels back down the nerve, making more copies. When the virus reproduces, you are potentially infectious, and this process is called viral shedding. Reactivation can result in a painful blister or ulcer close to the original site of infection, but reactivation may also have no symptoms and simply be viral shedding.

Understanding initial infections and reactivation is an important point because the first time you have an ulcer (sore) does not mean this is your first infection; it is the first visible infection. The first ulcer could be a new infection, but it could also be the first visible reactivation of a virus acquired months or even years ago. It is not possible to tell the difference by looking if the ulcer is an initial infection or a reactivation.

The Basics About HSV-1 and HSV-2

We used to believe HSV-1 only infected the mouth and HSV-2 the genitals, but now we know that about 50 percent of new genital herpes infections in North America are due to HSV-1. This is likely because fewer people are exposed to HSV-1 as a child, and so their first exposure may be during receptive oral sex as opposed to day care or the playground (kids and oral secretions go hand in hand).

If you catch HSV-1 orally as a child or before you become sexually active, you will not get genital HSV-1 because you have antibodies that will protect you. There are only two scenarios where people can have both oral and genital HSV-1. The first is if you have both oral and genital contact when you are exposed, so both your mouth and genitals get the infection at the same time. The other scenario is during your initial infection, before antibodies develop, you can technically spread the infection to other body parts; this is called autoinoculation.

HSV-1 prefers the mouth. While recurrent oral herpes sores are common, recurrent painful outbreaks of HSV-1 on the genitals are not. This is one of the reasons that knowing the type of genital herpes can be helpful: if you know the outbreak that you had was HSV-1, you are less likely to have painful outbreaks and also less likely to get recurrences where you shed the virus, so genital-to-genital transmission of HSV-1 is uncommon. There is some data that suggests HSV-1 is more likely to cause a visible genital ulcer with an initial infection than HSV-2.

Having a previous infection with HSV-1, either oral or genital, doesn't protect you from getting HSV-2. However, if you have HSV-1 before you get HSV-2, you are less likely to get painful (visible) outbreaks of genital HSV-2, although you will still shed the virus. So having HSV-1 modifies the severity of HSV-2.

How Many People Have Herpes?

Worldwide, about 67 percent of the population has antibodies to HSV-1, meaning evidence of a previous infection (prevalence). In North America, that number is around 50 percent. The global prevalence of antibodies to HSV-2 is about 11 percent, but is almost double in women versus men (15 percent versus 8 percent). In the United States, 15.5 percent of people ages 14–49 have antibodies to HSV-2, 20.9 percent of women and 11.5 percent of men. This number has been slowly dropping over time, but primarily among populations with the greatest access to preventative health care.

What Are the Consequences of a Genital Herpes Infection?

Most people, approximately 80 percent, who are positive for herpes don't know. The classic herpes sore is a blister that ulcerates and then crusts over. There may be swollen lymph nodes in the groin, muscle aches, or a temperature. However, many people, especially women, never have a sore, and if they do it may appear vaginally, and the symptoms are easily mistaken for a different infection. The sores or lesions of herpes can also be misdiagnosed, for example as an ingrown hair.

While a sore means the infection is active—meaning a new virus is being produced and can be transmitted—the virus is also produced from time to time when there are no sores, and this is called shedding. This is how herpes is typically transmitted, as most people do not have sex with an active sore because they are in pain. Shedding happens more often with genital HSV-2 infections than HSV-1. Overall, the risk of transmitting or catching herpes in a heterosexual relationship without condom use is approximately 10 percent a year.

An important consequence of HSV-2 infections for women is the increased risk of acquiring HIV if exposed. The break in the skin from the ulcer is part of the risk, but even shedding HSV-2 causes local changes that increase the chance of contracting HIV if exposed.

Women with genital HSV have unique issues during pregnancy. If a woman sheds the virus during a vaginal delivery, her newborn can acquire neonatal herpes. There are approximately 1,500 cases a year in the United States, and 50 percent of affected newborns develop a serious infection that involves the nervous system. Even with aggressive therapy there can be devastating consequences, even death.

About 75 percent of cases of neonatal herpes occur among women who contract genital herpes during their pregnancy, and the rest are from reactivation of a previous infection. There are strategies to minimize this risk which are beyond the scope of this book, but if you have had a history of genital herpes, make sure to tell your OB/GYN, family doctor, or midwife and report any new genital symptoms during a pregnancy so you can be evaluated and treated appropriately.

Diagnosing Herpes

Clinical diagnosis means your provider looks at the sore and says, "That looks like herpes." This is often inaccurate, and so the recommendation is a swab from the lesion (this will be painful, but should only take a few seconds). The most common test is a nucleic acid (DNA) test, which is very accurate. Culture is also an option, but it can miss the virus, especially if the sore has started to crust over. Both the nucleic acid test and culture can distinguish between HSV-1 and HSV-2. This is important. If you have HSV-1, you are much less likely to have recurrent lesions and viral shedding than if you have HSV-2.

Blood tests identify antibodies, meaning they tell you if you have previously been infected. The guidelines vary a lot, with some medical organizations recommending against testing and the Centers for Disease Control and Prevention (CDC) not recommending for or against, just noting that blood tests can be considered.

Herpes antibody tests must be type specific, meaning they are able to distinguish between antibodies for HSV-1 and HSV-2. There are several on the market in the United States (HerpeSelect and Uni-Gold HSV-2 are two). The gold standard is called a Western blot, offered by the University of Washington.

There are two kinds of antibodies to herpes, IgM and IgG. IgM antibodies develop quickly after an infection, and IgG antibodies can take several months. There is no reliable IgM test for herpes, so it should never be ordered.

Whether or not you decide to get a blood test for herpes depends on how you and/or your health care provider will act on the results. Think about how the results will change what you do. Some scenarios where blood tests might be useful include:

- **A RECURRENT GENITAL ULCER THAT HAS ALWAYS GONE BY THE TIME YOU HAVE AN APPOINTMENT:** If your IgG blood test for HSV-2 is negative, then it is unlikely herpes. Just keep in mind if the test is positive, it doesn't mean that it is herpes.
- **YOUR SEX PARTNER TELLS YOU HE OR SHE HAS A HISTORY OF GENITAL HERPES:** If you test negative for HSV-2, how will you navigate these results? Will you ask your partner to take measures, such as always using condoms and taking medication, to reduce their risk of transmitting the virus to you?
- **YOU HAVE A NEW ULCER AND THE NUCLEIC ACID (DNA) TEST IS POSITIVE FOR HSV-2:** You really want to know if this is a new infection. If the blood test is negative for HSV-2, then you likely contracted the virus relatively recently.
- **YOU JUST NEED TO KNOW:** If you test positive for HSV-1, this does not tell you if it is oral or genital. If you test positive for HSV-2, it is genital. Will you disclose this information to your partners? Will you insist on condoms? Will you take antiviral

medication to reduce the risk of transmitting herpes to other people?

Treatment

There are three drugs to choose from, and they are very similar: acyclovir, famciclovir, and valacyclovir. There is a very low risk of resistance among people who are HIV negative.

The first outbreak of herpes, meaning the first time you have a sore, the options are one of the following:

- Acyclovir 400 mg orally three times a day for 7–10 days
- Acyclovir 200 mg orally five times a day for 7–10 days
- Valacyclovir 1 g orally twice a day for 7–10 days
- Famciclovir 250 mg orally three times a day for 7–10 days

These medications can also be taken during recurrent outbreaks but must be started within one day of the onset of the lesion or during tingling or burning before the outbreak. This shortens the duration of the lesion by about twenty-four hours. There are multiple different regimens, anywhere from 1–5 days depending on the drug and the dose.

Instead of waiting for recurrences, there is the option of suppressive therapy, meaning taking a medication every day. This strategy reduces outbreaks 70–80 percent, reduces shedding, and also reduces the risk of transmission by about 50 percent.

The doses for suppression are as follows:

- Acyclovir 400 mg orally twice a day
- Valacyclovir 500 mg orally once a day (may be less effective if you have ten or more outbreaks a year)
- Valacyclovir 1 g orally once a day
- Famciclovir 250 mg orally twice a day

Other prevention strategies include condoms, which are more protective for women than men. Consistent condom use could reduce new cases of HSV-2 for women by 300,000 each year. Pubic hair removal may also be associated with an increase in genital HSV infections.

Emotional Consequences

One of the hardest conversations to have with a patient can be giving the diagnosis of genital herpes. Many women feel they have been given a scarlet H, so how you will feel if you test positive is an important consideration before a blood test. Once the shock is over, studies tell us that most women find they have few long-lasting emotional consequences. A lot of women are also reassured when they learn herpes does not cause cancer, recurrent sores are uncommon, and there are medications to reduce outbreaks as well as strategies to reduce the risk of transmission and minimize any harm in pregnancy.

I always point out that when we see someone on the street with a cold sore, which is very likely due to HSV-1, we don't all collectively point and shout, "Pariah." Most people do not give it a thought, but if they do it is usually a brief but empathetic, "Ouch!"

BOTTOM LINE

- HSV-1 can cause both oral and genital herpes; recurrences of HSV-1 on the genitals are uncommon.
- In the United States, 20 percent of women have antibodies to HSV-2, which only causes genital infections.
- Of people with positive blood tests for HSV-2, 80 percent have never had a sore.
- The most serious consequences of genital herpes are an increased risk of HIV transmission and risks to a pregnancy during vaginal delivery.
- Antiviral medications are effective at reducing outbreaks and transmission.

CHAPTER 28

Gonorrhea and Chlamydia

GONORRHEA (*NEISSERIA GONORRHOEAE*) AND CHLAMYDIA (*Chlamydia tra-chomatis*) are bacterial sexually transmitted infections (STIs). Chlamydia is the most common reportable infectious disease in the United States and gonorrhea is the second—there are approximately 1.6 million cases of chlamydia reported every year to the Centers for Disease Control and Prevention (CDC) and another 1 million that likely go undetected. Chlamydia is more common in younger people. Two thirds of new cases are in people ages 15–24, and the CDC estimates that for every 20 sexually active women ages twenty-four or younger, 1 has chlamydia. There are fewer cases of gonorrhea, but there are still over 500,000 a year, and unfortunately gonorrhea is on the rise. In 2018 there were 20 percent more cases than in 2016.

There are disproportionately higher rates of gonorrhea among African American versus white women in the United States—seventeen times higher. This is believed to be due to inequalities in social and economic conditions that affect access to quality health care.

Both gonorrhea and chlamydia can only live in specific kinds of skin (epithelial) cells called columnar and transitional cells. These cells are found in the cervix, in glands at the vaginal opening, the urethra, and the rectum. This is why after a hysterectomy, if the cervix is removed, a vaginal infection is extremely unlikely; a positive test would almost certainly be from the urethra or the glands at the opening. Columnar cells are also found in the throat, so oral infections are possible, and in the eyelids, so a baby can get an eye infection during delivery.

Women are very likely to become infected with gonorrhea if exposed—the risk of transmission from an infected male partner is 50–70 percent per episode of vaginal sex. Transmission from women to men in vaginal-penile sex is approximately 20 percent per encounter. Fellatio (performing oral sex on a man) is also a more efficient means of transmission than cunnilingus (performing oral sex on a woman). The risk of transmitting gonorrhea between women with finger play or shared toys is not known.

Statistics regarding transmission of chlamydia are not as well known, because there are so many people without symptoms, but the best estimate is about 10 percent per act of vaginal-penile sex, with the rate likely being higher for women getting infected than men. Women are also more likely to get oral chlamydia from fellatio than cunnilingus. One study looking at women twenty-four years and younger (the group with the highest risk for chlamydia) found equal rates of infection among women who have sex with men and women who have sex with women.

Chlamydia may be easier to transmit via secretion exposure. While anal sex is believed to be necessary for gonorrhea transmission to the rectum, chlamydia in the rectum has been reported due to contamination with secretions from the cervix when they get on the skin and are pushed back towards the anus with wiping. Infants can also acquire vaginal and rectal chlamydia during birth from exposure to infected vaginal secretions.

What Symptoms Do Gonorrhea and Chlamydia Cause?

Typically none—this is why screening is so important. Some women may have vaginal irritation or burning, more so with gonorrhea than chlamydia, but even then only 20 percent of women with gonorrhea have symptoms. Some women may have a heavy, thick, greenish or yellow discharge that looks like pus—because that is what it is (pus is a secretion filled with white blood cells). Chlamydia can also cause a low-grade inflammation of the cervix that can cause spotting after penetrative sex.

Left untreated, both gonorrhea and chlamydia can cause pelvic inflammatory disease (PID), a serious infection of the uterus and fallopian tubes. The consequences of PID include scarring of the fallopian tubes that can lead to ectopic (tubal) pregnancy, infertility, and pelvic infections, which also increases the risk of chronic pelvic pain. Chlamydia is often silent, meaning it can lead to significant tubal damage that causes infertility with no symptoms at all.

Who Should Be Screened for Gonorrhea and Chlamydia?

Women who are sexually active and twenty-four years and younger should be screened every year, as early treatment of infections reduces the risk of severe pelvic infections. This screening includes all women— straight, bi, lesbian, and trans. Trans men having vaginal sex should also be screened.

In general, the incidence of gonorrhea and chlamydia are much lower after the age of twenty-four, even among high-risk populations. That doesn't mean it doesn't happen, but it is possible the way women have sex over twenty-four differs. The columnar cells on the cervix that are the cells at risk for infection are more prominent for younger women (this is called an ectropion), so it may be biologically easier for a younger woman to become infected with gonorrhea and chlamydia if exposed.

Women over twenty-four years of age or who have had a new partner within the past year, have had multiple partners in the past year, and those who have had chlamydia or gonorrhea before should be screened. Some experts suggest sexually active women aged nineteen and under should be screened every six months. Pregnant women should also be screened, as both chlamydia and gonorrhea are associated with complications during pregnancy and for the baby after birth.

As gonorrhea and chlamydia are associated with other STIs (they tend to travel in packs), if you screen positive, it is generally a good idea to get tested for syphilis, trichomoniasis, and HIV as well, and make sure your cervical screening is up to date.

When Did I Get Chlamydia or Gonorrhea?

Everyone wants to know the answer to this question. The incubation period, meaning how long from exposure to a positive test for gonorrhea or chlamydia, is not known with certainty.

Does Dormant Chlamydia Exist?

Many women in heterosexual relationships ask specifically how long they can be positive for chlamydia without symptoms. This question does not seem to come up as often with gonorrhea, possibly because 80–85 percent of men with gonorrhea have symptoms, versus 30 percent of men with chlamydia.

There are not many quality studies to tell us how long a woman can have chlamydia without knowing. It would be unethical to do the study. Pulling data from older studies, researchers have found the following very soft conclusions (a medical "educated guess") regarding the number of women who will still test positive for chlamydia when they were never treated: 50 percent at one year, 17 percent at two years, 8 percent at three years, and 5 percent at four years.

It is also possible that this chlamydia represents a new infection, and someone has had a sexual encounter outside the relationship. In supposedly monogamous heterosexual relationships, approximately 23 percent of men and 19 percent of women admit to sexual infidelity.

Whether a chlamydia infection was acquired recently, months ago, or years ago is not possible to know. How you interpret that data in the context of the infidelity statistics is up to you.

How Should I Get Tested?

The tests for gonorrhea and chlamydia are all nucleic acid (DNA) tests (see chapter 22). They can be done from urine, a swab collected during a pelvic exam (with a speculum), and even with a self-collected vaginal swab.

Only some tests can be used for the rectum. If you have only had receptive anal sex, tell your provider so they can make sure they have the appropriate test.

What Is the Treatment for Chlamydia?

A single 1 g dose of the antibiotic azithromycin or 100 mg of doxycycline twice a day for seven days are the two preferred regimens. If these medications are not available or you cannot take them for other reasons, the CDC has guidelines for other options.

What Is the Treatment for Gonorrhea?

This is more complicated, as gonorrhea is a master at developing resistance to antibiotics. Since sulfa-based antibiotics were first introduced in the 1930s, gonorrhea has defeated multiple classes of antibiotics, including sulfa drugs, penicillins, tetracyclines, some types of cephalosporins, and quinolones. The emergence of resistance has often been very rapid, taking less than twenty years for some classes of antibiotics. The pace at which gonorrhea is defeating antibiotics far outstrips our ability to develop new classes of antibiotics.

We now have very few treatment options for gonorrhea. It is important to know what works locally, as resistance patterns can vary from country to country. In the United States, the recommended treatment is an injection of 250 mg of ceftriaxone and a single dose of 1 g of azithromycin by mouth together on the same day, preferably one right after the other. If ceftriaxone is not available, a 400 mg dose of cefixime can be substituted, but this has a lower cure rate and so is not preferred.

Follow-Up

No sex for seven days after treatment is completed for both gonorrhea and chlamydia. Sex partners within the past sixty days should be treated, and if there has not been a partner within sixty days, the last sex partner should be treated. In some states, partner-expedited therapy for chlamydia, meaning giving prescriptions to you to give to your partner, is legal and recommended. Gonorrhea exposure requires a visit.

The nucleic acid tests for gonorrhea and chlamydia can be positive for up to fourteen days after treatment, so retesting in this time frame is never indicated. Repeat testing at three months is recommended to make sure there is no reinfection.

BOTTOM LINE

- Sexually active women under the age of twenty-five are at the highest risk for gonorrhea and chlamydia.
- Gonorrhea can cause a heavy discharge or burning with urination, but only 20 percent of women have symptoms.
- Spotting after sex can be a symptom of chlamydia.
- As symptoms are uncommon with both gonorrhea and chlamydia and untreated infections have serious consequences, screening is essential.
- Gonorrhea resistance is a significant problem, and treatment options are limited.

CHAPTER 29

Trichomoniasis

Trichomoniasis is an infection caused by a protozoan, meaning a single-celled microscopic animal. formally known as *Trichomonas vaginalis*, although it is often referred to as trichomonas or even "trich" for short.

Trichomonas have five tiny whips called flagella that propel them around, so under the microscope they look somewhat like tiny squids. They are not parasites, as they reproduce outside human cells, but trichomoniasis is a parasitic infection, meaning it gets its nutrients from the host—in this case, the storage sugar, glycogen, that is found in the vagina. It attaches to the cells with a barb in the tail and causes an intense inflammatory reaction.

Trichomonas is uniquely adapted for the vagina, so it can't infect the mouth or anus, although it can infect the urethra (in men, it infects the urethra and prostate). It requires a high pH to live and grow. Normally, the vaginal pH is 3.5–4.5, so a rise in pH, for example with a vaginal infection like bacterial vaginosis or due to low levels of estrogen, can make it easier for an infection to be established if exposed.

How Common Is Trichomoniasis?

This is not a reportable infection, so the true incidence is unknown. Worldwide, approximately 8 percent of women are infected, although in some communities it can be as high as 20 percent. In the United States, approximately 2–3 percent of women of reproductive age (ages 14–49) are positive for trichomoniasis.

The incidence, meaning new cases, of most STIs drop with age, but this is not the case with trichomoniasis. As expected, the rates are high among teens and young women (ages 15–24) and then they steadily decrease, but what is different about trichomoniasis is that there is a significant spike in cases for women over age forty. One hypothesis is that as estrogen levels start to drop and vaginal pH starts to rise, it is easier to become infected with trichomoniasis if exposed. Trans men who have vaginal sex will also be at increased risk if they are on testosterone, as they will have reduced levels of estrogen.

What Are the Symptoms of Trichomoniasis?

Incubation, meaning the time from exposure to establishing an infection, is 4–24 days.

The most common symptoms are a yellow-green discharge, pain with urination, odor, itching, and irritation (of the vulva and/or vagina). Some women can have so much inflammation that they can have a small amount of bleeding from the vaginal walls, which presents as spotting. The most common symptoms of trichomoniasis are symptoms seen with many conditions, so they are nonspecific, meaning it is very hard to tell based on your symptoms if the cause is trichomoniasis or something else.

It is important to know that 85 percent of women with a trichomonas infection have no symptoms and by six months only 40–50 percent of women have symptoms, so relying on symptoms to identify trichomoniasis is not sufficient. How long a woman can have trichomoniasis with no symptoms before she tests positive is not known.

What Are the Consequences of Trichomoniasis?

Trichomoniasis increases the risk of acquiring other STIs and of pelvic infections (pelvic inflammatory disease). The intense inflammation of trichomoniasis particularly facilitates the transmission. In the United States, it is estimated that 6.5 percent of HIV infections in women happen because of trichomoniasis.

Trichomoniasis is also associated with premature delivery and lower birth weights.

How and When Do I Get Tested for It?

Trichomoniasis is often not routinely included in STI testing, so if you ask to be "tested for everything," ask specifically what that includes. There are no recommendations for who should be screened for trichomonas, meaning testing without symptoms. If you have symptoms, for example a heavy discharge or odor, or inflammation on exam, then diagnostic testing is definitely recommended.

There are several tests for trichomoniasis, and some are more accurate than others, so knowing what test you are getting matters.

- **LOOKING UNDER THE MICROSCOPE:** Also called a "wet mount," this test is very dependent on skill. Your provider takes a swab from the vagina and looks at the secretions under the microscope. The test can miss trichomoniasis 30–50 percent of the time. If inflammation is seen, trichomoniasis should be considered. If the wet mount is negative, that does not rule out trichomoniasis.
- **VAGINAL PH:** Trichomoniasis requires an elevated pH to grow. There are many things that can raise the pH, but it is rare to see trichomoniasis with normal pH. If your vaginal pH is normal, there is approximately a 95 percent chance you don't have trichomoniasis.
- **AMINE TEST:** A sample of fluid from the vagina is mixed with potassium hydroxide (KOH), and if there is an overgrowth of a type of bacteria associated with trichomoniasis, a fishy smell is released. The other cause of a positive amine test is bacterial vaginosis (BV, see chapter 30). A positive test means you should be evaluated further for trichomoniasis, and a negative test means trichomoniasis is less likely.

Putting these three tests together, if your doctor feels that your exam is normal, meaning no redness or inflammation, a normal-appearing vaginal discharge under the microscope, a pH less than 4.5, and a negative amine test, it is unlikely you have trichomoniasis.

Other tests for trichomoniasis

For many women, the tests described above (wet mount, pH, amine test, and exam) are a cost-effective screening option. If they are negative, then the risk of trichomoniasis is low. However, not all doctors have the ability to do a wet mount and test pH. Sometimes those tests are not definitive; for example, the pH may be elevated but no trichomoniasis is seen under the microscope. Finally, women at high risk for trichomoniasis who have negative office screening may want additional testing.

There are several very accurate ways to test for trichomoniasis that don't require a microscope and the ability to test vaginal pH. They include the following:

- **OSOM:** An office test that takes ten minutes. It will identify about 83 percent of cases of trichomoniasis. False positives, meaning erroneously telling you that you have an infection, are uncommon.
- **AFFIRM III:** A swab that is sent to the lab, it can miss 35 percent of cases of trichomoniasis, but if it is negative then you likely do not have the infection.
- **INPOUCH:** A culture, this can miss 20–30 percent of cases, as trichomoniasis can be hard to grow in the lab. If you test positive, then you definitely have the infection.
- **NUCLEIC ACID TESTS:** The most accurate, but also the most expensive. They require a swab from the vagina or cervix. There are two currently on the market: Aptima, which only tests for trichomoniasis, and BD Max, which also tests for yeast and BV.
- **PAP SMEAR:** The liquid-based sample is very accurate. The older method of Pap smear, where the cells are placed directly on a slide, is less accurate. In this scenario, it is recommended that you retest with a nucleic acid test unless you are in a population at higher risk of trichomoniasis.

Whether every woman who wants full STI screening but doesn't have symptoms should have a nucleic acid test has not been definitively answered. If you are concerned about trichomoniasis or want to be definitively tested for everything, then a nucleic acid test is the way to go.

Can You Catch Trichomoniasis Sitting on a Toilet Seat or Other Nonsexual Activities?

There is a pre-internet urban myth about catching trichomoniasis from a toilet seat. It is such a specific myth—I can't recall anyone asking about catching another STI, like herpes or gonorrhea, from a toilet seat.

Trichomoniasis can live for a few hours outside of the vagina or urethra. There are reports of it being transmitted between young women who are using the same basin for washing their vulvas. It likely can be transmitted between women who are sharing vibrators or other vaginal sex toys.

The toilet seat myth is likely very old, as in 1950 a study was performed where vaginal secretions from women with trichomoniasis were placed on an enamel surface (so like a toilet seat) and left to dry. At one hour, 96 percent of the trichomonas seen were active (this was taken as a proxy for capable of causing an infection), and at three hours 56 percent were active. It was not until seven hours later that no active trichomonas were identified. Whether an infection can happen this way is not known, as the vaginal opening and urethra do not typically make contact with the toilet seat.

One study suggests trichomonas when placed in 500 ml of chlorinated water from a community swimming pool may be viable for several hours; however, considering the volume of dilution in a pool (or a river), swimming seems like an unlikely method of transmission.

There are have been reports of women transmitting trichomonas to their daughter's vagina during birth, but this likely involves direct exposure to vaginal fluid.

If you have not been sexually active and are diagnosed with trichomoniasis, it is important to remember that false positives with most testing methods can occur. The chance of a test being a false positive is less than 1 percent with nucleic acid tests and 0 percent with a culture.

Treatment and Follow-Up

The recommended treatment is antibiotics, either metronidazole 2 g orally in a single dose or tinidazole 2 g orally in a single dose. This latter antibiotic may be slightly more effective and better tolerated nausea-wise, but is usually more expensive. Another option is metronidazole 500 mg orally twice a day for seven days. Topical metronidazole does not work. Alcohol has to be avoided while taking either oral medication.

Sex partners should be treated, and if you live where expedited partner therapy (meaning you can give the antibiotic to your partner) is an option, then ask your provider about this. This helps reduce reinfection from sex partners. Avoid sex for seven days after treatment. In addition, do not use any vibrators or sex toys you may have used when you had the infection until they have been adequately cleaned.

Resistant trichomoniasis is increasing, so if your symptoms persist after treatment you should be retested. The nucleic acid tests should not be repeated sooner than 14–21 days after treatment, as they can be falsely positive. Repeat testing at three months after treatment is recommended to ensure there has been no reinfection. In one study, 17 percent of women were reinfected at three months.

If you fail treatment, there are two possibilities: the treatment worked but you were reinfected, or you have trichomoniasis that is resistant to antibiotics. If you and your provider are sure this is not a reinfection, the CDC has specific guidelines for providers to follow, and referral to someone who has experience managing trichomoniasis that is harder to treat may also be recommended.

BOTTOM LINE

- Approximately 3 percent of women in the United States ages 14–49 have trichomoniasis.
- Unlike other STIs, the risk of acquiring trichomoniasis increases for women over forty years of age.

- Trichomoniasis can cause a heavy and/or irritating discharge, but for many women it has no symptoms.
- Testing for trichomonas is often not included in standard STI screening, so if you want to be tested ask specifically.
- While technically it is possible to catch trichomonas from nonsexual activity, this requires very close, wet contact—such as sharing a basin for washing the vulva.

CHAPTER 30

Pubic Lice

PUBIC LICE ARE INSECTS CALLED *PTHIRUS PUBIS*, commonly called crabs due to their crab-like appearance under the microscope. Technically they are parasites, meaning their entire life cycle is dependent on the host (in this case, a human). They live on and around the pubic hair, although they can also infest any coarse hair such as eyebrows, eyelashes, armpits, chest hair, and beards. They have specific hair preferences due to the spacing of the hair follicles—pubic hair follicles (and other coarse hair follicles) are about 2 mm apart, which is the distance between the louse's hind legs, allowing it to crawl from hair to hair. Lice also like a humid environment, so pubic hair is the ideal habitat.

Pubic lice have to crawl to get where they are going, so they are spread by close genital touching (transmission to eyelashes and eyebrows happens during the close contact that occurs with oral sex). Pubic lice can also be transmitted by sharing clothing or bedding. You cannot get lice from a toilet seat—they can't grip the smooth surface—and you can't get it from pets. I'm not sure why people ask specifically about catching pubic lice from pets, but they do.

There is also an incorrect belief that pubic lice are associated with being dirty or unclean. They are not.

As a gynecologist, you get a lot of panicked emergency middle-of-the-night consult requests from friends, and the person who needed the most talking off the ledge was a friend with pubic lice. A physical parasite on the outside is more bothersome to a lot of people than a bacteria or parasite on the inside.

A Really, *Really* Bad Itch

Lice feed on blood, and the reaction to the bite causes intense itching—essentially an allergic reaction. Even reading about this might be making you feel itchy—itch is contagious that way.

The first time you catch lice, the itching may be delayed for up to four weeks, as it takes a few weeks after first exposure to get sensitized and develop the reaction. Some people get a gray-blue spot where they have been bitten, which may be a reaction to the louse saliva. Tiny drops of blood from the bites may be seen on underwear.

Most people seek medical care because of the itch, although occasionally people notice adult lice (about 1–2 mm in length) on their hair. The eggs (also called nits) are smaller, typically 0.5–0.8 mm in size, and are pearly like a tiny grain of rice stuck to the hair. They are harder to see unless combed out with a nit comb (a very fine-tooth comb that can snag the nits and pull them off).

The One STI That Is Decreasing

The incidence of pubic lice used to be around 2 percent, but the number of new infections is dropping dramatically and now less than 0.1 percent have an infection. In the past fifteen or so years, I have seen one case. Before that, I saw several cases a month, so my experience is definitely reflective of the data. One proposed explanation for the decrease is the increasing popularity of pubic hair removal. If you remove the habitat, you cannot catch or spread the infection.

Getting Rid of Lice

The treatment for lice involves killing the adults and removing the nits. The medications recommended by the CDC (Centers for Disease Control and Prevention) are a 1 percent cream rinse of permethrin (sold in the United States as Nix) or pyrethrin and piperonyl butoxide (RID). Avoid contact with your vestibule (the vaginal opening), vagina, and anus.

After you have rinsed the medication off, try a nit comb to remove any surviving nits and eggs, although combing pubic hair can be frustrating given the nooks and crannies and the difficulty seeing all the areas you need to comb. This is why another treatment in a week is usually recommended to kill any of the newly hatched nits that were missed before they become adults and are capable of laying eggs. Depending on how long you have been infected, there can be hundreds of nits. Nix is supposed to kill the nits, but many people do a second treatment anyway. Rid does not kill nits, so a second treatment a week later is recommended.

An alternative therapy is 0.5 percent malathion lotion. You have to leave it on for 8–12 hours versus ten minutes for the methods just described, so it is a lot less convenient. It also smells terrible. There is an oral medication called ivermectin. It definitely does not kill nits, so you have to repeat the treatment two weeks later.

Another important aspect of therapy is getting screened for other STIs, as studies tell us if you have acquired pubic lice, you have a higher risk of also being exposed to other STIs.

If you suspect you have lice on your eyelashes or eyebrows, see a doctor, and if you are pregnant or breast-feeding, talk with your doctor before starting therapy.

How can I kill the pubic lice around my house?

It is easy to go a little over the top. The first time my kids had hair lice, I went overboard throwing things away (culling their herd of stuffed animals proved medically unnecessary, but the one welcome side effect) and buying powders to kill lice that I imagined had fallen onto the carpet and were lying in wait, ready to reinfect us.

After all, they sell those powders for a reason, right? It is so easy to be swayed by what we see on the store shelves. Turns out, none of them are necessary.

To kill lice on your clothes, towels, and bedding, machine-wash everything and anything that has been worn or slept in for the past 2–3 days in hot water (50° C or 122° F) and/or machine-dry on hot. Dry cleaning is also an option. Place any clothes or bedding that cannot be washed in a sealed plastic bag for three days (European guidelines). The U.S. guidelines still recommend putting items that can't be washed away for two weeks, but that seems excessive as pubic lice can't live for more than two days without blood.

BOTTOM LINE

- Pubic lice are parasites uniquely adapted for pubic hair.
- The incidence is decreasing significantly, likely due to trends in pubic hair removal.
- The most common symptom is a terrible vulvar itch. It may take four weeks after infection to develop symptoms
- There are over-the-counter treatments—you have to make sure you get all the nits as well as killing the lice.
- Wash and dry bedding, towels, and clothes in hot water and dry on hot to prevent reinfection.

Conditions

CHAPTER 31

Yeast

YEAST IS PROBABLY ONE OF THE MOST misunderstood conditions of the vagina and vulva. It is often overdiagnosed, meaning women are told they have yeast when they do not. Many women are plagued for years with a seemingly untreatable yeast infection, when they really are suffering from something else. And paradoxically, it is also underdiagnosed, as providers can miss it during testing.

The yeast-industrial complex, in both Big Pharma and Big Natural, is big business, complicating the information factor even further. Over-the-counter (OTC) yeast medication is heavily advertised, and there are more "natural" remedies for yeast than any other gynecological condition, from anti-yeast diets and detoxes to supplements and suppositories. The misinformation online is astounding, and while some may be well intentioned, most of the bad information is to move product.

The antidote? Yes, facts.

The Yeast-Vagina Connection

Yeast is a single-cell, microscopic organism, and there are many species of yeast that live normally on our body without typically causing harm. If I checked one hundred random women on the street who had no, vaginal symptoms and they gave me a vaginal culture, about 20 percent would have yeast at that single point in time. If I used nucleic acid technology that can identify smaller quantities of yeast and sampled these same women, 65 percent would have yeast.

Colonization by yeast (so yeast is present, but there are no symptoms) drops with menopause for women who do not use estrogen. At first this seems counterintuitive, as one would think the loss of lactobacilli (gatekeeper bacteria) typical of menopause would favor overgrowth of yeast. This is a good example of the complexity of the vaginal ecosystem. A reason why GSM may protect against yeast is that the elevated pH makes it harder for yeast to cause infections. The lower glycogen stores may starve the yeast (glycogen is an energy source for yeast as well as lactobacilli). Low estrogen levels in the vagina may be one reason why infants do not get vaginal yeast infections despite having diaper rash, which is a skin infection with yeast.

It is normal for a premenopausal woman to have yeast. It is not *whether* you have yeast, it is *whether* that yeast is causing your symptoms. Any test that is positive for yeast must be put in context. Some women can have symptoms with low levels, and other have no symptoms with high levels.

Women who develop yeast infections are more likely to be colonized, and the reasons some women are colonized and others are not is not well understood. We also do not understand why some women transition between normal yeast not causing any mischief to raging inflammation and itch. Some theories include:

- **AGGRESSIVE YEAST THAT IS ABLE TO EVADE THE VAGINA'S DEFENSE MECHANISMS.**
- **A WEAKENED VAGINAL MICROBIOME THAT ALLOWS NORMAL YEAST TO OVERGROW:** This may be lactobacilli that are unable to control yeast or another mechanism.
- **CONDITIONS THAT FAVOR THE GROWTH OF YEAST:** For example, high sugar levels in the urine or high estrogen levels favor yeast.
- **IMMUNE SYSTEM ISSUES:** Women who are on medications that suppress the immune system or have AIDS are at higher risk for yeast infections.

- **MICROTRAUMA:** Causes include scratching or from sex. For yeast to cause symptoms, it has to avoid the defense mechanisms and stick to cells. Microtrauma damages surface defense mechanisms that prevent yeast from attaching.
- **ATYPICAL RESPONSES TO NORMAL LEVELS OF YEAST:** A good analogy is the variation in responses to seasonal allergies. Some people can tolerate any amount of pollen and never get a runny nose, some people are only bothered occasionally, while others are very symptomatic with the smallest exposure.
- **LOW IRON:** Studies have linked this with yeast infections. Two possibilities include scratching (trauma), as low iron can cause an itch, and a direct impact of low iron on some part of the immune system.

With recurrent infections, some additional factors may be involved:

- **RESISTANCE:** Some yeast cannot be treated by the commonly available prescription and over-the-counter medications.
- **BIOFILMS:** These are complex structures that allow yeast or bacteria to form protective coatings and adhere to tissues and even to devices, such as IUDs and the contraceptive ring. This allows the yeast to avoid detection and capture by the immune system and medications and may thus be a source of reinfection.

Other cofactors for yeast colonization are cigarette smoking and the use of cannabis. For more information on the role of underwear (or lack thereof) see chapter 8.

How Common Is Yeast?

Approximately 70 percent of women have at least one lifetime yeast infection, and 5–8 percent experience recurrent infections, meaning four or more a year. The most common yeast species is *Candida albicans* (about 90 percent of infections). Other species that can cause symptoms are collectively called non-*albicans* and include *Candida glabrata* (second most common), *Candida parapsilosis*, *Candida tropicalis*, and *Candida krusei*. They are less likely to produce vaginal and vulvar symptoms— approximately 50 percent of the time when they are identified, they will not be the cause of the symptoms.

Non-*albicans* species are, however, increasing. Many are resistant to the regular medications used for yeast, and the widespread use of yeast medications has changed patterns of colonization, favoring the growth of yeast that is inherently resistant to the medications.

What Is a Yeast Infection?

When yeast overgrows, it causes an inflammatory reaction, which causes swelling, redness, itching, burning, and pain. A feeling of vaginal dryness and pain with sex are other common symptoms. Some women describe a thick, white, curdy discharge, but that is an unreliable sign of infection. One study tells us that women who do not have a yeast infection are just as likely to have a thick, white, curdy discharge.

The itching caused by yeast can be intense. If you feel as if you need to scratch or that you are scratching in your sleep, then yeast has to be considered. For other women, the itch is less intense and burning is the predominant symptom.

Self-diagnosis with yeast is notoriously inaccurate. The classic symptoms are also the classic symptoms of irritant reactions, allergic reactions, and some skin conditions (see chapter 35). Some women with bacterial vaginosis (BV) do not perceive any odor and may mistake their vaginal irritation and burning for yeast.

In one study, women who were planning on buying an OTC medication for yeast were tested, and it turned out only 40 percent of them would have been treating themselves correctly had they bought the medication. Besides the expense, repeated exposure to yeast medication that you do not need can lead to resistance and the emergence of yeast that cannot be killed by these medications. There is also the aggravation of treating yourself, often repeatedly, without success. Many women who have tried these medications, often for years, tell me it makes them feel broken when a therapy that is supposed to work does not.

How to Diagnose Yeast

Yeast on the skin causes a red rash that may be itchy or tender to the touch. The rash classically has what we call satellite lesions—small islands of rash next to the larger area. This is diagnosed by looking at the skin. Unless the rash is atypical, a biopsy (a small sample of cells cut from the skin) is rarely required.

Your provider might see vaginal swelling and redness, but as women can have different responses, it is possible to be very uncomfortable with very little objective evidence of inflammation on exam. Your provider should test your vaginal pH, which should be less than 4.5.

Tests for yeast include the following:

- **LOOKING AT A SWAB UNDER THE MICROSCOPE:** A test that's very inexpensive and has immediate results. *C. albicans* can be identified this way, but the non-*albicans* species are too similar to distinguish from each other. The disadvantage is that even experienced providers can miss yeast 30–50 percent of the time.
- **A CULTURE:** A swab is sent to the lab, and any yeast is grown and identified. This is the gold standard. A culture identifies the species of yeast, which can be helpful for women who do not respond to therapy or who have recurrent infections. A culture is more expensive than microscopy; however, microscope skills are not needed. Results take 3–5 days.
- **A NUCLEIC ACID TEST:** There are at least two on the market: BD MAX and NuSwab. They can identify several species of yeast. The advantage is these swabs can test for other infections if needed, such as trichomoniasis or BV. They also take microscope skills out of the picture. Their disadvantages are that they are typically more expensive than cultures and not all insurance covers them—they can be as much as $75–100. Results may take several days.

You do not need to be screened for yeast

Many women want to get checked for yeast, but you should only be tested if you have symptoms.

When an Exam Is Just Not Possible

In an ideal world, every women would get an accurate diagnosis from their provider before starting therapy. That reality does not exist for every woman. It may be reasonable to consider buying an over-the-counter (OTC) yeast medication or calling in for a prescription if you meet these criteria:

- Not menopausal or menopausal and using estrogen: women who are menopausal and are not on estrogen have a very low chance of having yeast.
- Intense vaginal itching: you want to scratch high inside.
- No odor.
- No blood in discharge.
- No need to be seen for STI testing.
- No history of recurrent infections, meaning three or fewer infections a year.
- When you have treated identical symptoms before, they have resolved within a week and did not return sooner than two months.

Treatment for *C. albicans*

The class of drugs is called the azoles. This is the medication in the OTC creams and ovules, and they come in one-day, three-day, and seven-day regimens. They are all equally effective. Many women find the creams very soothing, but if you are very inflamed, any product may burn on application. Some lower-quality data suggests that clotrimazole might be the best tolerated with the least irritation.

The oral medication that is widely used is fluconazole (trade name Diflucan, but a generic is available). A single 150 g dose is fine for mild to moderate infections. Two doses spaced seventy-two hours apart may be more effective for severe infection when there is a lot of redness and swelling. The medication works for seventy-two hours, so giving a second dose sooner is not necessary.

The oral and topical medications are equally as effective—they both cure a yeast infection due to *C. albicans* 90 percent of the time. I know many women and even many providers have a hard time believing this, but no study has demonstrated superiority. The Centers for Disease Control and Prevention (CDC) suggests that either the topical or oral is appropriate; however, the Infectious Diseases Society of North America (IDSA) recommends the topical therapies first, as they will not affect the yeast in your bowel. I favor this approach, and where possible and practical it is best to treat with the medication that will cause the least collateral damage to other tissues.

Oral fluconazole has a lot of drug interactions, so that is a consideration when choosing a therapy. Fluconazole can affect some blood thinners, and there is a possibility of serious drug interactions with some cholesterol medications as well as trazodone, a medication often used for sleep. Always tell your provider and your pharmacist about your medications. The vaginal medication is absorbed in a very minor degree and is not believed to have the potential for serious drug interactions.

I tell women about the IDSA recommendations, but ultimately if there is no concern about drug interactions, I let them choose. Many cannot stand the creams, and others find the pill makes them nauseous.

Some other treatment tricks:

- **START AN ORAL ANTIHISTAMINE:** Such as cetirizine (Zyrtec) or loratadine (Claritin), the generic version is just fine. This helps to reduce the itch and you will feel better faster.
- **A TOPICAL STEROID ON YOUR VULVA:** Will help reduce inflammation and itch.

Be realistic about how long it will take to feel better. You should start to feel better by seventy-two hours, but it may take a week for all of the inflammation to subside.

Recurrent *C. albicans*

This is generally well treated with 150 mg of fluconazole once a week for six months. The idea is to suppress the yeast, giving time for whatever mechanism that allowed the yeast to occur to resolve. While on the therapy, most women do well and have no symptoms. Once it is stopped, the yeast returns for 30–50 percent of women. If this is you, it is time to see a specialist.

I Used a Yeast Medication, and My Symptoms Did Not Go Away

This is a common scenario, as 50–70 percent of women who self-diagnose with a yeast infection actually have a different diagnosis.

Let's break this down because it is important. We will be generous (also the math is easier) and say that 50 percent of women who self-diagnose with yeast are correct. We know both the OTC medications and prescription fluconazole work 90 percent of the time.

We will start with one hundred women who think they have a yeast infection and used either an OTC medication or fluconazole that was prescribed over the phone or that they had at home—fifty will have yeast and fifty will not. Of the fifty who have yeast, forty-five will get better and five will be medication failures. The fifty who never had yeast to begin with will not get better. Of the original one hundred, fifty-five women will still have symptoms, and only five (or 9 percent) have yeast. If you are in that 9 percent you need to be seen, because there is a chance you could have the type of yeast not treated by the medication you took. That takes an exam, and you need a culture. There is a 91 percent chance you do not have yeast, and so you should be seen so you can get the correct diagnosis. Either way, you need an exam.

For women who fail treatment, I always recommend a culture and not a nucleic acid test. If you have *C. albicans* that has become resistant, we can only get that information from a culture. Some of the nucleic acid tests do not distinguish among all yeast species, and that may be important in this treatment-failure scenario.

Non-*albicans* Species

As at least 50 percent of the time non-*albicans Candida* is not the source of the symptoms, the first step is excluding other causes of your symptoms. You may need a specialist for this.

Some of these species can be treated orally with fluconazole, others topically, and some require 600 mg of boric acid in a gelatin capsule vaginally once daily for two weeks. The cure rate is approximately 70 percent.

If your provider is not comfortable managing non-*albicans Candida*, then a referral to a specialist is recommended.

Boric acid is covered in more detail in chapter 22. From a yeast standpoint, it should only be used in very specific situations: *C. albicans* that is resistant to the azole medications and certain non-*albicans* strains.

Do I Have a Systemic Yeast Infection?

Not if you are reading this book.

A systemic yeast infection means the yeast is in your bloodstream, and in that situation, you would be very ill and in the hospital. You might even be in the intensive care unit.

Therapies That Do Not Work for Yeast or Are Not Recommended

Home DIY therapies for yeast are medical whack-a-mole—just when I think I have heard it all, another one pops up. Here are some that I have heard about that you should *not* use:

- **GARLIC:** Apart from the burning sensation on inflamed tissue, it has never been tested. The antifungal property is the chemical allicin, but you have to crush or chop the garlic to release it, so a whole clove is worthless. Garlic may have soil bacteria, and the crushed garlic will be pretty near impossible to retrieve. Did I mention it will burn? Wrapping it in gauze has been recommended, but that makes no sense as the allicin is not liquid and will not seep through to the tissues.
- **TEA TREE OIL:** This can cause nasty allergic reactions on the vaginal mucosa. It is also an endocrine disruptor and has not been tested for vaginal yeast infections.
- **HOMEOPATHIC PRODUCTS:** A common one has mistletoe leaf and boneset. Neither ingredient has been studied for yeast, but this is the one time it does not really matter, as homeopathic products contain no active ingredients and are a waste of money.

- **THE CANDIDA DIET:** This is based on the false premise that eating sugar increases the sugar in your vagina. It is all kinds of wrong. See chapter 7 for more.

What about probiotics?

They are covered in detail in chapter 22, but they can be best summarized as expensive products that may not contain what they claim, and whether they prevent yeast infections is highly questionable.

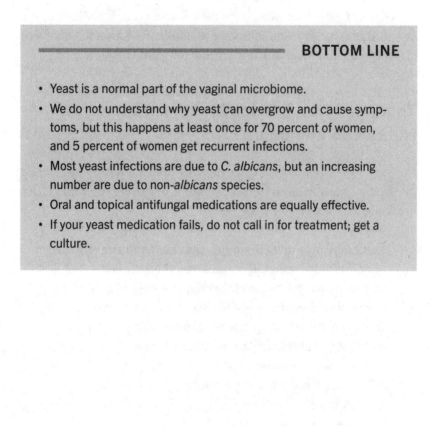

BOTTOM LINE

- Yeast is a normal part of the vaginal microbiome.
- We do not understand why yeast can overgrow and cause symptoms, but this happens at least once for 70 percent of women, and 5 percent of women get recurrent infections.
- Most yeast infections are due to *C. albicans*, but an increasing number are due to non-*albicans* species.
- Oral and topical antifungal medications are equally effective.
- If your yeast medication fails, do not call in for treatment; get a culture.

CHAPTER 32

Bacterial Vaginosis

BACTERIAL VAGINOSIS, OR BV, is a bacterial imbalance in the vagina. It is the result of a reduction in lactic acid–producing bacteria (primarily lacto-bacilli), which leads to an overgrowth of pathogenic bacteria, such as *Gardnerella vaginalis, Mobiluncus curtisii, Mycoplasma hominis,* and others.

The symptoms can vary from an increase in vaginal discharge to an odor and irritation, although technically women can have BV and have no symptoms. Odor after a male partner ejaculates is often reported. This is because BV is associated with an increase in bacteria that produce compounds called cadaverine and putrescine that have a musky, fishy smell. When they mix with the alkaline (or elevated) pH of ejaculate, these compounds become volatile and are much easier to smell.

Approximately 30 percent of women will have an infection with BV at one point in time, and BV is the most common cause of an acute vaginitis, even though most women and doctors mistakenly ascribe that status to yeast. It is important to get treatment for BV because it increases the chance of acquiring an STI—such as gonorrhea, chlamydia, or HIV—if exposed. In addition, women with BV are more likely to develop pelvic inflammatory disease, a serious infection affecting the uterus and fallopian tubes. BV also increases a woman's risk of developing a pelvic infection after a pregnancy termination and after a hysterectomy.

Why some women get BV and others do not is likely a complex combination of their microbiome and environmental exposures. Some reasons include the following:

- **LESS LACTIC ACID PRODUCTION:** Some women may have microbiomes that simply can't produce enough protective lactic acid, and so the pathogenic (harmful) bacteria overgrow.
- **ENVIRONMENTAL EXPOSURES:** Vaginal infections, spermicide, some antibiotics and vaginal products, douches, and cigarette smoking can all impact lactobacilli. The link between douching and BV cannot be overemphasized.
- **MENSTRUAL BLOOD:** Lactobacilli bind to red blood cells. This may be why many women report their symptoms return right after their period, as their lactobacilli counts are the lowest. Women with heavier bleeding may lose more lactobacilli this way. Irregular bleeding may chronically impact the lactobacilli counts, or the chronic exposure to blood may elevate the pH and/or provide nutrients that allow more pathogenic bacteria to grow.
- **COLONIZATION WITH MORE AGGRESSIVE STRAINS OF PATHOGENIC BACTERIA:** Some strains of *Gardnerella* and other harmful bacteria are harder to kill.
- **BIOFILMS:** These are complex communities of bacteria that produce a film-like plastic wrap protecting them from lactic acid and other natural defense mechanisms as well as antibiotics. When biofilms develop, they may serve as a reservoir for reinfection. One study suggests that 90 percent of women with BV may have biofilms.

Several studies have shown that birth control with estrogen (the pill, the ring, or the patch) is protective against BV. The exact mechanism is unknown, but this may be because estrogen increases glycogen deposition, providing more nutrients for lactobacilli or other beneficial lactic acid–producing bacteria. Hormonal contraception typically results in lighter periods, so there is less loss of lactobacilli with menstrual blood.

Sex and BV

BV is primarily associated with sex, so much so if you have never been sexually active then you do not have BV. Studies following virginal women and the impact of exposure to sexual activity show that once women become sexually active, their lactobacilli start to risk compromise. The reason(s) are not clear. Ejaculate itself or the temporary elevation in pH may have a direct impact on lactic acid–producing bacteria, or there may be another mechanism.

The more male sexual partners, the greater the risk of BV. Many women also report no issues with BV until they encounter one specific male partner. There is some data that suggests some men may have biofilms with *Gardnerella* and other pathogenic bacteria on their penis and theoretically could be transmitting this bacteria, the biofilm, or the ability to make biofilms to their female sexual partners. Studies treating male partners with antibiotics have been discouraging; this could be because the antibiotics were ineffective due to the biofilms.

Condoms protect against BV, and any woman struggling with BV who partners with men should consider using condoms. Whether this protects her lactobacilli from effects of ejaculate, protects her from biofilms, or protects against something else is unknown.

Women who have sex with women are also at risk of BV. This may be because shared vaginal secretions transmit biofilms or exposure to a lactic acid–deficient microbiome could lead to your vagina being colonized with this new bacteria.

We have known that it takes more than exposure to bacteria to cause BV ever since Dr. Gardner's original work in the 1950s. In what I can only describe as a horrific experiment that would not be approved today, he inoculated women with the bacteria that would eventually bear his name, *Gardnerella vaginalis*. These women did not develop BV. He then inoculated women who were healthy with vaginal secretions from women with BV—the women developed BV.

These women were all white women in Dr. Gardner's private clinic, and how they actually consented and whether they truly, freely understood the implications of being inoculated with bacterial vaginosis discharge is not clear.

Pregnancy and BV

The role of BV in pregnancy complications, specifically miscarriage and premature birth, is not well understood. Some studies suggest an association, but treatment has not significantly improved outcomes. Screening is not recommended for women at low risk for a premature delivery. For women with a moderate to high risk of a premature delivery, for example a woman with a previous premature delivery, there are some conflicting recommendations. If you are at high risk for a premature delivery, talk with your doctor and ask their advice.

Diagnosis of BV

There are several ways to make the diagnosis of BV. The methods endorsed by the Centers for Disease Control and Prevention (CDC) include the following:

- **AMSEL'S CRITERIA:** This involves four tests, and you must be positive for three to have BV. The criteria are a classic discharge, a positive amine test (an odor when the discharge is mixed with potassium hydroxide), a vaginal pH greater than 4.5, and an evaluation of discharge under the microscope for clue cells, which are vaginal skin cells studded with bacteria. Inflammation seen under the microscope excludes BV.
- **NUGENT'S CRITERIA:** A swab is sent to the lab and scored for the ratio of lactobacilli-type bacteria to BV-associated bacteria. This is the gold standard used in studies. It is not as widely available.
- **AFFIRM VP III:** This tests for high concentrations of *G. vaginalis*. It can also test for trichomoniasis.
- **OSOM BV BLUE TEST:** This detects sialidase, an enzyme produced by the bacteria associated with BV.
- **NUCLEIC ACID TESTS:** NuSwab and BD Max can also identify yeast and trichomoniasis. They are the most expensive. They look at several types of bacteria associated with BV.

A Pap smear is not a reliable test for BV, and cultures looking for bacteria such as *Gardnerella* are also not recommended, as they are not reliable enough, either.

Testing for BV can be frustrating. Not all providers can offer the more cost-effective Amsel's criteria testing, and some of the other tests, which do not require a microscope, can be very expensive.

A good strategy is to triage testing based on vaginal pH. In my opinion, if your provider cannot do a vaginal pH, they should not be managing vaginitis. It is an easy test, pennies to do, and provides a lot of information. The amine test also does not require a special skill.

If your vaginal pH is less than 4.5 and you do not have a positive amine test, then there is almost a 0 percent chance you have BV. These tests are not specific, meaning you can have an elevated pH and an odor from other causes, but they may be a cost-effective way for screening when a microscope evaluation isn't an option. If your pH is less than 4.5 and the amine test is negative, paying for expensive BV tests may not be a good use of resources.

Women with BV are often asymptomatic—up to 50 percent. If you are getting screened for an STI, it is worth adding screening for BV as it is a risk factor for STIs. Again, these additional tests are expensive, so if you are screened with a pH and an amine test you can get a lot of information. If you are planning on a hysterectomy or a pregnancy termination, then screening for BV and treatment if positive are also recommended.

Treatment of BV

The treatment is based on killing the pathogenic (harmful) bacteria. The recommended treatment is one of the following antibiotic regimens:

- **METRONIDAZOLE 500 MG BY MOUTH, TWICE A DAY FOR SEVEN DAYS:** This can cause a serious reaction (vomiting) if taken with alcohol, so avoid alcohol for the duration of treatment and for twenty-four hours afterwards.
- **METRONIDAZOLE 0.75 PERCENT VAGINAL GEL, ONE FULL APPLICATOR (5 G) INTRAVAGINALLY ONCE A DAY FOR FIVE DAYS:** Alcohol consumption

with the vaginal metronidazole gel, which results in about 2 percent of the blood levels seen with the oral medication, has not been studied. Whether this is enough to cause a reaction with alcohol is unknown. It can produce a clumpy discharge that may be confused with yeast, although the actual risk for yeast is low. Get tested if you think you have a yeast infection.

- **CLINDAMYCIN CREAM 2 PERCENT, ONE FULL APPLICATOR (5 G) INTRAVAGINALLY AT BEDTIME FOR SEVEN DAYS:** This has the highest risk of causing vaginal yeast infections (see chapter 22). It's oil based, so it will impact condoms for seventy-two hours after use.

Other treatment options include the following:

- **SECNIDAZOLE GRANULES 2 G IN A SINGLE ORAL DOSE:** This may be an option for women who cannot swallow pills and who do not want a vaginal therapy.
- **TINIDAZOLE EITHER 2 G ORALLY ONCE DAILY FOR TWO DAYS, OR 1 G ORALLY ONCE DAILY FOR FIVE DAYS:** Tinidazole stays in the bloodstream longer, so alcohol must be avoided for seventy-two hours after finishing the medication. Tinidazole is typically more expensive, but some studies (low quality) suggest it may be more effective for the pathogenic bacteria. If there is a BV recurrence shortly after completing therapy, tinidazole might be an option.
- **CLINDAMYCIN 300 MG ORALLY TWICE DAILY FOR SEVEN DAYS:** This has the highest chance of causing antibiotic-associated diarrhea and yeast infections.
- **CLINDAMYCIN OVULES 100 MG INTRAVAGINALLY ONCE AT BEDTIME FOR THREE DAYS:** This is oil based, so it weakens condoms.

Recurrent BV

The recurrence rate is high—20–40 percent of women will have a recurrence of BV within three months of treatment, and in some studies almost 60 percent by twelve months. This is not because the treatments don't work; rather, the antibiotics reduce the pathogenic bacteria, but they do not increase the amount of lactic acid–producing bacteria. Antibiotics also cannot penetrate biofilms to treat evasive organisms, and they don't destroy the biofilm.

Strategies for recurrent BV suppress the pathogenic bacteria while trying to encourage lactic acid–producing bacteria to grow. For women with three or more recurrences in twelve months, there are two recommended regimens:

- **ORAL METRONIDAZOLE OR TINIDAZOLE 500 MG TWICE A DAY FOR A WEEK FOLLOWED BY VAGINAL 0.75 PERCENT METRONIDAZOLE 5 G GEL TWICE WEEKLY FOR 4–6 MONTHS:** I reduce the metronidazole gel to once a week at four months and then stop at six months.
- **2 G OF METRONIDAZOLE AND 150 MG OF FLUCONAZOLE (PREVENTATIVE THERAPY FOR YEAST) ONCE A MONTH.**

Women who fail the above regimen or who recur quickly after stopping likely have a biofilm, and intravaginal boric acid 600 mg daily for twenty-one days after the oral medication (the first regimen) but before the vaginal metronidazole is recommended. The boric acid does not work by changing the pH; it is disruptive to the biofilm.

Weekly boric acid is not recommended, and neither is boric acid alone for BV.

Other complementary therapies to consider for recurrent BV or to reduce the risk of BV include the following:

- **CONDOMS FOR WOMEN WHO PARTNER WITH MEN:** For at least six months, but longer if possible. Make sure they do not have spermicide.
- **WOMEN WHO PARTNER WITH WOMEN:** Do not share sex toys and consider having your partner tested for BV and treated if appropriate.
- **CONTRACEPTION WITH ESTROGEN:** The pill, the ring, or the patch. Several studies show a protective effect against BV. If one of these is an option for you, consider using it continuously so you don't get a period.
- **CONSIDER THE ROLE OF YOUR IUD IF YOU HAVE ONE:** A couple of studies have suggested an association. Biofilms have been identified on IUDs, and the risk increases the longer the IUD is in place. This mirrors what I have seen—women reporting they were fine

for years and then developing recurrent BV 4–5 years into their IUD. Admittedly, it is not clear, and so this could be correlation, not causation. Another way the IUD could contribute to recurrent BV is with spotting (typically seen with the levonorgestrel IUD). IUDs are expensive, and for many women insertion is painful, so an in-depth discussion may be needed with someone who is an expert before recommending removal. If an IUD is removed, we don't know how long it needs to be out to clear any vaginal biofilms. When insertion of a new device is medically recommended is unclear.

- **VAGINAL HYGIENE:** No douching, no petroleum jelly vaginally, no spermicide, and no lubricant that is damaging to lactic acid–producing bacteria (see chapter 9).
- **MENSTRUAL CUPS:** I don't know of any association, but biofilms have been identified on diaphragms, so if you have recurrent BV it would not be an outrageous hypothesis to think your menstrual cup could be a source of reinfection, especially as blood may have a role. Switching to pads or tampons might be a temporary consideration to see if there is an association for you.

BOTTOM LINE

- BV is a common cause of vaginitis—classic symptoms include irritation, discharge, and an odor.
- There are several tests for BV. There are pros and cons for each one.
- BV has a high recurrence rate. The reasons are not well understood and may be due to issues with lactic acid–producing bacteria and biofilms.
- Condoms and estrogen-containing contraception are protective against BV.
- Recurrent BV can be a challenge—this is a time to see a practitioner with extensive experience.

CHAPTER 33

Vulvodynia

Vulvodynia is a pain condition—the pain can be anywhere on the vulva, including the vestibule, but it stops at the hymen. When the pain is widespread on the vulva we use the term vulvodynia, when it is confined to the vestibule we call it vestibulodynia (the older name is vulvar vestibulitis), and when the pain is confined to the clitoral glans and hood we call it clitorodynia. The most commonly used word to describe the feeling of vulvodynia is "burning," but other symptoms include irritation, pain, and pain with sex.

Provoked vulvodynia means the pain is not noticeable until the area is touched or provoked in some way. The provoking stimulus can be intercourse or a tampon, but it can also be the light touch of clothes or even underwear. Spontaneous vulvodynia means the pain is constant or comes and goes with no relation to a triggering touch.

The hypothesis is that vulvodynia is nerve pain, meaning there is no obvious visible cause on exam; rather, something microscopic has triggered the nerves to produce pain. This does not mean your pain is not real—pain is a microscopic process. At a cellular level there is inflammation and miscommunication with neurotransmitters. Many pain conditions have no visible physical findings. The pain from migraines is a good example.

A good analogy for vulvodynia is a sound system that is malfunctioning. Signals that do not typically cause pain, like light touch or underwear, are amplified and/or misinterpreted. Why this happens is not known. The location of the miscommunication in the nervous system is also not known. A pain signal from the vulva involves the nerve endings that pick up the signal, the nerves that transmit that signal to the spinal cord, the nerves in the spinal cord that relay that signal to the brain, the area in the brain that processes the signal and turns it into what we feel as pain, and then a similar relay system that sends a dampening signal back down to reduce pain. The issue could be anywhere in this pathway, or it could be at multiple points.

Chronic pain can also alter this pathway to favor pain.

How Many Women Have Vulvodynia?

Approximately 8–15 percent of women have or have had vulvodynia symptoms. That doesn't mean 8–15 percent of women have severe vulvar pain all the time; for some women, the pain may be present for months or years, and others may have it for a time and then the pain goes away. The annual incidence, meaning new cases, is approximately 4 percent, and it is more common among younger women. Hispanic women have the highest incidence, followed by white women, and African American women have the lowest.

Many women suffer in silence. Approximately 70 percent of women with vulvodynia have seen a health care provider in the past two years for their pain but were not diagnosed. Over 50 percent of women with vulvodynia have seen at least three providers before getting the right diagnosis.

Many women are misdiagnosed, sometimes for years, with chronic yeast infections. While yeast can cause burning, just like vulvodynia, it is almost always associated with itch, and vulvodynia is not. This is another reason why an accurate diagnosis of yeast is essential—meaning a test like a culture (see chapter 31)—so as not to mistake vulvodynia for yeast. Many of the topical yeast therapies are soothing, and so women with vulvodynia may feel a temporary benefit from anti-yeast medication and erroneously think their diagnosis of yeast was correct.

How Do I Know If I Have Vulvodynia?

This is a diagnosis of exclusion, meaning other causes of pain are ruled out and the diagnosis that remains, if the symptoms fit, is vulvodynia.

Symptoms that should make you consider vulvodynia include the following:

- Pain at the vaginal opening for at least three months
- Burning vulvar pain
- Knifelike vulvar pain
- Pain with touch such as tampon insertion, masturbation, exams in the doctor's office, and sex

Itching makes vulvodynia less likely, but there is a caveat. As women with vulvodynia may have increased sensitivity in their nerves, they may be more likely to feel symptoms of yeast—meaning a small amount of yeast that may not produce symptoms for most woman could be a big neon sign of pain for women with vulvodynia. That is part of what makes pain complex—it is often more than one thing.

A gentle physical exam is needed to rule out other causes of vulvar pain. The most common are GSM, yeast, and skin conditions. If you have GSM, most providers recommend treating that adequately before making a diagnosis of vulvodynia.

The most reliable sign on physical exam of vulvodynia is the cotton swab test—touching the vestibule (vaginal opening) with a cotton-tipped swab. If that causes severe pain, there are no skin conditions to explain the pain, and testing for yeast is negative, then the diagnosis of vulvodynia should be considered.

The cotton swab test is not 100 percent accurate—some women have pain only on their labia or their clitoral glans, but the majority of women with vulvodynia will have a positive result.

It is also important to check for pelvic floor muscle spasm (PFMS, chapter 34), as there is an increased incidence among women with vulvodynia. Pain of PFMS can sometimes feel as if it is coming from the skin.

There is a strong mind-body connection, so depression and anxiety are important cofactors for pain. They don't cause it, but they are accelerants. Think of whatever causes your pain as the match that started a fire. Depression and anxiety are fuel on that fire. It is hard to put out a fire while someone is dousing it with gasoline. Therefore, it is a good idea for women with vulvar pain to be screened for depression and anxiety and to seek treatment if they screen positive.

What Is the Underlying Cause of Vulvodynia?

Some women report their pain was triggered by a painful event, such as surgery or a series of yeast infections. Others report that the onset of their pain was associated with a stressful situation. Stress is bad for every medical condition—many of the chemical changes in the nervous system with stress can lower the threshold for pain conditions. However, most women report no triggering event.

Why the vulva develops this unique pain condition is not known. There are a lot of sensory nerves in the vulva. However, chronic pain is more often about genetic risk. Consider the physical trauma of a vaginal delivery, which often involves tearing of the vulva. Most women, even those with significant injuries, do not develop chronic vulvar pain. I have also seen women survive massive pelvic trauma due to car accidents, even pelvic fractures, who never develop chronic pain. People can also develop severe, crippling pain from something as seemingly innocuous as a yeast infection. And of course, chronic pain can happen spontaneously, much in the way that some people develop high cholesterol from diet and others get it spontaneously despite adhering to a lifelong healthy diet.

Many women with vulvodynia report a history of chronic yeast infections. We don't know if these women have increased sensitivity to low levels of yeast, if yeast triggers an inflammation-pain cascade that becomes vulvodynia, or if these women were misdiagnosed for years with yeast given the symptom overlap between yeast and vulvodynia.

Some people have wondered if birth control pills may play a role in vulvodynia. The hypothesis is that the estrogen of birth control pills suppresses testosterone activity and that is somehow a triggering mechanism. The studies that make this claim are of lower quality. A large, well-done study found no connection between oral contraception and vulvodynia.

It is true that hormones have a role in pain; this is one of the reasons women have more chronic pain syndromes than men. Many women also report their pain is different right before their period. It is not unreasonable to see if for you there is a change in your pain without hormonal contraception, but there is no good data to say you should do this, and women should not worry based on the information that we have that their hormonal contraception caused their pain.

Women with other genital pain conditions, such as chronic bladder pain or irritable bowel syndrome, are more likely to develop vulvodynia. Women with chronic pain in areas that clearly do not share the same nerves as the vulva, for example temporomandibular joint pain (or TMJ) and migraines, also have a higher incidence of vulvodynia, as do women with fibromyalgia, a widespread pain condition associated with extreme fatigue.

Some studies also suggest that women with vulvodynia are not only more sensitive to pain at the vulva, but when tested with a painful stimulus at sites not connected with the vulva, for example a finger, they report higher pain levels than expected. All of this suggests vulvodynia is not a medical condition confined to the vulva, but involves widespread changes in how the nervous system processes pain. Whether these changes are the cause or the result of the pain is not known.

One exception may be women with localized pain at the vestibule, or vestibulodynia. For some of these women, some or all of their pain condition may be due to local nerve changes.

Therapies

Just getting a diagnosis can help women with vulvar pain. One study found a class that provided the kind of information found in this chapter lowered pain scores. Having painful symptoms and being told by providers that it is "nothing" or erroneously being diagnosed with a chronic yeast infection is disempowering and distressing. Giving women a name for their condition and validating that it is real is empowering and can be very helpful.

As women with vulvodynia may have heightened sensitivity to products, it is important to make sure irritants, like soap and wipes, are not being used (see chapters 9, 11, and 12).

Common therapies for vulvodynia include the following:

- **TOPICAL LIDOCAINE:** An anesthetic. It temporarily blocks the pain signal, providing short-term relief. The less pain you have, the less stimulation to the nervous system, so this may also help long term.
- **ESTROGEN CREAM AT THE VESTIBULE:** Can help some women with vestibulodynia.

- **ORAL NERVE PAIN MEDICATIONS:** These affect neurotransmitters that may be imbalanced and contributing to the pain. We have more data on these medications for other pain syndromes, like migraines or fibromyalgia, so much of what we recommend is based on this data. These medications are more effective for women who have unprovoked pain. Some common options are nortriptyline, venlafaxine, gabapentin, topiramate, and pregabalin. There is no data that one works better than the other. There are services that offer testing to identify the best nerve pain medication for individuals with pain, but none of this has been tested clinically. The most common mistake with these medications is not going high enough dosage-wise.
- **PHYSICAL THERAPY FOR THE MUSCLES OF THE PELVIC FLOOR:** This can be very helpful for women who also have muscle pain.
- **NERVE BLOCKS:** This involves injecting an anesthetic and steroid medication around nerves. There is very little good data on how to use these therapies, and most of the recommendations are based on expert opinion and not high-quality studies. For some women they can help with diagnosis, meaning if the anesthetic temporarily takes your pain away you know those nerves are somehow involved. The steroid may reduce inflammation, and pain at a cellular level is typically inflammatory (we called it neuroinflammation). Two nerve blocks that are used are pudendal nerve block and ganglion impar block.
- **BIOFEEDBACK:** A technique where you learn to control your body's functions, typically heart rate and breathing. You are connected to sensors that identify your body's signals, and you use that biological feedback (hence biofeedback) to relax muscles or reduce pain.
- **WORKING WITH VAGINAL DILATORS:** This is a form of desensitization therapy. Vibrating dilators may also help; vibration travels to the brain faster than pain, and the brain processes the faster signal preferentially. Some women find incorporating vibration into sex helpful. Not all women can tolerate touching with dilators.
- **A PAIN PSYCHOLOGIST:** This does not mean the pain is in your head. Pain causes suffering, and working with a pain psychologist has been shown to reduce suffering. A pain psychologist may also be helpful in identifying accelerants such as depression, anxiety, and

post-traumatic stress disorder (PTSD). Some women with vulvo-dynia have a history of sexual abuse, and working with a therapist for support can be helpful. A pain psychologist can also be helpful because many people treat their chronic pain like acute pain. A pain psychologist can suggest ways that in the long term may be more helpful pain-wise. For example, pacing, which is the fine art of living like the tortoise instead of the hare. Not overdoing it when you feel good prevents setbacks, and in the end you accomplish more. Think of this as constantly taking a half step forward. A psy-chologist can also offer cognitive-behavioral therapy.

- **SURGERY:** Some women with pain localized to their vestibule (women who only have pain with sex or tampons) may benefit from surgical removal of that portion of the vestibule. Women who have the best outcome with this surgery have provoked pain, and they had pain-free sex for a period of time before de-veloping vestibulodynia.

The low-oxalate diet

Restrictive diets, the most common being the low-oxalate diet, are widely reported for treatment of vulvodynia. In one study, 41 percent of women with chronic vulvar pain reported trying a low-oxalate diet. How this diet became almost mainstream is a testimony to lack of evidence, desperation of patients, inadequate evidence-based therapies, snake oil, and something called the illusory truth effect (meaning mistaking repeti-tion for fact). Basically, a perfect pseudoscience storm.

The idea that oxalates had a role in vulvodynia stemmed from a single case report published in 1991 in which a woman with refractory vulvody-nia was found to have periodic hyperoxaluria, and calcium citrate, which binds oxalate in the urine, preventing it from irritating the skin, relieved her symptoms

Science tells us that dietary oxalate consumption and urinary oxalate levels are the same among women with vulvodynia compared with women without chronic vulvar pain. In studies, a low-oxalate diet helped 2.5–24 percent of women—equivalent to or worse than the placebo response rate.

What is the harm? The exasperation from trying multiple interven-tions that can't work or work temporarily due to the placebo effect cannot be underestimated, never mind the money spent on dietary changes, cookbooks, and twenty-four-hour urine samples for oxalate that are not indicated and not covered by insurance. The low-oxalate diet is also very restrictive, and many patients get stressed about sticking to it or feel bad when they find it too hard.

BOTTOM LINE

- Vulvodynia is a common and frequently undiagnosed cause of vulvar pain.
- If you have vulvar pain, make a list of the causes and work through them with your provider. If you exclude them all, then vulvodynia is likely (see chapter 41).
- Pelvic floor muscle spasm is a common co-diagnosis.
- Depression and lack of sleep are accelerants that can make the pain worse.
- The most common treatments for vulvodynia include nerve pain medication and topical numbing medication.

CHAPTER 34

Pelvic Floor Muscle Spasm and Vaginismus

THE MUSCLES OF THE PELVIC FLOOR (meaning the muscles that wrap around the vagina, see chapter 2 for a review) can develop pain conditions due to muscle spasm. The term is pelvic floor muscle spasm, or PFMS, when the muscles are constantly tight, and this can cause vaginal pain, pain with sexual activity, and the urge to empty your bladder. When the muscles contract only in anticipation of penetration, the term is vaginismus, and the only symptom is pain with sexual activity. Vaginismus is considered a type of PFMS.

Think of a clenched fist. PFMS is your fist clenched all or most of the time, and vaginismus is clenching only when someone tries to shake your hand.

PFMS is understudied. For many years, medicine did not emphasize this as a pain condition. Many doctors ignored the muscle spasm that was obvious on exam or were not taught to recognize it as abnormal. Others were taught this was a psychiatric problem or a woman just being "unable to relax."

PFMS is also rarely discussed publicly, so when I diagnose a woman with PFMS or vaginismus it does not surprise me that she has never heard of it before.

How Do You Get PFMS?

There are two main categories of PFMS: spasm that seems to have been present from the very first attempt at penetration and spasm that developed sometime later, after pain-free vaginal penetration (this could be intercourse, finger play, or tampon use, etc.).

Some theories regarding the cause of PFMS include the following:

- **AVERSIVE SEXUAL MESSAGING:** A belief that sex will hurt, sex is shameful, or something that one does only for procreation.
- **PAINFUL MEDICAL EXPERIENCES:** Pain primes the nervous system for more pain. Part of this is a result of microscopic changes to the nervous system, and part is anticipation. This does not mean it is in your head; pain is assembled by the brain, and emotions or responses such as fear or anxiety change the chemical signaling and the pain experience.
- **PAINFUL CONSENSUAL SEXUAL EXPERIENCES:** Many women with pain do not tell their partners and simply tolerate the experience. This leads to anticipation, which only worsens the pain. If every time I offered you chocolate I hit you with a hammer, you would begin to cringe every time you saw chocolate. You may even start to hate chocolate. Anticipating negative experiences causes muscles to spasm and primes the nervous system to experience more pain.
- **MEDICAL PROCEDURES/SURGERY:** This can be a big surgery, like a hysterectomy, or a vaginal delivery, or something that might medically seem minor, such as an IUD insertion or a cervical biopsy. Stimulating nerves can produce pain in unpredictable ways.
- **CHRONIC CONSTIPATION:** Straining to empty your bowels can lead to uncoordinated muscle contractions. The reverse is also true; having PFMS can lead to constipation as the muscles have a harder time relaxing for a bowel movement.
- **OTHER PELVIC PAIN SYNDROMES:** There is a higher incidence of PFMS for women with other pelvic pain syndromes, like vulvodynia (a nerve pain of the vulva, see chapter 33), painful periods, endometriosis (a condition where the lining of the uterus grows in the pelvis, causing painful periods and pelvic pain), and bladder pain syndrome (see chapter 36). This may be due to shared nerves

allowing pain to travel between organs. In addition, if something hurts, reflexive muscle spasm is a protective mechanism.
- **PREVIOUS SEXUAL TRAUMA:** This can have devastating consequences for many women.

For many women, PFMS can be a combination of many or even all of these factors; and for some women there may be one or two underlying causes. That is part of the complexity.

Symptoms of PFMS

The symptoms can vary depending on many factors that we do not yet understand. For example, it is not known why some women can have very tight pelvic floor muscles all of the time and only have pain with penetration, and others have daily pain. Pain is very complex, and much of the pain experience—meaning what you feel—depends on how your nervous system processes pain signals and not about what medicine can find on exam or with imaging studies like as X-rays and ultrasounds.

The pain experience of PFMS can include some or all of the following:

- **VAGINAL PAIN PRESENT SOME OR ALL OF THE TIME:** Women often describe this pain as pressure, cramping, or a feeling like the insides are falling out or that there is a stick or a bowling ball in the vagina.
- **PAIN WITH SEXUAL PENETRATION:** Either initial penetration or deep inside.
- **PAINFUL PERIODS:** The first layer around the vagina is smooth muscle, and this contracts to help push menstrual blood to the vaginal opening during your period. When this muscle activity is uncoordinated, it can cause pain. This may trigger the next layer, which is the pelvic floor muscles, to spasm.
- **FEELING TOO TIGHT:** The spasm can functionally narrow the vaginal opening, preventing insertions.
- **FEELING A "ROADBLOCK":** Deeper spasm can be so tight that it feels as if attempts at insertion are hitting a wall.
- **PAINFUL ORGASM:** Orgasm is contraction of the pelvic floor muscles.

- **A SENSATION OF AROUSAL:** As orgasm is contraction of the pelvic floor muscles, when the muscles are tight it can fuel a state of arousal. Women with persistent genital arousal disorder, or PGAD, a rare condition with a sensation of constant sexual arousal, should be evaluated for pelvic floor spasm.
- **INABILITY TO USE TAMPONS OR MENSTRUAL CUPS COMFORTABLY:** Some women can never insert them, others describe the tampon coming back out, and others report it never feels right inside (when in correctly, tampons and menstrual cups should not be felt).
- **CONSTIPATION:** For some women, the pelvic floor muscles are unable to relax sufficiently for a complete bowel movement.
- **URINARY HESITANCY:** A feeling of incomplete bladder emptying and/or difficulty starting the urine stream.
- **PAIN DURING PELVIC EXAMS AND/OR PAP SMEARS:** Stress about the exam or anticipation of the pain can make the pain worse. Some women with PFMS have trouble letting their legs flop open for an exam.

How to Diagnose PFMS

If any of the above symptoms are present, then PFMS should be considered.

The most important part of an evaluation of PFMS is to do as little as possible to trigger spasm and pain. The more pain you have, the more you will anticipate pain, and so painful exams can feed the pain experience. Painful exams are also emotionally traumatizing for many women, and if they create muscle spasm, less information can be obtained from an exam. Painful exams are also mean.

Listening to women speak about their pain experiences, what we in medicine call the medical history, offers many clues about PFMS. If a woman tells me she feels too small or too tight, feels as if her insides are falling out, she feels as if she has a bowling ball in her vagina, or it feels as if she has a roadblock inside, then she almost certainly has some degree of PFMS.

In reality, we need very little to make the diagnosis of PFMS. When doing a gynecological exam for pain with sex, your provider should reassure you that they will stop if you seem uncomfortable or if you want them to stop. If you don't get that kind of control over the exam, then they may not be the provider to help you with this condition. A speculum exam is also not needed to diagnose or treat PFMS. I find telling many women this before the exam helps reduce anxiety significantly.

If you are having menstrual periods, or had them at some point, then an internal obstruction is very unlikely to be the cause. If you have never had a period, then your provider needs to consider other diagnoses as well, and that is beyond the scope of this book.

During an exam, you doctor needs to consider a few things to help make sure the pain is from PFMS and not another painful condition:

- **RULING OUT A SKIN CONDITION:** Lichen sclerosus and lichen planus are painful skin conditions (chapter 35). Trichomonas, an STI (chapter 29), can cause so much inflammation that there is pain with sex. If you have always had pain with sex, these diagnoses are unlikely. A skin condition can almost always be ruled out by looking at your vulva, and a vaginal swab can be performed to rule out trichomoniasis if necessary.
- **MAKING SURE YOU DO NOT HAVE GSM:** The pain of GSM can trigger PFMS. An exam is helpful, but not necessary, to consider GSM (see chapters 18 and 19).
- **EVALUATION FOR VULVODYNIA:** This is a nerve pain condition of the vulva (chapter 33). It could be mistaken for PFMS, but some women have both. An internal vaginal exam is not needed to diagnose vulvodynia.
- **EVALUATING FOR MUSCLE SPASM:** If you are having trouble keeping your legs open on the exam table or are lifting your buttocks, you have PFMS and no further exam is needed. If you are able to keep your legs flopped open, then your doctor should ask permission to touch with a gloved finger at the vaginal opening, and if you tolerate this then they should get permission to check the muscles internally with an exam.

If your provider is unable to rule out a skin condition or wonders about the possibility of an imperforate hymen or another cause of an obstruction and you cannot tolerate the exam in the office, then it is better to do the exam with some sedation, even if that means the operating room, than causing pain and trauma in the office. We have modern anesthesia for a reason.

If Sex Hurts, Should I Keep Having it?

This is a question only you can answer. If sex is excruciating, it will likely feed into the cycle of pain, muscle spasm, and anticipation. Sex is also supposed to be pleasurable. Some women tell me the physical bonding is worth the pain, but many have not been able to tell their partners about their pain. A sex therapist or other psychologist may be helpful in explaining the pain situation to a partner.

If you continue to have sex while you are working through PFMS, then make sure you are getting adequate foreplay. If sex is "twist a nipple and stick it in," that would hurt most women. Use plenty of lubricant and focus on areas that do not hurt, such as the clitoral glans and labia. Aim for an orgasm (or more than one) before any penetration. If you have a male partner, consider giving him the book *She Comes First*—the title itself is great advice. Some women find after an orgasm or two their pelvic floor begins to relax, and then penetration is easier.

If penetration is too painful, many women who partner with men find that masturbation and oral sex are not painful. Taking penetration off the table while you are working on your pelvic floor muscles still allows you to have satisfying sexual contact without the pain or with much less pain.

Treatment Options

There are a variety of considerations, and what works for you may depend on what is available locally and what you are comfortable with.

Vaginal dilators help desensitize the nerves and muscles. You proceed at your own pace in your bedroom with no pressure. They come in sets of four or five. You start with the smallest, inserting as far as you can go and stopping when you feel pain, and then holding it in place for five minutes. Focus on slow, deep breaths to help relax your pelvic floor. Some dilators are vibrating, and many women find that helpful. Dilator exercises depend on forming muscle memory; it is more important to do them 5–10 minutes a day every day than thirty minutes once a week.

Pelvic floor physical therapy can be very helpful. These are specialized physical therapists with advanced training. There are a variety of techniques. For women who cannot tolerate any insertion, the therapy should start externally. Some use biofeedback machines that give a visual representation of the muscle spasm on a computer screen; this can be a helpful aid for some women. A pelvic floor physical therapist will eventually work with her gloved fingers inside your vagina and should prescribe a home exercise regimen. There are some bodywork practitioners who claim to treat PFMS, but I would advise against seeing anyone who is not a physical therapist certified by the APTA (American Physical Therapy Association).

Working with a psychologist to address trauma, anxiety, and any relationship issues may be part of the treatment plan. This doesn't mean that your pain is in your head, it means that pain affects your life. Addressing this impact can help reduce suffering. Women who have extreme anxiety responses to the thought of or attempts at penetration may find working with a therapist especially helpful.

Managing constipation if you are overworking your pelvic floor muscles is also important, as straining will feed the cycle of spasm.

Another option is botulinum toxin injections. Yes, Botox for the vagina. This is done with sedation, as it is painful. Botulinum toxin treats muscle spasm—that is its mechanism of action. While approved by the FDA for some types of muscle spasms, it is not FDA approved for PFMS. For some women, botulinum toxin injections can help break the cycle of pain and spasm. The medication wears off after 10–12 weeks, and so this is most effective when combined with dilators and physical therapy.

What doesn't work?

Oral muscle relaxants are largely ineffective. They sometimes are used to treat acute spasm (think sudden-onset back pain), but they are not very good for chronic muscle spasm. Some people advocate for vaginal diazepam (Valium); however, two studies show that it is ineffective. Diazepam works on the spinal cord and brain—there are no receptors for the medication vaginally, so if any benefit is felt it is because the medication is absorbed into the bloodstream, which negates the point of using it vaginally.

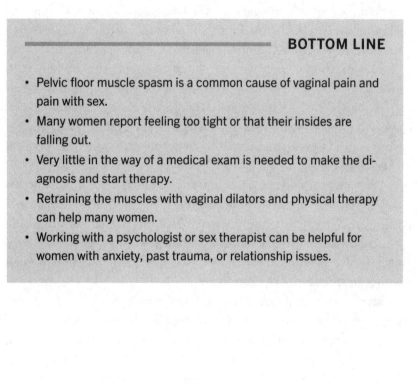

BOTTOM LINE

- Pelvic floor muscle spasm is a common cause of vaginal pain and pain with sex.
- Many women report feeling too tight or that their insides are falling out.
- Very little in the way of a medical exam is needed to make the diagnosis and start therapy.
- Retraining the muscles with vaginal dilators and physical therapy can help many women.
- Working with a psychologist or sex therapist can be helpful for women with anxiety, past trauma, or relationship issues.

CHAPTER 35

Skin Conditions

THE VULVA IS AT INCREASED RISK of skin conditions. It is more prone to irritant reactions, and there are some unique skin conditions that only or preferentially affect the vulva.

Getting a correct diagnosis can be a challenge. Symptoms can be non-specific, meaning they could signify a number of conditions and the diagnosis is not clear even to an experienced provider. Some skin conditions are mistaken for other diagnoses. And then there are women who have their symptoms and physical concerns completely ignored.

This is where self-advocacy comes in (see chapter 38 for more information on how to advocate for yourself medically). If you know these skin conditions exist and what you read here sounds similar to what you are experiencing, you can ask specific questions about how your provider reached their diagnosis or about treatment options not discussed by your provider. I am happy when patients do research. In addition, an opportunity to revisit my diagnosis is welcome. If your provider is sure of the diagnosis, they should be able to confidently reassure you about what they believe you have. That is part of the job.

Many gynecologists do not get an opportunity to manage the wide range of vulvar skin conditions during their training, as many affect 1–3 percent of women or even less. A general gynecologist may only see a few cases a year, whereas a specialist may see 2–3 women a day with these conditions. Do not be shy about advocating for a referral to a specialist if your symptoms are not improving.

A Word on Biopsies

Many times we are able to make a diagnosis without a biopsy because the skin condition has a classic appearance. In this situation, initiating the treatment and then assessing the outcome is typically the recommended approach. If initial attempts at treatment do not provide the expected results, then a biopsy may add more information.

What most people do not realize is that biopsies are not always definitive. You would think they should be—after all, they are looking at tissue under the microscope—but as far as skin conditions are concerned, a biopsy does not give a binary "yes" or "no" answer. With a biopsy, a pathologist looks at the tissue and is essentially doing microscopically what we do macroscopically. When I look at the vulva, I look at the pattern of redness, thickness of the skin, and whether there are ulcers or erosions. I assemble that information and say, "This looks like condition X." The pathologist does the same thing, just microscopically, by looking at the type and distribution of inflammatory cells, the thickness and appearance of the epidermis (skin), and many other features. Sometimes what they see is classic—meaning only ever seen with one condition—but often what they see is a little bit of this and a little bit of that, just like we do looking at your skin. To make matters even more confusing, sometimes two skin conditions coexist.

Think of a biopsy as a piece of the puzzle, not the whole picture. A dermatopathologist (pathologist who specializes in the skin) once told me that up to 50 percent of biopsies, even when the skin appears to have classic changes, can have nonspecific results. This doesn't mean biopsies are not useful; it is just important to know their limitations. Many women are disappointed after a biopsy, not because the result did not prove they had a condition but rather because they were not advised of the possibility the information might not be diagnostic or definitive proof.

A biopsy is definitely indicated when there is a concern for cancer. Some general (not definitive, though) guidelines for when a biopsy may be indicated to rule out a cancer are the following:

- **A SUSPECTED CONDYLOMA (WART) FOR A WOMAN OVER FORTY:** Early skin cancers can look just like a wart.
- **A WART THAT RETURNS DESPITE THERAPY:** Many therapies for warts can also make the visible part of a skin cancer go away, but as that is incomplete therapy, the cancer returns.
- **A PIGMENTED LESION THAT IS RAISED OR LARGER THAN A CENTIMETER:** Skin cancers can have pigment. One exception is a classic raised lesion called seborrheic keratosis. It can look like stuck-on brown wax.
- **A NONHEALING ULCER:** Also a potential sign of cancer.

Lichen Simplex Chronicus

This is an eczema-like condition of the vulva. It often starts as an irritant contact dermatitis, meaning a product or ingredient has irritated or damaged the skin's acid mantle or even the top few layers of cells. This can be from a single exposure or after repeated exposures. Some common irritants include solvents and alcohols, which are in many skin care products. Detergents and plants/botanicals can also be irritants. A yeast infection or other infection may also be a trigger. Pubic hair removal may increase the risk of the initial reactions due to the microtrauma or the loss of the physical protective barrier of hair. Women who have urinary incontinence and wear menstrual pads for protection instead of incontinence pads may develop irritation.

What happens next is feeling itchy, which leads to scratching or rubbing. This further traumatizes the skin and primes the nervous system to feel even itchier. Scratching and rubbing can produce redness and thickening of the vulvar skin. The itch can be intense, and some women develop significant skin trauma, like fissures, from scratching. Itch is often worse at night, and some women may scratch in their sleep.

Lichen simplex chronicus does not involve the vagina, so the symptoms will be external or at the vaginal opening, not deep inside.

There can be enough skin changes from scratching that sometimes a biopsy is needed to rule out cancer. Scratching, when deep enough, can damage the bottom layer of skin cells (the basal layer). This can lead to scarring, and it can cause the melanocytes to release pigment, leading to flat, dark areas called melanosis. This can look like melanoma, a skin cancer.

The treatment is removing all potential irritant triggers, treating the inflammation, and no scratching or rubbing. This can be hard. Recommendations include stopping all cleansers or soaps, incontinence pads where indicated, wearing loose clothing (as even very light friction can trigger itch), and stopping hair removal. Some women may need to sleep with socks on their hands at first.

The medication to reduce itch and inflammation is typically a high-dose topical steroid ointment. Once the itch is controlled, it can be tapered down and stopped. Coconut oil or petroleum jelly can increase moisture and may be helpful in protecting the skin barrier. Oral antihistamines can help with the itch and may be sedating, so when taken at night they may help reduce scratching. Once the scratching has stopped and the itch has gone away, medications can be tapered off. Some women may need to use a topical steroid 1–2 times a week to keep the itch away.

If the initial therapy is ineffective, the next step is a gynecologist or dermatologist who has experience managing vulvar skin conditions. Sometimes a longer course of topical steroids or even an injection of steroids may be needed. There are also other topical medications, called calcineurin inhibitors, that can be helpful for itch. Occasionally oral medications, similar to those we use for nerve pain, may be needed to help reduce the itch at the level of the nervous system.

Lichen Sclerosus and Lichen Planus

These are autoimmune skin conditions that affect 1–3 percent of women. Lichen sclerosus only affects the vulva, so it will stop at the vestibule. Lichen planus can involve mucosa so can affect the vulva and vagina (it can also affect the mouth). The conditions can also coexist. Lichen planus is less common than lichen sclerosus.

Lichen sclerosus and lichen planus can cause itching, pain, pain with sexual activity, ulcerations, fissures, and skin changes. The impact on sex life and how women feel cosmetically about their vulva is significant. Both conditions increase the risk of squamous cell cancer of the vulva—over a ten-year period, the risk of developing this cancer is approximately 6 percent. This does not mean you will get this cancer; rather, you need to be followed closely so if there are early changes a diagnosis and treatment can be made, hopefully before the cancer spreads.

I always ask women if they want to see the changes on their skin. I use a selfie-stick mirror so I can describe what I am seeing and also show where medication should be applied. For many women, this can be very helpful so they know what is happening and how to correctly apply their topical products. However, for others it is too upsetting. If you want to see your vulva, let your doctor know, but if you would rather not, that is okay, too.

Lichen sclerosus causes the skin to become white and thin. The classic appearance is around the vulva (labia minora) and anus like a figure 8. As the disease progresses, the labia minora can atrophy and even disappear, the clitoral prepuce (hood) can fuse, trapping the clitoris, and if left untreated there can be enough scarring that the vaginal opening closes, preventing penetration and even, when very severe, blocking the flow of urine.

Lichen planus typically does not cause the same intense white changes seen with lichen sclerosus and does not classically involve the anal area. The same cosmetic and functional changes, loss of the labia minora, and fusion of the clitoral prepuce can occur. Lichen planus can produce vaginal erosions and ulcerations, which can be very painful and lead to scarring that can severely narrow and even completely close the vagina.

Women should be screened for thyroid conditions, as they are more common among women with lichen sclerosus. Women with lichen sclerosus and lichen planus are at increased risk for yeast infections. The reason is not well known, but may include the increased vulnerability to microtrauma, physical changes to the skin, and the topical medications.

The mainstay of therapy involves reducing trauma as this can trigger the conditions to become active. Women approaching menopause and those who are menopausal may benefit from topical estrogen, as reducing physical changes of GSM will add moisture and help increase tissue elasticity, reducing trauma. Restoring the lactobacilli may also be helpful. Soap is drying and should be avoided. Creams and ointments may not be adequately removed with water, so using a cleanser with a pH close to 5 every few days may be helpful at preventing odor from product buildup.

High-dose topical steroids (called Class 1 superpotent steroids, these include clobetasol propionate 0.05 percent and augmented betamethasone dipropionate 0.05 percent) are the recommended therapy. Typically, an ointment is preferred because they have better skin penetration and tend to be less irritating, as they usually do not need preservatives. A start-ing dose is a pea-sized amount twice a day for 6–12 weeks and then tapered down to twice a week. This should be guided by an experienced provider. Petroleum jelly or coconut oil may be helpful for both the emol-lient and barrier properties. Lichen planus involving the vagina can be treated with vaginal steroids and dilators to prevent scarring.

There are other therapies, and for these it is best to see a gynecologist or dermatologist who has experience. Labia minora loss is permanent, and surgery cannot reverse those changes. Scarring at the vaginal opening that prevents intercourse or impedes the flow of urine, scarring of the cli-toral hood, and vaginal scarring can be treated surgically. This should only be done by a gynecologist who has experience with these conditions and these techniques.

Molluscum Contagiosum

This is an infection with a virus called a poxvirus. It produces pearly papules about 3–4 mm in size (a papule is a small, solid, raised bump with no visible fluid). The bump or papule has a small central depression like a belly button that we call an umbilication. Most people only have a few, but sometimes there can be large crops. A biopsy is rarely needed, as the appearance is classic. The virus only infects the top layer of skin above the basement membrane and does not go dormant and reactivate in the way herpes or human papilloma virus (HPV) can.

Molluscum can appear anywhere on the body exposed to the virus. On the vulva, molluscum can be sexually transmitted from skin-to-skin contact and possibly by sharing towels. Scratching and microtrauma of hair removal can spread the virus.

Molluscum often goes away on its own, so avoiding mechanical trauma may be enough for many women. Realistically, spreading the virus is common (not touching yourself or avoiding an occasional scratch is practically not possible), so it can often take 8–12 months to clear. Rea-sons for removal include not wanting to wait, the lesions being itchy or bothersome, or it has been long enough and they are still present.

There are a variety of treatment options including (but not limited to) the following:

- **PHYSICAL DESTRUCTION:** The lesions are scraped away (curettage) or frozen off (cryotherapy). This can be painful, but if there are only a few lesions this may be a good option. Don't try to do this at home; you might spread the virus or get a bacterial infection.
- **TOPICAL THERAPIES:** Trichloracetic acid applied by a provider in the office, using the wooden end of a cotton swab. This may need to be repeated every two weeks until the lesions disappear. Podophyllotoxin cream applied at home (a cycle of applying twice a day for three days then off for four days, repeated every week for up to four weeks). Benzoyl peroxide 10 percent cream may be effective when applied twice daily for four weeks and is very inexpensive. Imiquimod cream, an immune modulator, applied 3–5 times a week for up to sixteen weeks, is another option.
- **ORAL CIMETIDINE:** A drug for acid reflux, you may know it by the trade name Tagamet. It may be an option for two months for situations where topical therapy is too painful to tolerate or unacceptable for other reasons. It has the potential for drug interactions.

Hidradenitis Suppurativa

Hidradenitis suppurativa is a painful, chronic inflammatory disorder of hair follicles with apocrine sweat glands. It affects about 0.3 percent of women in the United States ages 20–40 (the group with the highest risk). It is about twice as common among African American women and biracial women versus white women. Data from Europe suggests the incidence may be as high as 2–4 percent. It is not clear if that is a true difference, or if either the European or American data are incorrect.

Women develop painful red nodules (firm lumps of tissues beneath the skin) that when mild can look like acne or be mistaken for chronic ingrown hairs. More advanced cases have blackheads, abscesses, lesions that drain pus, and severe scarring. It can take women an average of seven years to get the correct diagnosis, and the psychological impact of having painful, chronic, draining sores that are misdiagnosed or never diagnosed cannot be underestimated. Fortunately, most women have a mild disease, but 4 percent of cases can involve a large portion of the vulva with abscesses and scarring.

The cause is not known, although a key step is blocking the hair follicle and buildup of secretions from the apocrine sweat glands, which cause the hair follicle to rupture. This results in bacterial infection and intense inflammation, which can trigger abscesses and scarring. Once the inflammatory response has developed, it can spread to adjacent hair follicles, making the condition harder to treat. Scarring cannot be reversed. Early diagnosis and treatment may give better long-term results.

Treatment involves minimizing inflammation. Underwear should be loose to limit friction and traumatic hair removal, such as waxing or shaving, should be stopped. Some data suggests laser hair removal may be helpful. Consult a board-certified dermatologist for this. Smoking is a known cofactor, so if you smoke, quitting can help. Weight loss has been shown to be helpful.

Specific treatments include estrogen-containing birth control pills or a drug called spironolactone (100 mg a day)—they both reduce the effect of testosterone on tissues (testosterone thickens secretions from the affected glands). Topical antibiotics and oral antibiotics are also useful. Disease that does not respond to initial therapies or is advanced with abscesses and scarring should be managed by an experienced gynecologist or dermatologist.

BOTTOM LINE

- Irritants and microtrauma worsen all vulvar skin conditions.
- Lichen simplex chronicus is a common cause of intense vulvar itch.
- Lichen sclerosus and lichen planus are autoimmune skin conditions that can cause significant pain and may need a specialist for appropriate treatment.
- Molluscum contagiosum is a virus that can cause small, sometimes itchy lesions on the vulva.
- Hidradenitis suppurativa is a chronic inflammatory condition of the hair follicle that, while uncommon, often goes undiagnosed— early intervention may improve outcomes.

CHAPTER 36

UTIs and Bladder Pain Syndrome

As MANY AS 11 PERCENT OF WOMEN have at least one urinary tract infection (UTI) each year, and for 20–30 percent of these women UTIs are a recurrent issue. A UTI is one of the most common reasons women are prescribed an antibiotic.

The classic symptoms include urgency as well as frequency of and burning with urination. Some women may also have pain in their bladder and blood in their urine. Some women may have incontinence or the worsening of preexisting incontinence. Not all women have classic symptoms, so that can also make diagnosis confusing.

A Word About Tests

There are three kinds of tests to help diagnose UTIs. They include the following:

- **A URINE DIPSTICK:** A quick test done on your urine in the office that provides information about blood, bacteria, and white blood cells. These are the urine strips that are sold over the counter. The test does not confirm or rule out a bladder infection, but it may raise or lower suspicion. The most helpful part is the nitrate reading, which is a sign of bacteria. While these tests are widely done, in most situations they add little useful information. If your symptoms are classic, a negative test should not prevent you from being treated. If your symptoms are not classic, you need a culture (the definitive test). Phenazopyridine, a bladder pain medication that turns your urine orange, affects the results of this test.

- **URINE MICROSCOPY:** Looking at the urine in the lab for white blood cells, bacteria, and blood—a more accurate version of the dipstick. If the microscopy identifies bacteria or white blood cells it makes the diagnosis of UTI more likely, but again, it doesn't add much over the dipstick. This test is not affected by phenazopyridine.

- **A URINE CULTURE:** Growing bacteria from the urine. This is the gold standard. If the report indicates 100,000 colonies of bacteria per ml of urine, this is traditionally considered an infection. There are some caveats. Up to 5 percent of premenopausal women and 10–15 percent of postmenopausal women will have that amount of bacteria and no symptoms, meaning they don't have a UTI. It is not whether the culture is positive—it is whether the positive culture matches your symptoms. We also know that some women can have a UTI when there are not enough bacteria for the culture to show growth. A culture is not affected by phenazopyridine.

Do I Have a UTI?

The general statement "I think they have a bladder infection" is accurate about 50 percent of the time. A few more questions can help narrow it down a lot, so you and your provider can decide if you qualify for treatment over the phone, if you need to drop off a urine sample, or if you need an exam. These guidelines apply to women with 2–3 bladder infections a year. Women with four or more infections a year have recurrent UTIs, and the management may be different.

There is a high likelihood of a UTI with an increase in frequency of trips to the restroom (really needing to go), dysuria (burning with urination), and no change in vaginal discharge. If there is no evidence of a kidney infection (flank pain, chills, high fever), it is reasonable to treat over the phone without a urine sample. If you do not get better with treatment, you should be seen by your provider, as you may have not had a UTI (meaning the diagnosis was incorrect) or you may have a bacteria that requires different therapy, and this can only be decided with a urine specimen.

If you have frequency, dysuria, and a change in your vaginal discharge or a new vaginal discharge, then the likelihood that you have a bladder infection is only about 45 percent, and you should be seen. This is where the urine dipstick test or microscopy may prove helpful. If there is no evidence of a vaginal infection on exam and the nitrate test is positive, the chance that you have a UTI could be as high as 80 percent.

If you think you have a UTI based on symptoms other than frequency and dysuria, then you should be seen and evaluated. This is a situation where an exam and office test (dipstick) might be helpful. You may also need a culture.

Women with recurrent infections, meaning four or more in twelve months, should have urine cultures. Pregnant women also need a urine culture.

Waiting for the Culture

It can be hard to wait for the culture, but if your symptoms are not classic or there is concern about a hard-to-treat bacteria, it is the right option. In addition to the complication of taking antibiotics that you may not need—diarrhea and yeast infections being two of the most common—we are slowly running out of effective antibiotics due to the problem of antibiotic resistance. Taking antibiotics when they are unnecessary or the wrong choice is a big cause.

A culture takes 1–2 days to get the results, one day to know if it is positive, and then another day to know the most appropriate choice of antibiotic. Depending on where you live (the type of bacteria and sensitivity to antibiotics varies significantly by region) and how many infections you have had, it may be appropriate to treat once you know the culture is positive, but it also may be best to wait for the results to limit collateral damage from exposure to an antibiotic that cannot work for your infection.

While waiting two days may be uncomfortable, taking acetaminophen and phenazopyridine can help. There is a possibility that pain medications like diclofenac and ibuprofen (the class of drugs called NSAIDs, or nonsteroidal anti-inflammatory drugs) could increase the risk of a kidney infection, so acetaminophen may be a better choice. However, waiting will not give you a kidney infection—in fact, after two days 20–25 percent of UTIs will have cleared spontaneously. While that seems low, reducing antibiotic use by 25 percent for UTIs would be significant, globally speaking. It is a reasonable strategy for women with atypical symptoms to get an antibiotic prescription while waiting for the culture and then only take the antibiotic if the culture is positive and you have the right antibiotic.

Treatment

For women who do not have a history of recurrent infections, the recommended initial choice of antibiotics are one of the following:

- Nitrofurantoin 100 mg twice a day for five days.
- Fosfomycin 3 g a single oral dose.
- Trimethoprim-sulfamethoxasole 160–800 mg twice a day for three days.

The other antibiotics are all broad-spectrum antibiotics, meaning they kill a wider range of bacteria and are more likely to have collateral damage in the form of diarrhea, yeast infections, and contributing to antibiotic resistance. One of these antibiotics is ciprofloxacin, and it can also cause damage to tendons. Ciprofloxacin should only be used when cultures indicate it is the best choice or there are other specific medical reasons, for example, allergy to other options.

Prevention of Bladder Infections

Women with GSM will likely benefit from vaginal estrogen, which has been shown to reduce UTIs.

Cranberry juice, widely touted for its ability to prevent UTIs, seems to be ineffective. Whether cranberry tablets and capsules are also as ineffective is not clear, but the studies are low quality. No one even knows if the compound in cranberries that is reported to prevent UTIs, proanthocyanidins, even makes it into the urine in quantities sufficient to prevent bacteria adherence (its supposed mechanism of action). Other options, also not well tested, are 1,000 mg of vitamin C three times a day and d-mannose 2,000 mg a day (divided into two or three daily doses). The theory behind these products is that, like cranberries, they prevent bacteria from adhering to the bladder lining. There is not likely to be any harm besides expense. If you do decide to try one of these options and see no reduction in UTIs in six months, then they are probably not effective for you.

Women who have UTIs that are triggered by sex can consider daily antibiotics or an antibiotic after sex. They have not been studied head-to-head, but seem similarly effective. The latter reduces the amount of antibiotic exposure.

A long-standing recommendation has been to empty the bladder immediately after sexual intercourse with a male partner. There are two studies that show this is ineffective and belongs in the "Journal of Old Wives' Tales" (chapter 47). I have heard of women who sprint to the bathroom seconds after her partner ejaculates and have heard from male partners, "You mean we can't actually have some cuddle time?"

I call these types of interventions, like wearing cotton underwear or emptying your bladder after sex, the burden of "well, it can't hurt." But they truly are a burden. Every time we make a woman jump through a useless hoop to get better, we add a burden, be it financial, or emotional, or the exasperation of doing so many things and yet realizing that you are running very hard but not getting anywhere.

I Feel as If I Have Recurrent Bladder Infections, but My Tests Are Always Negative

Frequency, dysuria (pain), and even blood in the urine are also symptoms of a condition called painful bladder syndrome (PBS). We used to call this condition interstitial cystitis, but PBS is a more accurate description. Many women are treated for years with antibiotics for bladder infections that they do not have when really PBS is the cause. Other symptoms of PBS include pain with sex and difficulty emptying the bladder after getting the urine stream started.

PBS is a clinical diagnosis that we make if there have been at least six weeks of pain related to the bladder, urinary urgency, and frequency, and other causes have been ruled out. The most important conditions to rule out are UTIs and bladder cancer. Bladder cancer is much less common in women versus men, and it is rare under the age of fifty-five. If you are forty or older and have symptoms suggestive of PBS, especially if you have blood in your urine, you should ask about being screened for bladder cancer.

The cause of PBS is unknown. Common theories involve inflammation in the bladder lining and/or nerve pain.

Women with suspected PBS should also be evaluated for pelvic floor muscle spasm (PFMS, chapter 34) and vulvodynia (nerve pain of the vulva, chapter 33). Looking inside the bladder, a procedure called cystoscopy, may be recommended to screen for bladder cancer, but it is not recommended to diagnose PBS. Most women with PBS have no bladder abnormalities that can be seen this way. A test called potassium instillation is no longer recommended, as it is also not helpful and can be very painful.

There are many therapies for PBS, but many of these recommendations are based on low-quality data. Some treatment considerations include the following:

- **PELVIC FLOOR PHYSICAL THERAPY:** The therapist treats any accompanying muscle spasm and may be able to perform biofeedback as well.
- **TIMED VOIDING:** This is a form of biofeedback, training the bladder to accept larger volume.
- **DIETARY MODIFICATION:** There are many reports of foods being irritating. Common bladder irritants are coffee, tea, soda, alcoholic beverages, artificial sweeteners, citrus fruits and juices, cranberry juice, tomato products, soy, and spicy foods.
- **PENTOSAN POLYSULFATE:** An oral medication that is supposed to help rebuild the bladder lining. It may take up to six months to have a visible effect. It may only help 30 percent of women, which is likely not much higher than placebo.
- **INSTILLATIONS:** Substances that reduce inflammation or repair the lining of the bladder are put into the bladder as a topical therapy. Some options are heparin, pentosan polysulfate, and high molecular weight hyaluronic acid.
- **PTNS:** This is a form of neuromodulation, meaning electricity to modify nerve function. An acupuncture needle is placed just be-

hind the ankle and an electrical impulse is delivered to the under-lying nerve, which connects in the spinal cord in the same place as the nerves from the bladder. Weekly treatment for twelve weeks can be helpful, followed by maintenance therapy every 2–4 weeks.

- **PHENAZOPYRIDINE:** The oral medication for bladder pain with UTIs. While the package says only take for three days, that is not because longer courses are harmful, it is so a kidney infection is not missed and for manufacturer liability. If this medication treats your pain, you can take it daily if needed or on an as-needed basis as long as the orange urine doesn't bother you.
- **ORAL NERVE PAIN MEDICATIONS:** Common options are nortriptyline and gabapentin, but there are several options.
- **ANTIHISTAMINES:** Some theories of PBS involve an abnormal his-tamine response.
- **HYDRODISTENTION:** Stretching the bladder in the operating room by filling it very full of fluid.
- **BOTULINUM TOXIN A INJECTIONS INTO THE BLADDER:** This can treat the overactive bladder component and sometimes the pain.

If PBS does not respond to initial therapies, a cystoscopy (looking in-side the bladder) may be helpful, as 5–10 percent of women have ulcers. With the knowledge gained from a cytoscopy, some specialized treatments may be recommended. Other options are beyond the scope of this book.

BOTTOM LINE

- UTIs affect 11 percent of women a year.
- Burning while urinating and the need to empty your bladder fre-quently in the absence of a new vaginal discharge are very reliable signs of a UTI.
- OTC dip tests are not useful.
- Emptying your bladder after sex does not reduce infections.
- Symptoms that feel exactly like a UTI but with repeatedly negative urine cultures may be painful bladder syndrome.

CHAPTER 37

Pelvic Organ Prolapse

THIS IS A BOOK ABOUT VAGINAS and vulvas, so why is there a chapter on pelvic organs? What we in medicine called pelvic organ prolapse (POP) is the descent or dropping of the vagina or uterus, which happens through the vagina. Sometimes the bladder or bowel can also come down. POP can also sometimes cause vaginal symptoms, and other times vaginal symptoms are erroneously blamed on POP, so a good basic knowledge is essential.

Wait—You Mean My Vagina Can Fall Out?

Can, yes, but the odds that it will fall outside of your body are very low.

The vagina is built to stretch—otherwise it could never deliver a baby—and gravity preferentially affects tissues with a greater ability to stretch. Whether this happens to you or not depends on multiple factors, including genetics, smoking (this weakens all tissues), menopause, previous vaginal deliveries, chronic constipation (straining is bad for the tissues), and weight (more pressure on the tissues means they are more likely to descend). It is not possible to predict with certainty who will get POP and who will not.

What Exactly Do You Mean by Prolapse?

The part that starts to drop can be the cervix (the bottom part of the uterus), the front wall of the vagina, the back wall of the vagina, or if you have had a hysterectomy, the top of the vagina. A good visual is pulling a sock partially inside out—the part you are pulling on is the prolapse.

What Are the Symptoms?

Approximately 40–50 percent of women have POP on exam, but they don't have symptoms. This means that some laxity or mild prolapse is normal. It is not whether you have POP, it is whether the POP is bothering you. If your doctor mentions that you that you have some prolapse after a pelvic exam, do not let that worry you; it just means you are like a lot of other women. POP is not a health problem in the sense that there are no severe consequences from simply leaving it alone, so if you are not bothered then your doctor should also not be bothered.

The main symptom of POP is a vaginal bulge, and this affects about 3–6 percent of women. This means a bulge of vaginal tissue is felt during activities like wiping, masturbating, or even while sitting. Another common symptom is pressure. Less common symptoms include interference with sex (the bulge gets in the way) and obstructing the flow of urine. Occasionally, some women have difficulty with bowel movements and need to insert their fingers vaginally and push backwards to provide support so they can have a bowel movement. This is called splinting. Symptoms not typically caused by prolapse are pelvic pain, back pain, or pain with sex. If your provider tries to explain those symptoms by prolapse, get another opinion.

The test for POP is a vaginal exam by a trained provider. POP is staged based on how close the part that is farthest down is in relation to the hymen. The length of the vagina, the width of the vaginal opening, and the perineal body (the connection of muscles between the vagina and anus) are also taken into consideration. There are five stages of prolapse from 0 to IV, and your doctor should assign a measurement called a POP-Q score to stage your prolapse. Knowing the score typically only matters when it comes to surgery.

Your provider should also assess the strength of your pelvic floor by asking you to squeeze your pelvic floor muscles (a Kegel exercise, see chapter 10). If you have bladder symptoms, other testing may be indicated.

If your main bothersome symptom is pelvic pressure or a feeling that something is falling out, then an evaluation of the pelvic floor muscles for spasm or tightness is also indicated, as pelvic floor muscle spasm can also cause these same symptoms (see chapter 34). A gynecologist or uro-gynecologist (a gynecologist who specializes in the bladder and prolapse) can evaluate your pelvic floor muscles. A visit with a specialized pelvic physical therapist may also be useful to help rule out muscle spasm.

What Treatments Are Available for POP?

It is important to make sure constipation is adequately treated, as straining will aggravate prolapse. Having 25 g of fiber a day in your diet will help prevent constipation for many people, although some may also need a laxative. Osmotic laxatives are very safe; they draw water into stool, making it softer and easier to pass. Polyethylene glycol 3350 powder is an osmotic laxative—the brand name in the United States is MiraLAX, but the generic is just fine. Elevating your feet on a small stool while you are sitting on the toilet can sometimes help reduce straining while you are having a bowel movement.

Kegel exercises (see chapter 10) and other exercises to strengthen the pelvic floor muscles can treat the symptoms of prolapse. Many women find a pelvic floor physical therapist very helpful.

A pessary is a device that sits in the vagina supporting the prolapsed tissues. Pessaries come in a wide variety of shapes and sizes—rings, discs with holes (to let discharge drain), and even one called a Gellhorn that looks like a large pawn from a chess set. Some may look uncomfortable, but just like a tampon, when they fit correctly they are not felt. A doctor or nurse practitioner should fit you in the office. They should have you empty your bladder, as a poorly fitting pessary can obstruct the flow of urine, and make sure you can insert and remove it yourself comfortably.

Pessaries can stay in for a month or more (even up to three months) between cleaning. If they are left in longer, they can injure the vaginal tissues. You can't have sex while wearing a pessary, but you just take it out and reinsert afterwards.

A pessary can effectively treat approximately 90 percent of women who are bothered by their symptoms of POP. There are very few therapies in medicine with that kind of success rate that you can simply remove if you are unhappy or uncomfortable. The higher the grade of prolapse the less effective a pessary gets, but even with advanced prolapse, a correctly fitted pessary will work 64–70 percent of the time.

What about surgery?

A review of prolapse surgery is beyond this book. Some are done vaginally and others abdominally with the operating telescope (laparoscope). The choice of surgery depends on the part that is prolapsed, the severity, the symptoms, whether you have had surgery for prolapse previously, future plans for sexual activity, the presence of incontinence, and a few other factors.

Prolapse surgery changes vaginal anatomy, and about 10 percent of women develop pain with sex afterwards. Fortunately, this can often be treated. This doesn't mean the surgery is bad—34 percent of women choosing this kind of surgery are not having sex because of their bulge—it is a reflection of the extent of surgery that is needed. Pain with sex after prolapse surgery is commonly due to muscle spasm (see chapter 34). Many women report prolapse surgery has a positive impact on their body image.

There has been a lot in the news about mesh and prolapse surgery. Mesh is material that looks like fine netting and is used when the tissues are felt to be too weak. It is associated with a higher rate of complications and can erode through the tissues into the vagina. Mesh is currently only recommended when the risk of the surgery failing without it is high. It's not wrong to use mesh; it is wrong to use it incorrectly. It may be advisable to get a second opinion if mesh is recommended.

Mesh has a troublesome history—many device manufacturers introduced different kinds of mesh for prolapse surgery with few, if any, studies. And many surgeons used them in a way that left some women with severe pain and scarring. This does not mean that all mesh is bad, it means that unstudied surgical therapies are bad. When we don't invest the time and effort to understand a novel therapy, there can be terrible, unanticipated consequences.

Even with correct surgical technique, some women may need more prolapse surgery as their tissues are inherently weak (that is why they prolapsed to begin with).

If you have bothersome prolapse that has failed to be improved by pelvic floor–strengthening exercises and you have tried at least two pessaries and they do not work or they are uncomfortable, then you may be a surgical candidate.

As prolapse surgery is typically a big surgery, it is wise to get a second opinion and consider seeing an OB/GYN or urologist who has done a fellowship in pelvic reconstructive surgery. This is three years of additional training after residency. Prolapse surgery is specialized, and you want a surgeon with good training and experience, who can discuss the risks and benefits of surgery.

BOTTOM LINE

- Pelvic organ prolapse means part of the vagina and/or the cervix/uterus is dropping down towards or even through the vaginal opening.
- The main symptom of POP is a bulge at the vaginal opening—POP does not cause pain with sex or pelvic pain
- The POP-Q grading system is used to accurately measure prolapse.
- Pelvic floor muscle exercises can help.
- A pessary can treat bothersome symptoms of POP for over 90 percent of women.

Symptoms

CHAPTER 38

Communicating with Your Provider

WOMEN KNOW THEIR OWN BODIES. They know what symptoms are typical for them and what is a change.

What is also true is that the vulva and vagina are unreliable narrators. By this I mean they have a very limited way of communicating illness and injury because of the unique wiring. There can be a lot of crossed signals, and symptoms are often not what they appear to be. In addition, many things that women have been taught about their bodies and medical conditions that affect the vulva and vagina are incorrect. This makes self-diagnosis (meaning a diagnosis based on symptoms or what you feel) or diagnosis over the phone a challenge. For example, as we have already discussed, 50–70 percent of women who think they have a yeast infection based on symptoms are incorrect.

Your Vulva and Vagina Have a Limited Vocabulary

In medicine, a symptom is the way you feel—for example, an itch or pain. The vulva and vagina only have so many symptoms to use to alert you to what is happening. The most common are the following:

- Irritation
- Sandpaper-like feeling
- Dryness
- Burning
- Itch
- Tingling
- Pain
- Pain with sex
- Tightness
- Pressure
- Vaginal discharge
- Odor
- Urgency for emptying the bladder
- Pain with urination

Making communication even more challenging, almost every condition has overlapping symptoms. For example, vaginal burning can be seen with yeast, skin conditions, muscle spasm, GSM, and urinary tract infections. Most vulvar and vaginal conditions are essentially pulling the same fire alarms.

Phenomenal pelvic power, crowded quarters

There is another layer of complexity—the wiring.

Orgasm, voiding, and defecating all require complex neural interactions. These actions depend on skin, muscles, nerves, the bladder, and the bowel all providing information to the nervous system and then responding accordingly. To do this, many of the pelvic structures, including the vulva and vagina, share the same nerves.

The nerves from the pelvic structures are very crowded in the spinal cord—the area of the spinal cord that handles the pelvis is tiny compared with other areas of the body. Think of the sacral spinal cord, the part that supplies the pelvis, as a power strip without enough outlets, so some outlets have splitters to accept a two-pronged or three-pronged plug. These tight connections facilitate cross talk and help everything run smoothly, but they can also lead to mixed messages.

To add another layer of confusion, the nervous system is not static. If you experience a painful symptom, your nervous system may turn the volume up on the nerves in the same region, so subsequent stimuli are more painful. This is called windup. It is a protective mechanism—you are more likely to protect an injury if every time you touch it you are in agony. Windup also causes the pain to spread beyond the original injury, widening the field of pain. Again, this provides protection. If the area close to the injury is out of proportion pain-wise, you are more likely to abort any painful activity that risks reinjuring healing tissues.

Symptoms can also spread. Pain, at a cellular level, is inflammation. If your bladder is painful, the pain can travel to the spinal cord and then, because of the tight connections, the pain can enter the nerves that supply the vagina or the skin and they can develop pain conditions and even signs of inflammation under the microscope. We know this because of intricate animal studies. When a caustic chemical is placed in a rat's rectum, the rat's bladder can become visibly inflamed. The injury isn't the chemical seeping through the tissues, because when the experiment is repeated with the nerves to the bladder severed, the bladder never develops the inflammation.

And there is one more thing. Itch, irritation, and pain—basically all bothersome symptoms—are transmitted to the brain using the same wiring. So something can start at your skin as an itch, but by the time it gets to your brain the perception is pain.

Basically, the wiring is very complex.

Tolerance

Many women have different levels of tolerance. For example, with a condition that causes itch, some women feel itchy immediately and for others it barely registers. This is a complex mix of biology and experience. For example, some itch is triggered at a cellular level by the release of the chemical histamine. Some women likely release more histamine than others. Others may have brains that respond differently to pain or itch signals.

Many women have also learned to put up with symptoms because they have been previously ignored. Other times it is like the frog being boiled by degrees—the symptoms come on so gradually they are not recognized until they are very bad. The opposite can also occur. Some women are overly vigilant, meaning they pay too much attention to symptoms—for example, evaluating their vulva daily with a mirror or inserting their fingers vaginally on a regular basis to check for odor. Many "feminine care" products make genital hypervigilance part of their advertising. If you remember back to our earlier discussion on vulvar and vaginal cleansing products, one product even suggests women can release a vaginal odor by uncrossing their legs!

Anxiety, stress, worry, relationship or financial issues, and lack of sleep can all lower tolerance and so symptoms become more bothersome.

Other Compounding Factors

The misinformation women are given about their reproductive organs, internet mythology, and the difficulty women face having non-sophomoric discussions about their vulvas and vaginas make accurate communication hard.

Another important factor is receiving an incorrect diagnosis. If the first time you have a vulvar itch you are misdiagnosed with a yeast infection, then of course every time you have a vulvar itch you will erroneously think you have yeast.

Even a Gynecologist Can Have Trouble Interpreting Signals

One night, while I was writing this book, I felt some discomfort in my left labia majora. I thought it must have been my underwear digging in—I had spent three hours sitting at the hair salon and was wearing ill-fitting underwear. I'd meant to throw it away, but you know how that goes.

I felt around, far out of my field of vision, and found a lump that hurt. A lot. This, I deduced, was either a bitch of an ingrown hair or an abscess. I got out the mirror and saw redness and swelling. Although it was hard to see, I was sure my initial thoughts about either an ingrown hair or an early infection, given the pain, must be correct. My attempts at removing the supposed ingrown hair were unsuccessful but did result in me traumatizing my skin, further increasing my pain. There are a lot of lessons here. For example, this is why you should never try to dig around your vulva at home. Doctors are the worst at taking good medical advice.

The pain worsened, and I imagined myself getting flesh-eating bacteria from my botched attempt at home surgery on an infection. I tried to figure out how this could have happened, and then I remembered the sugaring I did for this book—this was the side that was sugared! I wondered when I died from the resulting blood poisoning, what pithy headlines might appear.

The more I worried, the worse the pain.

I told myself to snap out of it. I took my temperature (normal, *phew*), swallowed an acetaminophen, and went to bed.

I woke up in a lot of pain. I made it to work and told my colleague I had a vulvar abscess. I mean, I am the expert, so telling her what was wrong seemed appropriate. She looked at my vulva and the look on her face told me she saw something completely unexpected. She brought out the selfie-stick mirror so I could see my own vulva. Clearly, I had an irritant reaction or contact dermatitis (an allergic reaction).

I was intensely red, equally on either side. Interestingly, I had no symptoms on the right side. The painful spot? Maybe a small ingrown hair that was amplified by the swelling and irritation from the skin condition, but it really was not clear. I had definitely traumatized my skin. There was no abscess. My colleague admonished me.

Both irritant reactions and contact dermatitis are typically itch or irritation predominant. When they cause pain, it is not typically confined to a pinpoint spot, but no one told my vulva, nerves, or brain.

Once I started thinking skin problem instead of infection, I realized I had run out of my free and clear detergent a few days before and popped down to the drugstore late one night and bought new laundry detergent. After topical steroids and rewashing everything in my regular detergent, in seventy-two hours I was fine.

It is a great example of how symptoms can be confusing. I'm an expert, and my symptoms were in no way classic. I couldn't do a proper self-exam, and my pain and recall biases led me to believe the sugaring was at fault. Thinking I had an ingrown hair or an abscess led me to make a bad decision with a pair of tweezers. The anxiety of my imagined obituary about how I died from a pubic-hair-removal experiment amplified my symptoms.

How to Think About Your Symptoms

The first step is to think about your bother factor and write it down or say it out loud so it sounds correct. Many women come to the gynecologist with bothersome symptoms, and then when we ask they have a hard time describing them. Some of this is the biological complexity that we have discussed. Some of this is the fact that in your brain, you know something is wrong or different, but you haven't yet assigned it a spoken word. Often when people say their symptoms out loud, they realize they were really thinking of something else.

Think about the list of symptoms at the beginning of this chapter and try to match one or more up with what bothers you the most. This is your *bother factor*. You can have multiple bother factors, but knowing the worst symptom can be helpful. Your bother factor can also be, "I am worried this is an STI or cancer." If you can't tell if one bothers you more, then simply say, for example, "My most bothersome symptoms are itch and irritation."

Consider the location of your symptoms: vagina (internal), at the vestibule (vaginal opening), or on the vulva (where your clothes touch your skin). Just remember, where you feel your symptoms may not be the actual source due to the wiring. Another option is to take a photo of the illustration of the vulva (image 11, opposite), mark on the image the location where you feel your symptoms, and then show the photo to your provider.

Don't use diagnoses to describe your bother factor to your provider. Remember how I prejudiced myself and my colleague by saying, "I have an abscess"? Many times, women say "I have yeast" or "I have bacterial vaginosis." You don't want to impose your bias on anyone else. Asking you to define your symptoms does not mean we do not believe your bodies, it means we know the symptoms are complex and we want to be accurate. Providers should not go by your self-diagnosis, but some do, and I am trying to give women a practical, real-world guide for self-advocacy.

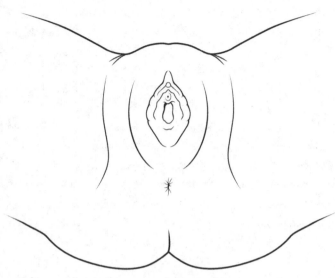

Image 11: Vulva. ILLUSTRATION BY LISA A. CLARK, MA, CMI.

You can absolutely still mention what you think is going on, but leave that for after you have discussed your symptoms or bother factor; don't lead with it. Do mention what you are concerned about diagnosis-wise before your exam because it may impact the testing.

If you can, be precise about how long you have been bothered by these symptoms and how often they occur. Many women say "a while" or "comes and goes," but a while could be one week, one month, or one year, depending on what that means to you. I have had women say "forever" and it means two weeks and other times say "not long" and it was five years. If symptoms are intermittent, or they come and go, do they last for seconds, minutes, or hours, and how many times a day or a week or a month?

Here's an example:

"I have a vaginal itch that is bothersome. I also have a fishy odor that appears after sex. The itch and odor started four weeks ago. The itch is there all the time, although it is worse at night. I only notice the odor after sex. I am concerned I have bacterial vaginosis because I had it last year and these symptoms are the same."

Your provider should ask more questions about other related symptoms to make sure they are considering all the possibilities; for example, they may want to know about new sexual partners, vulvar symptoms, pain with sex, and whether you have used any new lubricants or condoms.

- The biology of the vulva and vagina adds to the complexity of making a diagnosis.
- Almost every diagnosis can have identical symptoms.
- Because of the wiring, the location of the symptoms can add to the confusion; for example, bladder pain can be felt as vaginal pain.
- Think about your bother factor—say it out loud or write it down so the word choice feels correct to you.
- Lead with your symptoms when communicating with providers, not your suspected diagnosis.

CHAPTER 39

I Have Pain with Sex

PAIN WITH VAGINAL INTERCOURSE AFFECTS up to 30 percent of women. While for many women this is temporary, it can be very distressing. What is also upsetting is many women do not get a diagnosis, never mind therapy. Some women are led to believe that pain with sex is normal or that it is somehow their fault.

Pain with sex is a medical condition. It is not normal to have pain with sex. Many of the causes have treatments. Not every condition has a cure, but improving the pain is almost always possible. Many women tell me that knowing they are not the only one is very helpful. If you think you are the only woman to have pain with sexual activity, then it is easy to see how some women might erroneously think they are broken when what they have is a common diagnosis.

It is also very disempowering for a woman to have pain with sex and yet have no explanation or diagnosis. My analogy is providing someone with a destination, but no map, directions, or starting point. How can you possibly get anywhere?

There is data to suggest that just knowing pain with sex is common and has a diagnosis can help reduce pain scores. Anxiety, stress, and sadness all make pain worse. They don't cause it, but they are fuel on the fire, so taking away some of that pain accelerant can be helpful.

Some Questions to Think About Before You Start

Have you always had pain with sex or with tampons, or did that develop later in life? If you have always had pain with sexual touching or insertion, then the cause is not low hormones, unless your first sexual encounter was much later in life. The cause is also unlikely related to an event such as a vaginal delivery.

Do you only have pain with sex or with touch, or do you have pain at other times? Skin conditions, bladder pain syndrome, and endometriosis typically cause pain at other times, not just with sex.

Do you only have pain with one partner and not with others? If so, think about what may be different sexually. Has one partner been more into foreplay than another? Does your partner turn you on? This might suggest technique issues.

The Physical Exam

The most important part of the exam is to stop if you have pain.

A practitioner who is experienced in diagnosing and treating pain with sex can learn a lot from very little. Asking you about breastfeeding and your periods can tell us about low estrogen. Looking at your vulva without touching can help rule in or rule out most skin conditions.

It is also possible to diagnose most cases of muscle spasm without an internal exam. We can often visually see pelvic floor contractions. Touching with a cotton swab at the vaginal opening can help make the diagnosis of vestibulodynia (chapter 33). Testing for yeast, BV, and trichomoniasis can be done with a vaginal swab—no speculum needed.

A caring and attentive provider should be able to work with your comfort level to get enough information to get started. Some topical lidocaine (numbing medication) may help with part of the exam, but almost always a speculum exam is not needed—especially not at the first visit. If your doctor insists on one, then I would get another opinion. Traumatizing women with painful exams is wrong and just adds to the cycle of expecting pain. It's also not medically necessary, and so toughing it out is not going to help you find a solution any faster.

Low Estrogen/GSM

Consider low estrogen if you have one of the following:

- You are breastfeeding and your period has not returned.
- You are perimenopausal or menopausal.
- You are below your ideal body weight and your periods have stopped.

Hormone levels are not needed—if you are not getting a period for one of these three reasons, your estrogen levels are low. If moisturizers and lubricants are ineffective, starting with the estradiol ring or one of the estrogen creams is likely to be more effective. A complete rundown of the options can be found in chapter 19. Estrogen is safe while breastfeeding— we have extensive experience on safety from the use of estrogen-containing birth control pills. We have no data on the safety of vaginal DHEA or oral ospemifene while breastfeeding.

If there is no improvement after 6–8 weeks, you should follow up with your provider. It is not uncommon to see muscle spasm triggered by the pain of low estrogen, so if your pain persists this could be the cause.

Hormonal Contraception

Progestin-only methods of hormonal contraception can lower glycogen in the vaginal mucosa, affecting lubricant and causing pain. These methods include the levonorgestrel IUD, the medroxyprogesterone acetate shot Depo-Provera, the progestin-only birth control pill (sometimes called the minipill), and the etonogestrel implant (Nexplanon).

The changes are not typically as profound as with breastfeeding or GSM, but everyone is different. The treatment is a vaginal moisturizer, lubricants, and if needed a trial of low-dose vaginal estrogen. If the drop in estrogen is not as profound, the lower-dose options often suffice. If lubricants and estrogen do not work, then other causes should be considered.

Vaginal Infections

It is uncommon for vaginal infections to only cause pain with sex. Usually when they are producing enough inflammation to cause pain with insertion, there are other symptoms, such as itch or odor. However, everyone has a different level of tolerance, and sometimes people get accustomed to symptoms that come on gradually.

An infection is not likely to be the cause if you have always had pain with sex—although an infection could develop along the way that makes a preexisting pain-with-sex condition worse, so testing is always recommended.

The main infections that can cause pain with sex are yeast, bacterial vaginosis, and trichomoniasis. A less common condition, desquammative inflammatory vaginitis (DIV), is another cause. It is typically associated with a very heavy and irritating discharge.

Just because you have an infection doesn't mean that it is causing some or all or your symptoms. After treatment, you should be reevaluated to make sure the infection has cleared and your pain with sex has improved. See chapters 29, 31, and 32 for more detailed information on trichomoniasis, yeast, and bacterial vaginosis. Diagnosis and treatment of DIV are addressed in chapter 40.

Pelvic Floor Muscles Spasm

This is a condition where the pelvic floor muscles that surround the vagina are tightening with penetration (chapter 34). The typical description is a woman feeling too "tight" or feeling as if she is clenching with penetration. Some women say it feels as if their partner is hitting a roadblock. Pelvic floor muscle spasm (PFMS) can cause insertional pain, deep pain, pain with friction, or all three. The increased friction against the tight muscles can lead to vaginal soreness or burning afterwards—even for a few days.

Almost always, the spasm can be identified with a minimal exam. It can even sometimes be visible without touching. Vaginismus can be the only cause of the pain or it can develop in response to another pain condition, most commonly GSM or vulvodynia (nerve pain).

Vestibulodynia

This is a type of vulvodynia, a nerve pain condition at the vestibule (vaginal opening). Typically, it causes pain with insertion. Many women also have muscle spasm, as the intense pain with insertion causes the pelvic floor muscles to contract. This makes a smaller vaginal opening, increasing the force against the tissues, and can lead to a cycle of pain and spasm, each making the other worse.

Scar Tissue

Scar tissue from trauma can also lead to pain with sex. The cause of the trauma may be injury, childbirth, or surgery.

After a vaginal delivery, the most common situation is a tear or episiotomy that is slow to heal. It will be very tender to touch. Rarely, there can be an entrapped nerve. Other issues related to delivery can be scarring that narrows the vaginal opening, causing significant pain on contact. This may require surgery to correct.

If you have never had surgery or a vaginal delivery, then this is an unlikely cause. Sometimes with muscle spasm there can be so much pressure at the vaginal opening that it can lead to splits in the skin, which are painful. These splits or tearing can sometimes heal in such a way that a web of tissue forms and traction during sex is painful.

Women who have had female genital mutilation may also suffer pain from scarring. A hysterectomy can produce deep pain with intercourse if there is nerve pain related to the surgery along the scar at the top of the vagina.

Vulvar Skin Conditions

Lichen sclerosus and lichen planus (chapter 35) can cause significant pain due to erosions and ulcerations. Lichen planus can lead to vaginal scarring, and both can lead to scarring at the vaginal opening that can result in intense pain when the tissues are manipulated. Scar tissue around the clitoris can be especially painful.

It would be uncommon for these conditions to only cause pain with sex; most cause pain or irritation even when not touched. There should be visible changes. If the exam is normal, then skin conditions have been excluded—a random biopsy of normal-appearing tissue is not indicated.

Endometriosis

This is a condition where tissue that is like the lining of the uterus grows in the pelvis, on the uterus and ovaries and other tissues. It can cause pain. Most women with endometriosis have pain at other times—usually with their periods, but not always.

Endometriosis can lead to scarring behind the uterus and occasionally even scarring of the uterus to the top of the vagina. This can be felt on pelvic exam and is very painful. As pain with sex is related to this scarring, it is usually with deeper penetration. Women with endometriosis are also more likely to have pelvic floor muscle spasm.

Treatments can include medical therapy for endometriosis, physical therapy to address the muscle spasm, and sometimes surgery.

Bladder Pain

Bladder Pain Syndrome (BPS) is usually associated with a history of overactive bladder (always having to go—although muscle spasm can also be a cause), pain with urination, and a history of symptoms that are exactly like bladder infections but the testing is negative (chapter 36). BPS is rare as a sole cause of pain with sex, but pain with sex could be an initial sign. BPS may also coexist with other painful conditions, such as vulvodynia and PFMS.

On exam, the bladder will be the source of pain, although sometimes there can be muscle spasm which might cloud the picture. Studies tell us that treating the muscle spasm can help with bladder pain.

Mechanical or Technique Issues

If everything else has been ruled out and there is no pain on exam, then the possibility exists that pain with sex could be related to technique issues. The sad truth is many women do not get enough foreplay. Watching a video about the mechanics of good sex and female orgasm might be helpful. A sex therapist is another option.

If no cause is identified after a thorough workup, I generally recommend a consultation with a pelvic floor physical therapist before settling on the diagnosis or technique. Sometimes muscle spasm can be situational, and a more detailed muscle exam might bring more information to the table.

BOTTOM LINE

- Pain with sex is not normal—tell your provider, and if they don't listen get another provider.
- There are ten common causes of pain with sex. It is possible to have more than one.
- Of all the causes, muscle spasm is the most common because it can be the only cause or be triggered by any other condition that causes pain with sex.
- You almost never need a painful exam to get started—an experienced provider can get a lot of information from very little.
- If there is evidence of low estrogen, it is typically best to adequately treat that first and then see if any pain remains.

CHAPTER 40

I Have Vaginitis

VAGINITIS IS ONE OF THE MOST COMMON reasons women seek gynecological care, and in the U.S., more than a billion dollars are spent annually on the combination of self-treatment, office visits, and prescription medications.

Before we go any further, let's define vaginitis. It is one or more of the following symptoms:

- Abnormal vaginal discharge
- Odor
- Itch
- Burning
- Irritation

These are not just nuisance symptoms. Many of the causes of vaginitis are associated with disturbances in the vaginal ecosystem that increase the risk of acquiring a sexually transmitted infection (STI) if exposed.

Despite the discomfort, medical risks, financial impact, and emotional drain of vaginitis, misdiagnosis is common. Diagnosing vaginitis by symptoms is very inaccurate—approximately 50–70 percent of women are incorrect in their self-diagnosis. Diagnosing over the phone is no better. For these reasons, the American College of Obstetricians and Gynecologists (ACOG) recommends against diagnosis without evaluation except in resource-poor settings.

Misdiagnosis by a medical provider is unfortunately common as well. In one study, doctors correctly identified yeast and bacterial vaginosis (BV)—the two most common causes of vaginitis—less than 40 percent of the time. One glaring reason for this is about 50 percent of the time doctors make the diagnosis of vaginitis without doing the correct testing, and sometimes without any testing at all. Self-advocacy to ensure you are getting the appropriate tests is important.

Understanding Normal Discharge

There is a significant amount of confusion regarding the definition of normal discharge online. Women have even posted underwear challenges to brag about how little discharge they have, but remember that up to 3–4 ml of discharge in 24 hours can be normal.

Checking internally for discharge is not needed. It is not discharge until it leaves your body. You will always find mucus or secretions. This is a very important part of the vaginal ecosystem and defense mechanisms.

You may also see discharge on your partner's penis or fingers after sexual activity. It may seem like a lot, as your discharge will be mixed with secretions from arousal and friction will rub cells off from the vaginal mucosa (skin). This is normal. If you partner with a man and do not use a condom, there will also be ejaculate.

The problem with symptoms that is they often reflect tolerance. I have seen women who say they have no discharge, but when I do an exam there is so much discharge that it runs out onto the floor. They obviously have an abnormal amount of vaginal discharge, but it is not bothering them or, over time, they have become accustomed to it. In addition, many women put up with a lot of symptoms.

When is discharge concerning?

Whether discharge looks like cottage cheese or not is not predictive of a yeast infection. The same number of women with yeast and without yeast report having a "cottage cheese" discharge. If your discharge is or has any of the following, then medically we would consider it abnormal:

- Blood-tinged
- Green or dark yellow
- Odor

If you have a change that is concerning for you, then that is another reason for an exam.

Before the Appointment

If you are having your period, your provider cannot do a full assessment for vaginitis. It is hard to see the discharge when it is mixed with blood, and it may not be possible to see if there is discharge from the cervix. The vaginal pH may also be inaccurate from the blood and it may not be possible to look under the microscope.

Ejaculate and vaginal products like yeast creams can stick around in the vagina for up to three days, affecting pH and what we see under the microscope, so no sex and no vaginal products for three days before the visit if possible.

Think About Symptoms

Are they high up in the vagina or at the vestibule (vaginal opening)? If they also extend onto the labia or mons, then your symptoms are not confined to the vagina. Consider reading the next chapter on vulvar itch and irritation.

When did they start, and have you used any new products? Are your symptoms related to sex?

Do you feel like you want to scratch deep inside the vagina? This symptom is suggestive of yeast.

Ask About Tests

It is valid to ask what tests your doctor is going to do to diagnose your symptoms. This is your body, and you will be paying for the tests and the therapies. The bare minimum to evaluate vaginitis is a pH test and an amine test (evaluates the odor of the discharge, see chapter 32 for more detail). These are inexpensive tests that tell us whether you have enough lactic acid–producing bacteria or not. They also help decide what other tests are indicated.

Not every doctor has a microscope or feels comfortable using one. Fortunately, there are other tests, including cultures and nucleic acid tests, that do not require a microscope. However, every doctor who looks after women with vaginitis should be able to do a pH and an amine test. If they are not planning on doing a pH and an amine test as a bare minimum, then they are not equipped to evaluate vaginitis.

My pH Is Less Than 4.5

The good news is your lactobacilli are producing lactic acid. The causes of vaginitis in this situation are as follows:

- **YEAST INFECTION:** Yeast should be seen under the microscope, so a culture or nucleic acid test should be positive. See chapter 31 for treatment.
- **SKIN CONDITIONS:** Lichen planus can cause irritation and vaginal discharge. There may be redness and ulcers. Areas that are not bleeding will have a normal pH. (More in chapter 35.)
- **HERPES:** Not a common cause of vaginitis, but herpes can cause significant redness and discharge. It should resolve within 10–14 days even without treatment. There will be a lot of inflammation.
- **VULVODYNIA:** Nerve pain. Some women with vulvodynia believe their discharge is irritating their skin. What is happening is their skin is painful and so they are mistaking their normal discharge for the cause of the pain.
- **NORMAL DISCHARGE:** If the pH is normal, your yeast culture is negative, and your discharge looks normal under the microscope—

meaning no excessive white blood cells—then the discharge is normal. Nucleic acid tests can confirm the absence of BV if needed.

My pH Is Greater Than 4.5

This means a shift in bacteria with a drop in the lactobacilli that produce lactic acid.

The next step is the amine test—checking discharge for odor. If this is positive, then the diagnosis is trichomoniasis or BV. Testing is required to make sure that it is not trichomoniasis. Looking under the microscope is an inexpensive way to test this, and if there is no inflammation, then trichomoniasis is unlikely. Other tests to diagnose trichomoniasis may be done depending on your risk.

If the amine test is negative, there are several possibilities:

- **TRICHOMONIASIS OR BV:** The amine test isn't always positive, so further testing may be needed to make a diagnosis. (See chapters 29 and 32.)
- **GSM:** Low estrogen. This should be suspected based on your age. For example, if you are twenty-five and have regular periods, you can cross GSM off the list without any testing. Typically, there is some pain on exam and inflammation and specific changes under the microscope. (See chapters 18 and 19 for diagnosis and treatment.)
- **DIV:** Desquammative inflammatory vaginitis, this is a combination of inflammation and a bacterial overgrowth. The discharge can be very heavy—even soak onto clothes. It is uncommon; in a referral practice, about 2–3 percent of women have this, and a general gynecologist or nurse practitioner will see far fewer cases. The cause is unknown, but it is believed to be an inflammatory reaction. Vaginal clindamycin and vaginal steroids have similar outcomes. The therapy is two weeks with either product vaginally and then a reassessment to ensure the discharge has cleared.
- **CERVICITIS:** This is inflammation of the cervix and should be visible to your doctor on exam. Tests should be done for gonorrhea, chlamydia, and possibly mycoplasma.

Should I Get a Test of My Microbiome?

These are DNA tests that purport to give you information about lactobacilli and other bacteria in your vagina, as well as yeast. The problem is they are untested in clinical situations.

Your microbiome also changes day to day and even throughout the day. A snapshot once a day for several days does not really tell us anything. Also, if you are positive for yeast, that does not mean you have a yeast infection, and the results could lead some women to get treated when there is no need.

If you find out that some of your bacteria is elevated, how will that make you feel? We do not know how to interpret all the results that might come with a microbiome test. Also, how will you feel having information that can't or shouldn't be acted upon?

What About Cytolytic Vaginosis?

A few articles of lower quality have proposed a condition that is exactly like a yeast infection—low pH, vaginal itch, irritation, and discharge. Yet no evidence of yeast exists, and an abundance of lactobacilli can be seen under the microscope. The theory is that this excessive amount of lactobacilli is causing symptoms.

Several years ago, I had the opportunity to speak with one of the world's experts on lactobacilli, and she said that lactobacilli have too many self-regulating mechanisms to overgrow. The studies proposing cytolytic vaginosis are also lower quality and not convincing. And in thirty years of vaginitis work, I have never identified a case.

This does not mean women who are told they have cytolytic vaginosis do not have symptoms. They do; they are just caused by a different condition.

Help, I Have Recurrent Vaginitis!

The first step is to confirm your diagnosis. Women who have been diagnosed with chronic vaginitis are often misdiagnosed—only 37 percent of women with recurrent vaginitis have an infection (such as yeast or BV); the rest have GSM, vulvodynia (nerve pain), contact dermatitis, or skin conditions. Many women have their external vulvar condition, like lichen simplex chronicus, misdiagnosed as a vaginal condition.

If you truly have a recurrent issue then it may be time for referral to a specialist, if you have not already been.

BOTTOM LINE

- If you believe you have vaginitis, make sure you are not mistaking vulvar symptoms for vaginal.
- Up to 4 ml of vaginal discharge in twenty-four hours is normal.
- A vaginal pH and amine test are essential.
- If you meet strict criteria, you can consider self-treatment for yeast.
- A common cause of vaginitis is GSM.

CHAPTER 41

I Have a Vulvar Itch

ITCH IS OFTEN TRIVIALIZED AS a minor health problem. It is not. Many women are devastated by years of itching that medicine cannot seem to answer. Some of my happiest patients are women who have had their itch and the impact it has had on their life validated and then treated.

Itch and pain are very different sensations. Even though they travel along the same nerves, they use different signaling and interact in very complex ways. An acute itch, like an itch triggered by an allergen, is relieved by pain (this includes scratching). Chronic itch is not relieved by pain or scratching, and light touch as well as pain can all be perceived as itch, perpetuating the cycle.

Do not use any anti-itch products with benzocaine. If you have them at home, throw them away so you are not tempted to use them. They can cause contact dermatitis (an allergic reaction) for up to 10 percent of women who use them.

What Causes Vulvar Itching?

I like to start with a list and then rule in or exclude conditions as the evidence presents itself. A list of the main causes of itching includes the following:

- **INFECTIONS:** Such as yeast, bacterial vaginosis, trichomoniasis, or molluscum contagiosum. Herpes can occasionally itch, although usually pain is predominant. Yeast is typically the only infection that leads to an intense itch and scratching that you have a hard time stopping.
- **LICHEN SIMPLEX CHRONICUS AND IRRITANT REACTIONS:** We reviewed these in detail in chapter 35. The itching can be intense. The skin may or may not be red. There may be scratch marks. The annoying thing about irritant reactions is they are not predictable; one day a product may irritate you, and weeks later it may not.
- **CONTACT DERMATITIS:** This is a delayed allergic reaction and will reoccur with each exposure. Some common causes are topical benzocaine, Balsam of Peru, fragrance, and ingredients in body washes and intimate wipes. If you are allergic to poison ivy, always wash your hands well after eating mango, as mango skin contains the same allergen as poison ivy—urushiol. Typically, there is significant redness. It is possible to develop an allergic reaction after years of using a product, so contact dermatitis does not have to be new exposure.
- **SKIN CONDITIONS:** Lichen sclerosus and lichen planus, chapter 35. As the skin is fragile, even mild rubbing can lead to significant trauma. Intense itching is uncommon.
- **GSM:** The itch should be at the vestibule or inside the vagina. It is not typically intense.
- **LOW IRON:** This can lead to intense itching that can start on the vulva. This is also a cofactor for yeast infections.

Any new products?

While you can develop an irritant reaction or contact dermatitis (allergy) to any product at any time, anything newly introduced is the most likely culprit. Even airplane toilet paper or a new menstrual pad can be the cause. I experienced a pad irritant reaction firsthand while flying from San Francisco to Frankfurt, Germany. I had not had my period for five months so I assumed I was menopausal. Of course, two hours into the flight my period started, and I was forced to use a pad that looked one generation removed from an abrasive kitchen sponge. I wasn't even over the Atlantic Ocean when I started to itch.

Soaps, cleansers, lubes, condoms, spermicides (not all women who partner with men know if the condoms they use have lube or spermicide) are all possible triggers. Once an irritant reaction starts, it can be like a snowball rolling down a hill. The trigger may have been a small thing, but your skin, immune system, and nerves turned it into a bigger thing.

Is this an acute or chronic itch?

An acute itch, meaning a few weeks at most, is likely to be an infection, an irritant reaction, or contact dermatitis. Every chronic itch was once an acute itch.

Anal Itch

If you have anal itching and bleeding, you should not self-diagnose and treat without at least discussing your symptoms with your provider.

Some of the conditions that cause vulvar itch can affect the anus, most commonly irritant reactions, contact dermatitis, and lichen sclerosus. Yeast does not cause anal itching. In addition, there are some unique causes of itch for the anal area:

- **HEMORRHOIDS:** Dilated clusters of veins in the anal canal. They can be painful, but sometimes the main symptom is itch. There are over-the-counter treatments that shrink the veins. Preventing constipation (eating at least 25 g of fiber a day and taking a laxative if needed) and not straining are the most important prevention tools.
- **PINWORMS:** A parasitic infection of the anal canal. This is usually something acquired by people who are around small children.
- **PERIANAL DERMATITIS:** This is an irritant reaction around the anus that is a combination of aging skin and exposure to fecal material, which is an irritant and leads to bacterial contamination. Women who need to wear occlusive garments for incontinence are at increased risk. The classic presentation is anal itching (or irritation) and redness. The treatment is meticulous skin care

with prevention of fecal soiling, cleaning the area with a cleanser so no fecal material remains (a bidet works the best), a topical steroid to reduce inflammation if needed, and liberal use of an emollient and barrier ointment.

- **ANAL STIS:** Typically they don't cause symptoms, but women with anal itching who are at risk for anal gonorrhea or chlamydia may wish to be screened.
- **ANAL PRECANCER AND CANCER:** If there is persistent itching and no identifiable cause, then an exam to rule out anal precancer or cancer is indicated.

No Cause for My Itch Can Be Identified

If there are skin changes, like redness or ulcerations, then another opinion, and possibly a biopsy, is indicated.

If you have removed the products that you can from your life, it may be time to visit an allergist to make sure that an environmental allergen isn't being overlooked.

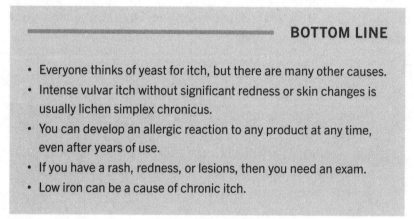

BOTTOM LINE

- Everyone thinks of yeast for itch, but there are many other causes.
- Intense vulvar itch without significant redness or skin changes is usually lichen simplex chronicus.
- You can develop an allergic reaction to any product at any time, even after years of use.
- If you have a rash, redness, or lesions, then you need an exam.
- Low iron can be a cause of chronic itch.

CHAPTER 42

I Have Vulvar Pain

MANY CONDITIONS CAN CAUSE VULVAR PAIN, and to make things a little more complicated, some conditions that are typically not painful for some women can be painful for others.

We all have different biology, so one woman may perceive a sensation as irritation and another woman may perceive it as pain. Previous experiences, anxiety, and worry can amplify pain. Sometimes there can be several symptoms, such as itch and pain, and it may be hard for the brain to perceive both. An analogy is a room with two radios playing: pain is typically the loudest one, and so other signals may be missed, so instead of perceiving both pain and itch, you only perceive pain. Finally, if you scratch an itch and break the skin, the pain may become the most bothersome symptom long after the itch has gone away.

Basically, pain has a lot of complexities.

I roughly divide vulvar pain into acute, lasting up to two weeks, and chronic, which is pretty much everything else. This is not a strict medical definition; it just helps me divide the causes of pain into manageable sections.

Keep in mind that every chronic pain was at one point in time acute pain, so having an open mind is important. For example, typically we think of GSM (low estrogen) as chronic, as it will not improve without treatment, but there was obviously a first day of symptoms, and so at one

353

point in time it was acute pain. If you get care early in the course of your symptoms (a good thing), what may be a chronic condition for someone else will turn out to be an acute problem for you.

Acute conditions can be missed and end up becoming chronic issues.

Acute Vulvar Pain

One day you were fine and then, ouch! Given the number of nerves in the vulva, anything that hurts can be more intensely painful here compared with elsewhere in the body. Also, you can't rest your vulva, as you do have to empty your bladder regularly. Swelling may be more prominent as the vulva is dependent (meaning lower than your heart), and it's not as if you can raise your vulva to reduce swelling like you can a sprained ankle.

The pain can be generalized, meaning affecting most of the vulva, or really discrete in one location.

Yeast infections, irritant reactions, and contact dermatitis typically present as itch, but occasionally they can be pain predominant. See chapters 31 and 35. They are both typically associated with redness of the skin.

Common causes of acute vulvar pain include the following:

- **HERPES:** The typical lesion is an ulcer, but it starts as a small bump. It is very painful. The lesions have typically crusted over by 7–10 days. The pain can extend beyond the lesion. The ulcer can become infected, increasing the pain even more.
- **INGROWN HAIR:** This is the result of the hair growing back on itself into the skin. This leads to inflammation and pain. Typically, the hair will work its way out (see chapter 13 for other suggestions). If you are not sure this is infected, contact your provider.
- **FOLLICULITIS:** Inflammation and infection of the hair follicle. The most common cause is pubic hair removal. Your provider may recommend a topical antibiotic depending on the number and the degree of inflammation.
- **BOILS:** Another name for an abscess. The most common cause is an ingrown hair or injury related to hair removal. Typically, a boil starts as a firm nodule that becomes increasingly painful as

the infection develops and fills with pus. The surrounding skin may be infected. Warm compresses are fine. If the boil drains on its own that is fine, but do not attempt to drain this yourself; you may introduce more bacteria and worsen the infection. If you have diabetes or a weakened immune system, you should contact your doctor immediately. If your pain seems out of proportion to what you see on your skin, then you should also be seen. If the overlying skin is red, this could mean the infection has spread to your skin, and so you should be seen.

- **BARTHOLIN'S ABSCESS:** The Bartholin's glands are small glands at either side of the lower vestibule (vaginal opening). A gland can get blocked, and the trapped secretions may get infected and cause an abscess—this affects 2 percent of women at some point in their lives. The result is a very painful lump, which can get fairly large—even as big as a Ping-Pong ball. This will be a very tender swelling in the lower labia minora. This needs to be drained. The most common technique involves leaving a small tube in the abscess called a Word catheter for up to four weeks so it can drain while a channel forms, preventing secretions from getting blocked again. The second option is going to the operating room and having surgery to open the gland and prevent recurrence. There are advantages and disadvantages to both techniques. Simply sticking a needle in to drain is not recommended, as the abscess often comes back.
- **TRAUMA:** This can be from sex, from using a sex toy, from riding a bike, or even from hair removal. Even if the skin has not broken, a large, typically painful bruise called a hematoma can form under the skin.

Chronic Vulvar Pain

When pain is present for a long time, many women worry about cancer, although typically cancer is not painful. If it were, we would identify it at an early stage more often. Cancer of the vulva is only painful once it gets large enough that it starts to ulcerate or grow into nerves.

The most common causes of chronic vulvar pain:

- Vulvodynia
- Muscle spasm (PFMS)
- Lichen sclerosus/lichen planus
- GSM
- Vaginitis
- Yeast infections
- Nerve injury (typically a one-sided pain, usually with a history of surgery or trauma)

BOTTOM LINE

- Ingrown hairs can become infected and cause significant pain.
- Pain with redness over both sides of the vulva with no breaks in the skin is most commonly yeast, an irritant reaction, or contact dermatitis.
- Chronic vulvar pain in the absence of redness or skin changes is typically vulvodynia, muscle spasms, or GSM.
- If there are ulcerations, breaks in the skin, and chronic pain, then autoimmune skin conditions must be considered.
- The discharge of trichomoniasis and DIV can be very irritating and cause vulvar pain.

CHAPTER 43

I Have an Odor

THERE ARE AN INCREASING NUMBER of women reporting abnormal genital odor. I am not the only OB/GYN to notice this. There has been no change in causes of genital odor over the past twenty-five years; what has changed is the proliferation of products designed to shame women about the normal smell of their body and tame the female genital tract for some misogynistic ideal. These products come from Big Pharma and are found on drugstore shelves in the form of douches and intimate washes, and they also exist in the realm of Big Natural, with vaginal steaming and vaginal herbal sachet packs, often called pearls.

With vulvovaginal odor, two thirds of the time a vaginal cause will be identified, and one third of the time the exam and testing will be completely normal and there will be no readily identifiable medical cause. Let's look at both of these issues.

What Are the Identifiable Causes of Odor?

Medically abnormal vaginal odors are typically related to changes in lactic acid–producing bacteria, the good bacteria. When lactobacilli levels drop, there is an increase in odor-producing bacteria. The most common causes are as follows:

- **BACTERIAL VAGINOSIS (BV):** Commonly associated with a fishy odor (see chapter 32). The odor is often worse after sex with a male partner. About 70 percent of women with a fishy odor will have BV.
- **TRICHOMONIASIS:** A sexually transmitted infection (chapter 29). Has the same bacterial imbalance and odor as BV.
- **GENITOURINARY SYNDROME OF MENOPAUSE, OR GSM:** As estrogen levels drop, so do lactobacilli (chapter 18). The odor is not fishy. Many women describe this in different ways, sometimes as musky or strong, but sometimes just "different."
- **DESQUAMMATIVE INFLAMMATORY VAGINITIS (DIV):** A bacteria imbalance that produces a profuse discharge. The only way to diagnose this condition is looking under the microscope at the vaginal discharge. The vaginal pH is elevated.
- **A RETAINED TAMPON OR OTHER FOREIGN OBJECT:** Can be fishy or musty or simply unpleasant. The odor is due to the overgrowth of bacteria.
- **SKIN CONDITIONS:** Such as lichen planus or lichen sclerosus (chapter 35).
- **INCONTINENCE:** Typically, smells of urine, but it could be pungent or musty. Not every woman is aware that she is leaking urine or that it could be causing odor.

What Are the Nonidentifiable Causes of Vaginal Odor?

Some women report a distressing odor, but we do not detect any abnormal odor on exam and all the testing is normal. It is important to not just "try" various antibiotics, as this can actually do more harm than good by adversely affecting the vaginal ecosystem, paradoxically increasing odor. It is very important to only treat when there is a firm diagnosis.

Causes of odor that we can't identify with tests include the following:

- **PREVIOUS ANTIBIOTICS, ANTIFUNGALS, OR VAGINAL CLEANSING:** Damaging lactobacilli can cause a shift in bacteria that may impact odor. It is not medically abnormal or harmful, but could be perceived as different.

- **BODY ODOR FROM THE VULVA OR GROIN:** The vulva and groin have sebum-producing glands as well as apocrine sweat glands. Bacteria digest the products that the glands make, and this produces body odor (it is the same in the armpits). Overcleaning may affect the surface bacteria, changing odor. Removing pubic hair may also have a role, as one function of hair is dispersal of odor. We also don't know if pubic hair removal affects skin bacteria. Sweating, blood flow to the genitals, and apocrine sweat gland secretions are hormonally dependent, and the ability to smell may also be affected by hormones, so some women may notice a subtle change in smell from their vulva and groin related to their cycle.
- **LONG-TERM HORMONAL CONTRACEPTION WITHOUT ESTROGEN:** Such as medroxyprogesterone acetate (Depo-Provera), the progestin-only birth control pill or "minipill," the etonorgestrel implant (Nexplanon), and the levonorgestrel IUD (e.g. Mirena, Skyla). For some women, these medications may affect vaginal glycogen, which affects good bacteria.
- **NONOXYNOL-9 SPERMICIDE:** Damages lactic acid–producing bacteria.

How to Investigate Odor

The most important thing is to be seen while you are having the odor. If it is normally worse at the end of the day, then schedule an end-of-day visit. If you do not have the odor when you see your doctor, there is a greater chance they will be unable to make a diagnosis.

The following initial tests should be done for odor:

- **VAGINAL PH:** Tells you about the presence of lactic acid–producing bacteria. Normal is less than 4. A pH of 4.5 and higher is seen with BV, trichomoniasis, GSM, and DIV.
- **AMINE TEST:** If this is positive, then the presence of an abnormal odor has been confirmed. Associated with BV and trichomoniasis.

An elevated pH and a positive amine tests suggest BV or trichomoniasis, and testing should be considered as appropriate (chapters 29 and 32). Looking under the microscope can help diagnose other conditions that cause odor. A yeast culture or nucleic acid may be considered, as some women report bothersome odor with yeast. An exam can help identify GSM or skin conditions.

Odor should not be managed over the phone, with two exceptions:

- **IF YOU ARE MENOPAUSAL, THE ODOR IS NOT FISHY, AND YOU ARE NOT AT RISK FOR A SEXUALLY TRANSMITTED INFECTION (STI):** It is reasonable to try a course of vaginal estrogen. If after eight weeks there has been no improvement, then an assessment is needed. If you are menopausal, have not had abnormal vaginal bleeding, and are not on aromatase inhibitors, there are essentially no health risks with trying vaginal estrogen. The downside is that in the United States vaginal estrogen is very expensive, possibly more expensive than an office visit, so there is a small chance you could be paying for unindicated therapy.
- **YOU ARE LEAKING URINE, THE ODOR IS NOT FISHY, AND YOU ARE NOT AT RISK FOR AN STI:** Make sure you are wearing incontinence pads and not menstrual pads, as they will not be absorbent enough. For some women the odor can go away with the use of the right protection. If you are unsure that you are leaking, you can take over-the-counter Pyridium. Pyridium is a pain medicine for bladder infections that turns urine orange. If there is orange on your pad, then you are leaking urine. Your doctor may be able to start therapies for incontinence over the phone.

What If My Workup for Odor Is Negative?

It is important to remember that one third of women who present with odor will have negative testing with no identifiable odor. Negative testing means the pH is less than 4.5, the amine test was negative, there was no inflammation under the microscope, testing for trichomoniasis was negative, there is adequate estrogen, and there is no incontinence. A swab like the BD Max can test for most of the major causes of odor without a microscope.

If your provider tells you that they don't find anything medically abnormal, ask them if they detect a smell. If they do not, it means the odor is not medically abnormal. It does not mean you do not have an odor that is different for you, but the therapy is not likely to involve antibiotics.

When I do not detect an odor, my next step to take a swab from the vagina, smell it, and then hand it to the patient to smell. This way we are both smelling the same thing. There are three possible outcomes:

- **THE PROVIDER THINKS THE SWAB SMELLS ABNORMAL:** In this case, the investigation has proven negative, but there is a medically abnormal vaginal odor. Referral to a vaginitis expert is indicated.
- **THE PROVIDER THINKS THE SWAB SMELLS NORMAL AND YOU DO NOT:** If your testing is all normal and you do not have GSM, or you do and it is being treated, then you may have had a change in your good bacteria, just not a medically concerning change that can be treated. Some women even develop an oversensitivity to their normal smell. Many aspects of modern life are geared toward vaginal hypervigilance. Some men make negative comments about the normal smell of a vagina, and there are shelves of products suggesting vaginal neglect is a concern.
- **THE PROVIDER DETECTS NO ABNORMAL SMELL AND THE SMELL ON THE SWAB IS NOT THE SMELL THAT IS BOTHERING YOU:** In this situation, the source is likely an external body odor.

When there is no medically abnormal odor, some options to consider include the following:

- **NOT WEARING POLYESTER UNDERWEAR:** The fabric is more likely to trap odor.
- **IF YOU REMOVE PUBIC HAIR, LET IT GROW BACK IN:** Pubic hair is involved with odor dispersal.
- **NO DOUCHES, FEMININE SPRAYS OR WASHES, OR ODOR CONTROL SUPPOSITORIES:** They can paradoxically affect odor.
- **IF YOU SMOKE, TRY TO QUIT.**
- **TRY SOME GOLD BOND POWDER OR DEODORANT IN YOUR GROIN:** This can help with body odor.
- **DON'T USE MEDICAL TREATMENTS WITHOUT A DIAGNOSIS:** Many of these products can kill good bacteria and paradoxically cause odor.

Some advocate douching with water if no other cause can be identified. A small study suggests there is no damage to the lactobacilli; however, other data suggests this practice is associated with an increased risk of contracting HIV, so it could be harmful to your good bacteria or the protective mucus. Give douching with water a pass.

BOTTOM LINE

- Two thirds of the time, a medically treatable cause for odor will be identified. The most common are BV, trichomoniasis, and GSM.
- One third of the time, the workup will be normal. This doesn't mean you are making anything up, just that the odor you smell is not medically abnormal (which is good!)
- If your testing is normal, ask to smell a swab from the side of the vagina. If you don't smell anything, the source could be body odor.
- Incontinence can cause odor. Make sure you are wearing incontinence garments.
- Antibiotics and antifungals (especially when not indicated), over-cleaning, douching, and odor-control products can paradoxically lead to odor.

CHAPTER 44

I Have Bleeding After Sex

BLEEDING AFTER SEX IS VERY SCARY. The first time it happens it is unantici-pated, so it is often a shock. It also almost always looks as if there is more bleeding than there is actually happening—even a few drops of blood can look like a lot.

We don't have the best data on how common bleeding is after sex, but it may affect around 5 percent of women at some point in their sexual life. It is very bothersome for many women.

What Are the Causes?

This chapter applies to women who are not pregnant. If you are pregnant and have bleeding after sex, you should contact your doctor or midwife immediately as there is a much different list of items to consider, some which can be very serious.

For women who are not pregnant, there are only a few conditions that cause bleeding after sex, so working through the list and coming up with a diagnosis and treatment plan should not be challenging. The blood is coming from one of four sources: vulva, vagina, cervix, or uterus. Some spotting or a light flow can happen after the first heterosexual penetrative sex with a penis due to tearing of the hymen, but this should be a onetime occurrence.

There is not a lot of literature on this subject, but based on what there is and my experience, here are the most common medical causes of bleeding with/after sex (from medically most urgent to least):

- **CERVICAL CANCER:** Approximately 11 percent of women with cervical cancer have bleeding after sex, so cancer must always be ruled out before another diagnosis is made. Fortunately, most women with bleeding after sex don't have cancer. If your last cervical screening was negative, cancer is very unlikely. Most experts consider a normal cervical screening within the past two years adequate. However, if you have a previous history of an abnormal Pap smear or are HPV positive, then more definitive steps may be needed to rule out cancer.

- **TRAUMA/INJURY:** A laceration (a tear) is more common with nonconsensual sex or consensual use of a sex toy, but it can happen simply from penile penetration (although rare). The vagina or the vestibule (vaginal opening) is usually the location of the injury. This can be very painful, but not always immediately as sexual arousal can blunt the pain response. The bleeding can be spotting, or it can be a heavy flow or even clots. Some women may even need surgery to repair the injury. Trauma is unlikely to be a recurrent cause, so if you have been spotting after sex for three months, then trauma is at the bottom of the list.

- **INFECTION:** Chlamydia and mycoplasma are bacteria that can cause inflammation of the cervix and can lead to spotting. Trichomoniasis can cause a bloody vaginal discharge because it causes so much inflammation.

- **GSM:** The vaginal mucosa (skin) becomes more fragile and can be traumatized very easily, even with a well-lubricated, gentle touch. Almost always there will be pain or burning that goes along with sex and/or bleeding afterwards. If you are having regular periods, you can rule this out without an exam.

- **SKIN CONDITIONS:** Lichen sclerosus and lichen planus (chapter 35) can cause ulcerations that bleed when touched. Typically, there is also pain.

- **A CERVICAL POLYP:** An overgrowth of tissue that hangs down from a stalk attached to the cervix. Almost always benign. When exposed to the acidic environment of the vagina, it becomes inflamed and bleeds easily with touch.
- **CERVICAL ECTROPION:** The cells that are typically inside the cervical canal (these are called columnar cells, and they produce the cervical mucus) are growing on the outside of the cervix. It is a normal variant, meaning some women have it and some women don't. As the columnar cells are typically inside the cervix, they are not as well adapted to the acid environment of the vagina. When exposed to the acidic vagina, they can become inflamed and bleed easily with touch. This is typically the reason why some women can bleed after a Pap smear or swab from the cervix. It is not medically harmful. An ectropion is very common in younger women (if you remember, this is one of the reasons women under twenty-five years of age are more susceptible to getting chlamydia) and higher estrogen levels, such as the estrogen-containing birth control pill and pregnancy, can also cause an ectropion.
- **UTERINE CAVITY SOURCE:** Sometimes the blood is coming down from the uterus courtesy of the ejaculate. It is also important to make sure you are not spotting at other times. If you are having irregular bleeding or spotting between periods, some of this blood may appear after sex. Irregular bleeding is managed very differently.

If There Is a Lot of Blood

In gynecology, a concerning blood loss is usually one soaked pad an hour for two hours. If this is the case, you should seek medical attention. If you are bleeding heavier than that or you don't feel comfortable gauging your bleeding (for example, there seems to be a lot of blood on the bedsheets), don't wait. If you think you may have been injured, you should also seek medical attention. While most people won't need stitches, medically it is always better to repair an injury within a few hours to lower the risk of infection.

When there is a lot of blood, the cause is almost always trauma or cervical cancer, although it is usually trauma.

The Next Steps

When the amount of blood doesn't lead to an emergency department visit, you should make an appointment with your doctor. You need an exam; this is something that can't be managed over the phone. Try to remember if you have had spotting or irregular bleeding, as that may signal a menstrual issue, not a bleeding-with-sex problem. Have a look at your vulva with a mirror to check for any lesions or sores that could be the source of the bleeding so you can show them to your doctor or make note, and tell your doctor if they healed before you get seen. One source of bleeding is a split at the bottom of the vestibule (vaginal opening), and often this heals quickly.

At your visit, ask when your last cervical screening for cervical cancer/precancer was performed. If it was more than two years ago, it should be repeated. Depending on what your doctor sees, they also may wish to repeat the test even if it was done recently.

During your evaluation, your provider should:

- **EVALUATE YOUR VULVA FOR ANY ULCERS OR FISSURES.**
- **PERFORM A SPECULUM EXAM:** To look for any signs of bleeding, such as trauma, sores, inflammation, or signs of low estrogen.
- **LOOK AT YOUR CERVIX FOR A POLYP, INFLAMMATION, OR ANY LUMPS OR ULCERATIONS:** A polyp can often be removed at the same time very quickly with minimal discomfort for most women. If there is a mass or lesion on your cervix, a biopsy may be recommended.
- **TAKE A SWAB FOR GONORRHEA AND CHLAMYDIA, MYCOPLASMA, AND TRICHOMONIASIS:** Not every lab can do the test for mycoplasma. If you don't have access to this test, get the other workup first, and then if everything is negative you can ask your doctor to help you get access to the testing if indicated.

- **EVALUATE THE VAGINAL DISCHARGE UNDER THE MICROSCOPE:** Helps in the diagnosis of low estrogen and trichomoniasis. The presence of a lot of white blood cells suggests inflammation or an infection.

What Are Mycoplasma and Ureaplasma?

They are bacteria that can be sexually transmitted, although in the United States they are not considered a true STI, meaning we don't recommend screening for them routinely in people who don't have symptoms. Many women can have ureaplasma without symptoms, less so for mycoplasma. In the United States, testing is recommended if you have inflammation of the cervix that could be causing bleeding after sex or an abnormal vaginal discharge.

The treatment is the same as for chlamydia: a single 1 g dose of the antibiotic azithromycin. Sex partners should be treated, and no sex for a week after treatment. It may be advisable to have your cervix reevaluated about three weeks after treatment to make sure the inflammation has gone. If your symptoms have persisted, you want to be retested—if you are still positive, you may have a resistant organism (assuming your sex partners were treated). The best tests for ureaplasma and mycoplasma are the nucleic acid tests, so you should not be retested sooner than three weeks after therapy.

My Tests Are All Negative—Now What?

The good news is the first round of evaluation is negative. If your skin is fine, there is no infection, and your cervical screening is normal, then the remaining possibilities are a cervical ectropion and bleeding from the uterus.

With an ectropion, there is no easy treatment, although the good news is that it often improves over time.

An ectropion is visible to your provider when they are looking at your cervix—it looks red and shaggy and will bleed easily when swabbed. One theory is that higher levels of estrogen are involved (hence why it can become an issue during pregnancy), although the true cause is unknown. Before the bleeding is explained by an ectropion, it is a good idea to have a colposcopy (a special exam of the cervix with a magnified lens) to rule out any cancers or precancers missed by the cervical screening.

If you are bothered by bleeding caused by an ectropion and you are on a birth control pill with estrogen, you could consider a birth control pill with a lower dose of estrogen (some pills have 30 or 35 mcg of the estrogen ethinylestradiol, but there are 20 mcg pills) or a birth control method without estrogen (if that is appropriate for your contraceptive needs). It may take six months or so after a switch to see a change.

Some providers have done laser surgery or cryosurgery (freezing) to kill the cells of the ectropion. These are the same therapies we use to treat precancer of the cervix, so you will be losing a small amount of tissue on the cervix. Whether that is advisable in the case of an ectropion is not known, as it is poorly studied. Surgery, even minor surgery, can have complications. If you get to this point, I would always consider a second opinion before a procedure.

The other possibility is the blood could be from the uterus. If all the testing is negative, it may be worth an ultrasound or another evaluation of the uterine lining to rule out a polyp (benign) or precancer as a cause.

I Have a Fissure That Keeps Reopening with Sex

The tissue at the base of the vestibule (vaginal opening) typically receives the most pressure with penetrative sex. If there is too much pressure or there is an underlying skin condition, the vestibule can split. There are a lot of nerve endings, so this is very painful. This tearing can be caused by poor sexual technique, lack of lubrication, nonconsensual sex, muscle spasm (chapter 34) that makes the vaginal opening smaller and results in more trauma to the tissues, GSM, and a skin condition (chapter 35) such as lichen sclerosus or lichen planus. Sometimes the splitting just happens, and we have no cause. In my experience, muscle spasm is one of the most common causes, so an evaluation with a pelvic floor physical therapist may be invaluable.

BOTTOM LINE

- Bleeding with sex happens to about 5 percent of women.
- Pay attention to your menstrual bleeding so you know this isn't a poorly timed irregular period or spotting.
- Make sure your cervical cancer screening is up to date.
- Infections that can lead to bleeding are chlamydia, mycoplasma, and ureaplasma.
- A cervical ectropion is a very common cause. This is a normal variant where the cells from the inside of the cervix grow on the outside and become inflamed.

Putting It All Together

CHAPTER 45

Medicine Cabinet Rehab

MANY PEOPLE ASK ME WHAT I USE for my own vulvar and vaginal maintenance. The answer is: as little as possible.

As far as the vulva is concerned, no expensive product performs better
than any other, and the vagina needs no regular care. I personally prefer
to spend my disposable income elsewhere (like shoes!). For example, I
use Old Spice Fiji (it's a men's deodorant) for my underarms. I can't stand
the flowery or "lady" scents of most deodorants made for women, and
the ones that leave a white powder residue are a source of much personal
aggravation. My Old Spice is a gel, so no stains on my clothing, it is inexpensive, and it makes me feel like a badass lady pirate, and that is a great
way to start the day!

There can be a variety of reasons that products bring us joy. Just be
careful not to mistake the pleasure you derive from such products for
medical benefit. If products in fancy jars are your thing, that is fine, as
long as the ingredients are safe.

Here is what is in my bathroom and why:

- **A FACIAL CLEANSER WITH A PH AROUND 5:** I use this sparingly on my
  vulva (and on my body and my face). Right now, I am using Cer-
  aVe Foaming Facial Cleanser for dry skin. The vaginal cleansers
  offer no benefit, and many have fragrance. I do not like my

shower crammed with bottles, so a single product I can use everywhere also appeals to me.

- **COCONUT OIL:** Menopause is a moisture suck. I use the off-the-grocery-shelf coconut oil on my vulva when I get out of the shower. I have really dry skin on my legs, so I use it there as well.
- **A TRIMMER:** I do not remove pubic hair from my labia majora. I actually did try it for this book and found it very irritating. Shortly after I developed an allergic or irritant reaction to laundry detergent, and I will always wonder if the temporary lack of hair or microtrauma from removal raised my risk.
- **A SILICONE-BASED LUBRICANT:** I dislike the feel of water-based products—the cellulose-based ones feel tacky to me, and the glycerin-based ones are too runny. I like Astroglide X, mostly because you can find it everywhere.
- **I DO NOT HAVE A RAZOR:** I cannot be trusted. I will not use good shaving technique, and I will keep that same razor for years if no one performs an intervention. It is important to know what you will and will not do—meaning not what you are planning to do in your head, but what you are actually willing to execute. (This is a work in progress for me in many domains, not just pubic hair removal.)
- **AN OVER-THE-COUNTER (OTC) TOPICAL STEROID:** Excellent for any little itches.
- **ANTIBACTERIAL SKIN WIPES:** I wax outside of my bikini line, and I use these cloths to prep my skin beforehand. These should not be used as a general cleanser and should not get on your vaginal mucosa or anus (they will hurt and irritate those tissues).
- **TOPICAL BACITRACIN OINTMENT:** To have on hand for folliculitis.
- **SALICYLIC ACID PADS:** These can be useful a week or two after hair removal to exfoliate and help prevent ingrown hairs. Pads allow for precise application and are cheap.
- **5 PERCENT BENZOYL PEROXIDE CREAM:** Spot treatment for ingrown hairs. I like the cream because I can also use it for that acne that comes back around again with menopause.
- **A CLEAN PAIR OF TWEEZERS:** I boil them after use to clean them, and when dry I put them in a sealable plastic bag. If an ingrown hair pokes through my skin, I will pull it out. If I have a pair of tweez-

ers roaming free that is in the back of my cosmetics drawer, it will be nasty with rogue cosmetic powders that have spilled and I will not take the time to clean them. I admit this is terrible and a great example of why doctors should not look after themselves. Never try to dig out an ingrown; the hair must have poked through the surface. If you are unsure, do not touch it and call your provider.

- **AN ORAL ANTIHISTAMINE:** Such as cetirizine or loratadine. They are great to reduce many causes of itch.
- **PETROLEUM JELLY:** It is a great emollient and barrier.

If I were still having my period, I would have an assortment of tampon sizes (for heavy and light days).

And when I get my bathroom renovated, I am getting a bidet—this is the superior method for cleaning after a bowel movement.

What are the Differences Between Lotions, Creams, and Ointments?

Ointments can have up to 20 percent water, but some are water free. As they are thicker, they stay put and are good for spot applications. They have emollient, protective, and occlusive properties, so the vehicle (what contains the medication) is helpful for a variety of skin conditions. Medication is absorbed more slowly from ointments and often penetrates better, so they are very useful for chronic conditions. Ointments are not a good delivery vehicle for the vagina. Many ointments do not need preservatives, so irritant and allergic reactions are less common. Lanolin can be a source of allergic reactions, so this would be an ingredient to suspect in the case of a reaction.

A cream is typically about 50 percent oil and 50 percent water. It will spread better than an ointment and have some emollient properties. To mix oil and water a solvent is often needed, and traces may remain. Typically, creams need preservatives. Drug delivery with a cream is faster. Many vaginal products are creams.

A gel is a semisolid water-based or alcohol-based preparation that is made with a gelling agent. If gels have alcohol, they can be drying and irritating, especially for the vagina and the vestibule (vaginal opening).

There are gels specifically formulated for vaginal use, but in general they are more irritating on the vulva than creams or ointments.

What I Would Remove from Your Bathroom

If you invited me over and asked me to check out your products, I would question or throw the following away:

- **DOUCHES:** These are cigarettes for your vagina.
- **ANTI-ITCH MEDICATIONS WITH BENZOCAINE:** A source of allergic reactions, and if you are itchy you do not need a topical anesthetic to numb the skin—you need a topical steroid and an antihistamine.
- **ANY DAILY PRODUCT WITH FRAGRANCE:** I am not a total fragrance nihilist. If you want the occasional bath bomb or bubble bath and it does not irritate you, then go for it.
- **INTIMATE WIPES FOR REGULAR USE:** They cause so much irritation. If you do not have fecal incontinence, let them go.
- **CONDOMS WITH SPERMICIDE.**
- **SINGLE MENSTRUAL CUPS:** If you use a menstrual cup, I will ask you why you do not have two cups, as proper cleaning is required before reinsertion, not a quick rinse.
- **DIRTY-LOOKING TWEEZERS:** so you are not tempted to use them for ingrown hairs.
- **LUBRICANTS WITH A HIGH OSMOLALITY AND THOSE THAT CAN DAMAGE LACTOBACILLI:** so no warming lubes and no lubes with chlorhexidine gluconate or polyquaternium. Not ever. I am a lactobacilli purist.
- **FEMININE ODOR ANYTHING:** that is choice patriarchy.
- **RAZORS (IF YOU DON'T HAVE SHAVING CREAM):** If I find razors, I will look for shaving cream. If I do not find any, I will throw the razors away.
- **DRYER SHEETS OR FABRIC SOFTENER:** I will peek into your laundry room on the way back from your bathroom and throw those irritant bombs away.

If you have soap, I am not going to take it away if you have no symptoms and you like what you are using. If you are using it sparingly then it is probably fine. However, you must promise to throw it away at the first sign of itch and irritation.

If you use condoms, I will suggest that you go out and buy your own, male or female as you prefer. Do not expect your partner to know this information. If it is your partner's contribution to buy condoms, tell them what you specifically want.

I will also ask if you are cleaning your vibrator(s) according to the manufacturer's recommendations.

BOTTOM LINE

- If you are a hair-removal devotee, give a trimmer a try.
- A topical steroid and an antihistamine are better for itch than a topical anesthetic.
- Ointments add moisture to the skin and also have a barrier function.
- Ditch the douches and odor-control products.
- Benzocaine and lanolin are two products in OTC medications that are well-known causes of allergic reactions.

CHAPTER 46

Internet Hygiene and Apps

MANY PEOPLE ASK: DOES IT BOTHER ME when patients look information up online?

Not at all.

I look up my own health concerns and those of my family. It would be hypocritical to suggest that was my privilege.

When a patient tells me she is researching her health online, I am excited. It means she wants to be engaged and learn. What I do is make suggestions—where and how she can find the best information.

Whether it is general information, self-diagnosis, investigating tests or therapies, or searching for alternatives not recommended by their provider, it's all valid as long as the information is accurate. No woman can be empowered about her health with false information, half-truths, and magic.

The problem when it comes to Dr. Google is that we have moved through the age of information without stopping, and the information highway has brought us to the age of misinformation. How can women find what serves them, and how will they know it is valid when the misinformation, lies, and bias are in competition with boring facts?

Sorting the good from the bad online can be hard even for a doctor with access to the medical literature as well as trusted colleagues who are experts in other fields. Just fact-checking a Goop post that is squarely in my field of expertise, like a post on tampons, can take several hours. I have to sort out quality studies from junk and make sure I do not get tripped up by predatory journals—medical publications that accept low-quality studies for profit. Then I cross-reference with guidelines from medical societies. If there is a product, then I also look up the requirements for submission to the FDA and I pull the related documents. Sometimes the legalese is so hard to understand I have to sidebar a lawyer.

How do you know if what you are reading has been sourced accurately? If the person behind the data has done their due diligence or if there are other motivations? Sometimes people are well intentioned, they just have dismal information. Other times, the intentions are financial.

There is also the problem of repetition. This is called the illusory truth effect: when incorrect information is repeated, it is more likely to be accepted as truth. Repetition of incorrect information is particularly problematic with our viral, story-obsessed 24/7 news cycle.

Sometimes the information online is just too good to resist. Let's face it; everyone, a physician included, is vulnerable to the lure of a quick fix!

Prep Work

Before you research one more thing online, go to the National Library of Medicine and do the tutorial "Evaluating Internet Health Information."

This is a great lesson in how to do your own research. While you are at it, bookmark the National Library of Medicine. It is a great place to start any health research. This is important because the first piece of information sticks the most, so you want to stack the odds in your favor and make sure the first thing that reaches your eyeballs is high quality.

When most people start researching online, they go to a general search engine, like Google. The problem is that what you get for your efforts is a result that is not generated by a medical expert, but by an algorithm based on popularity, relevance, and money. What comes up first may not be the best information, but most of us click anyway. It is rare for people to go beyond three or four entries, so less popular information quickly gets lost, and the articles with the most clicks stay at the top no matter how incorrect they may be. The most valuable piece of information may be on the second page of the search, which may as well be at the bottom of the ocean.

How to Search

Professional medical societies are a good place to start. They have experts who review the data, updating guidelines as new information comes to light. Many have excellent patient handouts written in easy-to-understand language. The American College of Obstetricians and Gynecologists (ACOG), The Society of Obstetricians and Gynaecologists of Canada (SOGC), and the Royal College of Obstetricians and Gynaecologists (RCOG) offer a wealth of information. Having more than one source of quality information on OB/GYN-related topics means you can compare their guidelines and recommendations with each other. Good sources for information on STIs (and a wealth of other sexual health topics) are the Centers for Disease Control and Prevention (CDC), the American Sexual Health Association (ASHA), and Planned Parenthood. The North American Menopause Society (NAMS) is a great resource for all things related to menopause.

I recommend searching one of two ways:

- **INTERNALLY ON THESE SITES:** For example, if you go to ACOG and enter terms in their search bar, you eliminate potential contamination from the general internet.
- **DO A BROWSER SEARCH:** Type in the name of the organization and the subject, and see what comes out. You can also add the term "patient handout." For example, if I want information from ACOG on vaginal estrogen enter: "ACOG vaginal estrogen patient handout."

In general, .gov sites have better quality information than .edu (university sites), as well as .org or .com sites. The .gov sites are typically curated by medical librarians who have no bias. I personally think librarians will save us all; we just need to give them the chance. They are the true superheroes of knowledge.

It surprises many people to hear that .edu sites are typically not much better than .com or .org. Universities have bias, whether they admit it or not. Every organization does. They want to promote their own work. That does not make them bad, just human, and you have to account for that in your research.

Other tips and tricks for separating the myths from the medicine

Does the site sell products related to the medical content? Then they cannot provide you with quality information. They have bias. This is true whether they are a doctor, a herbalist, or Gwyneth Paltrow.

Speaking of celebrities, ignore their medical advice unless they are telling you to get vaccinated and quit smoking. They have incredible financial privilege, never mind amazing genetics. They are also interested in attention. If they wanted to help women medically, they would go back to school and get a medical degree, or a PhD, or become a nurse practitioner, or a physical therapist, or... you get the picture. Health ventures are exactly that—ventures.

Does your doctor get money from Big Pharma? You can look them up on Dollars for Docs, a service from ProPublica. It does not mean your doctor is bad, but if they recommend a medication and they also get $30,000 a year from the company that makes that drug, they might be biased in their recommendations. My biggest issue with the ProPublica site is that it does not capture the money doctors make from their ventures with Big Natural, either promotions or from selling supplements. It also does not capture anyone else in the health industry, for example, naturopaths and physical therapists.

Does a doctor sell their own branded supplements? No studies have proven these products help, and there is potential for harm. I have a low opinion of anyone who abuses their medical privilege to push powders. If they have discovered some true medical miracle, why can you only buy it online for $39.95? If they are so devoted to health that they invented a miracle product, the studies showing benefit should be easy to find and they could help more people by proving their therapy works.

Just saying.

Does the site use words like "detox" and "cleanse"? If they do not know those are dubious concepts, what else escapes them? Do they use words like "pure," "clean," and "natural"? Women are constantly fed lies about toxins in their periods or that the vagina is dirty. "Pure," "clean," and "natural" are just modern riffs on that destructive messaging. They also do not mean anything medically. You want sound hypotheses and clinical evidence, not patriarchy's dog whistle.

Is homeopathy mentioned as a valid treatment option? Give them a pass. No study has proven homeopathy works, and the very idea is not compatible with the laws of physics. When there is one big information gap, there will be others. One study tells us that doctors who prescribe homeopathy are less likely to follow recommended medical guidelines.

Sensationalized content: Nothing is a miracle, and the world's first therapy belongs in a medical journal, not an online store. Throughout this book I have quoted success rates with therapies; the good ones have been in the 90–95 percent range. That does not mean medicine sucks; it means medical conditions are complex, and there are a lot of nuances. If there were cures, we would give them to you. The phrase "100 percent successful" means "high probability of scam."

Reliance on patient testimonials: This is not vetted, so you do not know if they had the medical condition or took the therapy they are supporting. You have no way of knowing.

Be wary of patient advocacy groups, especially any that are funded by the pharmaceutical industry. In 2015 in the U.S., patient advocacy groups received $114 million from the pharmaceutical industry.

Help Build a Medical Internet

How we interact with information online can have ramification beyond the actual facts. Here are some other safety tips:

- Do not read the comments. Ever. A negative comment about the author can change what you think of the quality of the information. Even one ad hominem attack in the comments changes a reader's perception of what they read.
- Do not share bad content, not even to laugh at it. Remember the illusory truth effect? If you see enough headlines in your Facebook feed about the HPV vaccine damaging the ovaries (it does not, so not to worry; it's just an example), you may start to believe there is a connection.

- Read to the end of an article. There will be information all the way through. Many news articles start with an empathetic story. If you do not read through to the end, you may miss an expert's information or refutation.
- Find a trusted resource and share its content. Find me on Facebook and Twitter and Instagram. I try to post vetted information, at least once a day, either original content or news stories that I find accurate and informative. There are other doctors, nurses, physical therapists, and other medical professionals out there as well.

BOTTOM LINE

- Take the National Library of Medicine tutorial "Evaluating Internet Health Information."
- Start your search with a professional medical society and expand outwards.
- Any site that sells product or uses nonmedical words, such as "detox" or "pure," is more heavily invested in selling you magic than providing useful medical information.
- Do not read the comments, and try not to share bad information.
- Avoid sites where there is any mention of homeopathy as a valid treatment for anything.

CHAPTER 47

Journal of Old Wives' Tales

BEFORE WE HAD MICROSCOPES AND TESTING, before we had X-rays or other imaging, we struggled to make real medical diagnoses. And of course, without knowing what is actually wrong, it is hard to prescribe the right therapy. For example, there was a time when people believed what we now know to be tuberculosis was caused by vampires. President George Washington, during his retirement, was killed in 1799 by bloodletting meant to reduce "bad humors" and inflammation. Washington had 40 percent of his blood volume removed in twelve hours and died.

These myths as they pertain to reproductive health care are particularly egregious. The ancient Greeks believed the uterus could wander. That's right—detach itself and roam around the abdomen, causing all kinds of medical mayhem, such as hysteria. If the womb wandered too high, a woman could feel sluggish, and if it went too low, it could cause death. Fortunately, there was a way to trick a shifty womb into submission: "Fragrant smells" could be used to coax that wanderer back into place. Pleasant scents applied to the vagina could lure the mischievous womb back into position, or you could drive it away from the upper body and back down where it belongs by putting a foul smell where the accursed womb had set up shop. So the uterus was basically a naughty sheep in need of herding.

It sounds ridiculous, right? Well, old wives' tales are remnants from these times. The best people could do with the little knowledge they had.

Certain remedies had some basis—for example, chewing willow bark for pain relief led to the discovery of salicylic acid, otherwise known as aspirin. (The name recalls that connection, as it is from the Latin *salix*, or willow tree.) However, most ancient remedies were discarded for good reason. They were harmful, or something better came along. Or we realized vampires didn't exist. Or that the uterus didn't wander aimlessly.

As women were denied an education and because of the social mores could not get an exam from a male physician, they often had to make do with female healers who likely did the best with what they had. I often wonder what these women would think of this modern trend of eschewing science for so-called "natural" and "ancient" remedies. I truly believe they would favor modern diagnostics and therapies such as vaccines and antibiotics as opposed to crystals and poultices. I believe they would look at antifungal medication for yeast and call it magic.

Undoing medical mythology is hard. We have been steeped in it generationally, and medicine has not done a great job of communicating or caring for women. If historically you have been dismissed, it seems only natural to turn elsewhere—especially if that person you turn to is welcoming and actually listens. Lack of trust is a huge barrier to quality medical care. In addition, we are exposed to these old wives' tales so often that we come to believe there must be some truth to them—the illusory truth effect (repetition being mistaken for accuracy) is real.

So here's a list of some old wives' tales, although some are not so old. After all, with old wives' tales, facts are more of a construct.

- **APPLE CIDER VINEGAR TO BALANCE YOUR VAGINAL PH:** Vinegar has approximately the same pH as stomach acid, so how a shot of vinegar could balance your pH but the acid floating around in your stomach doesn't is never explained. I mean, come on. You can't change your vaginal pH with food of any kind; vaginal pH is controlled by the vaginal bacteria. You can't change your blood pH with food because your kidneys and lungs control blood pH, and when they don't you get very ill and die. What drinking apple cider vinegar *will* do is damage the enamel of your teeth.
- **BIRTH CONTROL PILLS CAUSE WEIGHT GAIN:** This has been well studied, and the answer is no. This is not disbelieving women; this is the exact opposite. This is taking what women report about

weight gain and studying it. This data really reflects doctors listening to women. Several studies have shown no link between birth control pills and weight gain. One study even compared women who took birth control pills with women who had a copper IUD inserted—so no exposure to hormones. Both groups gained the same amount of weight. The life situation associated with starting new contraception may be associated with weight gain, but the pill is not.

- **COFFEE ENEMAS FOR ANYTHING:** Dear God, no. People, even some doctors, promote this to treat depression! I. Just. Can't. Even. First of all, this is a waste of good coffee. Medically speaking, to believe coffee in your rectum could treat anything is ludicrous. I mean, why doesn't drinking it have the same effect? It is a rabbit hole of epic proportions. This myth started relatively recently. The only medical reference is in the 1944 Royal Army Medical Corps training manual during World War II, and it was used to keep men awake. I'll say! Just don't, and run from anyone who tells you this will help.

- **DRINKING EIGHT GLASSES OF WATER A DAY:** Many doctors have tried valiantly and failed to kill this myth. It originated in the 1950s when a nutritional expert estimated that the total amount of water we consume in a day was equivalent to eight glasses. What everyone forgot is that calculation also included the water that we take in with food—which is how we get most of our water. Just drink when you are thirsty (there may be some exceptions for the elderly or people exercising or working outdoors in the heat). We have an intricate mechanism designed to tell us when we need to top up. Following your body's cues is the most natural thing of all. (I'm always fascinated how listening to your body is actually ignored when that is what modern medicine wants you to do. Sigh.)

- **ESSENTIAL OILS FOR ANYTHING:** "Essential oils" is an umbrella term for oils extracted from plants. Saying essential oils treat any condition is as vague as saying plants are a therapy. Um, okay. So there are a lot of plants, so like, which ones? In addition, many can cause irritation or allergic reactions when applied topically. If a scent pleases you, that is great. But using an essential oil for any medical condition is not backed by science. And no, they are not the "new antibiotics."

- **FANCY WATER:** The latest is so-called "alkaline water." Water has a pH of 7, and alkaline water has been modified so the pH is 8 or 9. This is an extension of the so-called alkaline diet, which has been promoted to "neutralize the acid in your body" (medical gibberish, by the way) to treat just about everything, even as a treatment for cancer. IT'S NOT. Why all caps? Because people have followed the alkaline diet for cancer and died. The man who wrote the book that started the alkaline trend received jail time for practicing medicine without a license. This is a grift of epic proportions, and that has not stopped celebrities and even some doctors from getting on the useless alkaline bandwagon. The latest version of it is this "special" alkaline water. There is no such thing, and anyone promoting the diet or so-called alkaline water is, in my opinion, unethical.

- **GARLIC FOR YEAST INFECTIONS—VAGINALLY, OF COURSE:** Nope. Garlic does have allicin, and in the lab this does have some anti-yeast properties. To release allicin, you have to crush the garlic, and the idea of small chunks of garlic on inflamed vaginal mucosa just makes me cross my legs. We have no idea if garlic works or if it damages the mucosa or the good bacteria, so stick to scientifically tested cures!

- **HORMONAL CONTRACEPTION CAUSES "INFERTILITY":** Nope, but the patriarchy trying to scare you away from controlling your reproductive health is invested in this myth. Sadly, many "natural" health proponents capitalize on this fear as well. Many people weaponize the patriarchy; whether it is based in ignorance (misinformation) or intent (disinformation) you will have to ask them. With the injection, there can be a delay of several months of return to fertility, but by one year all women are back to baseline. With all other methods of contraception, once stopped or removed, you are good to go pregnancy-wise the next month.

- **IODINE TO SUPPORT THE IMMUNE SYSTEM:** Some people (not people whose medical advice I recommend you follow) promote iodine supplements to "support" the immune system and kill bacteria and viruses. Iodine will do neither of these things. It is true we need iodine, but the only part of the body that uses and stores iodine is the thyroid. Most people in Western societies will get more than enough iodine from their diet. The recommended daily intake for a nonpregnant adult is 150 mcg (micrograms) a day—one teaspoon of iodized salt has 400 mcg. Iodine is also found in foods such as eggs, milk, soy milk, saltwater fish, and seaweed. Paradoxically, taking excessive doses of iodine can cause thyroid disease.

- **JADE EGGS FOR YOUR "YONI":** Popularized by my pal Gwyneth Paltrow. The idea is that you put an egg-shaped jade rock in your vagina, and it puts you in tune with your feminine energy or something. Goop's feminine energy, from what I saw at one of their *cough* "health conferences," is hopelessly heteronormative and conforms to the patriarchal ideal. A vagina does not make you a woman, how you feel inside does. Jade eggs were promoted as an ancient secret of Chinese concubines and queens. I researched this and published my data in a peer-reviewed medical journal—they are not. Promoting jade eggs like this is Orientalism, not health care or female empowerment. The only thing ancient about it is the scam.

- **KAVA, A DIETARY SUPPLEMENT TO ALLEVIATE ANXIETY AND STRESS:** Kava is made from *Piper methysticum*, a plant that is in the pepper family. It is found in supplements to reduce stress and anxiety; however, supplements may not be labeled correctly, and you really have no idea what it is in what, so you could be exposed to kava and not be aware. It can cause severe liver disease as well as heart and eye problems and skin discoloration. Don't. Take. Kava. Or listen to anyone who suggests it.

- **LIFTING YOUR ARMS OVER YOUR HEAD WHILE PREGNANT WILL CAUSE THE CORD TO WRAP AROUND YOUR BABY'S NECK:** Nope. This isn't a vagina myth, but OB/GYNs hear it all the time so I thought I would include it. This is just not biologically possible, and if pregnancies were that fragile, we would have died out years ago. I wonder if this myth serves the patriarchal ideal of the "delicate woman" or if it is simply born out of pregnancy fears.

- **MAGNETS NEXT TO YOUR VAGINA FOR HOT FLASHES:** Just clip in your underwear and go! Therapeutic magnets are a multibillion dollar industry and there is no evidence they do anything but lighten your wallet. The people who sell them make claims about the autonomic nervous system that sound good, but are medically meaningless—such as "balance." Medicine is not gymnastics. In addition to the dearth of studies showing that magnets have medicinal value, if magnets worked for anything we would already know because people would be liberated (at least temporarily) from pain and inflammation and hot flashes and whatever else magnet grifters say magnets work for, by an MRI scan, as that is one big-ass magnet. The magnetic field of an MRI is so strong it causes all the axes of your hydrogen protons to line up and yet it offers no respite for hot flashes (or incontinence, or trouble sleeping or, well, you get the point). Researchers have even done MRIs on women who suffer from hot flashes to try to understand how they impact the brain, and no one has reported their therapeutic effects. Sometimes I worry I am going to sprain my neck with my eye rolls writing about these and the "science" *cough, cough* behind them.

- **ONION APPLIED TOPICALLY FOR WARTS:** Applying slices to the warts or making onion juice to apply or sleeping with an onion in your socks for plantar warts on your feet. I mean, don't! It may shock you to know there are no studies. Just think about it—onions are super cheap and available almost everywhere, so if they worked no one would have warts.

- **PARSLEY IN THE VAGINA:** The sprig. Stuffed up the vagina each night for three to four nights to induce a period. Look, I don't make this stuff up, I just report on it. Apparently some people — people who are wrong—think it could stimulate uterine contractions. There is no evidence vaginal application of parsley can do that to the uterus, but even if it could that would not make you have a period. Progesterone withdrawal causes a period, not uterine contractions. Please don't put parsley in your vagina.

- **RAINBOW DIET:** Eating different colored foods will balance your seven chakras and even make you want to wear more colorful clothing. Literally, you will take off your black yoga pants and wear more colorful clothing. I heard that at the Goop "health" expo in New York. It made me look around and wonder if everyone else realized this was bordering on cult indoctrination? I also read it on the Goop website. Maybe it's not a true old wives' tale and more a California fusion version, a new old wives' tale, or essence of old wife. Eat a balanced diet. Wear what makes you happy. Next (definitely No Thank U).

- **STEAMING THE VAGINA:** This is promoted to "cleanse" the uterus. This ties into a destructive myth that the uterus is unclean or that a period is cleaning the uterus. The idea of a toxin-filled uterus is literally used by many cultures to exclude women from society—it's a defining characteristic of the patriarchy. So telling women this exists is promoting a patriarchal idea. Many "vegan bloggers" (I don't make up the terminology, I just report on it) promote losing weight to the point that periods stop to prevent the accumulation of so-called "toxins." This is harmful on so many levels. If you are dieting to the point your periods have stopped, you may be underweight, and if that continues you could suffer real health consequences, such as osteoporosis (thinning of the bones).

- **TEA TREE OIL FOR YEAST INFECTIONS:** Tea tree oil is an endocrine disruptor and a common cause of irritation. There are no published studies showing that it is effective, and the impact on the health of vaginal bacteria is unknown. Because that is what you want for your vagina, right?—an endocrine disruptor with an unknown effect! Seriously, that tea tree oil is offered as a cure-all is predatory and, frankly, enraging. And it shows how little research many people put into their "miracle" "natural" cures.

- **URINE SMELL INDICATES A BLADDER INFECTION:** Nope. Not sure how this started, but strong-smelling urine doesn't indicate anything, bladder health–wise. There are some medical conditions that can change how urine smells, but a bladder infection is not one of them.

- **VAGINAL TIGHTENING STICKS:** These are promoted as Japanese in origin; whether they are or not I don't know. However, there is a lot of Western exoticism regarding other cultures, so I would be wary when a specific culture or country is used as part of a marketing strategy. Anything offered to tighten your vagina is an astringent and will damage the mucosa and your mucus. It is also part of the patriarchal idea that a "used" vagina stretches and is undesirable. This mythology harms women medically and emotionally, and people who promote it should be ashamed of themselves.

- **WIDESPREAD YEAST OR "CANDIDA" THROUGHOUT YOUR BODY:** Yeast in the bloodstream, what medicine calls systemic yeast, is usually fatal without prompt, aggressive medical care. "Candida" is the wellness-industrial complex's Emmanuel Goldstein (the character from *1984* by George Orwell)—popping up everywhere, causing mayhem. That is just not how it works. At all.
- **YOGURT FOR YEAST INFECTIONS:** It doesn't contain the strains of lactobacilli that are important for vaginal health. When a woman puts yogurt in her vagina, she is putting other bacteria there, as yogurt has live cultures, and the consequences are unknown. It may feel soothing because it is cream-like, but the risks are unknown and it will be ineffective.
- **ZINC TO INCREASE YOUR LIBIDO:** Zinc is apparently appearing in neutraceuticals intended to increase libido. In one study, zinc supplementation made male rats thrust more during sex (sexxxy!) and generally increased their "sexual competence." However, injecting zinc directly into dog testicles contributed to subfertility. I am going to have to go with a big no on this one, as there are no studies in women—although Sexual Competence of Rats could be the name of a punk-rock band that never made it out of their parents' basement because their first single, "Thrusting," failed to chart.

Final Thoughts from Jen

Power and health are inseparably linked.

You can't be an empowered patient and get the health outcomes you want with inaccurate information and half-truths. You also can't be empowered when you are getting correct information but the person or source informing you is making you feel bad or is not listening to your concerns.

I've been attacked for coming out against the misinformation and disinformation that are presented to women as worthy of consideration. To me, the idea that women can take away what serves them from the morass of half-truths and lies about their bodies is the greatest perversion of choice. True choice—weighing your personal risk-benefit ratio and making a decision for your body based on that information—requires facts. And it is this quest to give women facts that keeps me up at night. It is why I keep fighting.

I want every woman to have the power that comes with knowing how her body works and how to look for help when her body may not be working as she hoped it would. I want all women to know when there is bias and medical subterfuge, when there are lies, and when the patriarchy is just invested in keeping them frightened about their own normal (and I might add, glorious) bodily functions.

The patriarchy and snake oil have had a good run, but I'm done with how they negatively affect and weaponize women's health. So I am not going to stop swinging my bat until everyone has the tools to be an empowered patient and those who seek to subjugate women by keeping them from facts about their bodies have shut up and taken a seat in the back of class.

That's my vagenda.

References

Chapter 1: The Vulva

Yeung, J., Pauls, R.N. Anatomy of the vulva and the female sexual response. *Obstet Gynecol Clin N Am* 2016; 43: 27–44.

Di Marino, V., Lepidi, H. *Anatomic Study of the Clitoris and Bulbo-Clitoral Organ*. Switzerland, Springer International: 2–14.

Kobelt, Georg Ludwig. Die männlichen und weiblichen Wollust-Organe des Menschen und einiger Säugethiere: in anatomisch-physiolog. *Beziehung*. Freiburg i.Br., 1844; digi.ub.uni-heidelberg.de/diglit/kobelt1844/0001/thumbs, accessed November 8, 2018.

O'Connell, H.E., DeLancey, J.O.L. Clitoral anatomy in nulliparous, healthy, premenopausal volunteers using unenhanced magnetic resonance imaging. *J Urol* 2005; 173: 2060–63.

Chapter 2: The Vagina

Luo, J., Betschart, C., Ashton-Miller, J.A., DeLancey, J.O.L. Quantitative analyses of variability in normal vaginal shape and dimension on MR images. *Int Urogynecol J* 2016; 27: 1087–95.

Levin, R.J., Wagner, G. Orgasm in women in the laboratory—Quantitative studies on duration, intensity, latency, and blood flow. *Arch Sex Behav* 1985; 14: 439–49.

Anderson, D.J., Marathe, J., Pudney, J. The structure of the human vaginal stratum corneum and its role in immune defense. *Am J Reprod Immunol* 2014; 71: 618–623.

Vaneechoutte, M. The human vaginal microbiology community. *Research in Microbiology* 2017; 168: 811e825.

Chapter 3: Vulvas and Vaginas in Transition

lgbthealtheducation.org/wp-content/uploads/LGBT-Glossary_March2016.pdf, accessed November 11, 2018.

ACOG. Committee opinion no. 512 health care for transgender individuals, December 2011.

Chipkin, S.R., Kim, F. Ten most important things to know about caring for transgender patients. *Am J Med* 2017; 130: 1238–1245.

Peitzmeier, S.M., Reisner, S.L., Harigopal, P., Potter, J. Female-to-male patients have a high prevalence of unsatisfactory Paps compared to non-transgender females: Implications for cervical cancer screening. *J Gen Intern Med* 2014; 29: 778–784.

Chapter 4: Female Pleasure and Sex Ed

Pauls, R.N. Anatomy of the clitoris and the female sexual response. *Clinical Anatomy* 2015.

Vaccaro, C.M. The use of magnetic resonance imaging for studying female sexual function: A review. *Clinical Anatomy* 2015: 28; 324–330.

Shirazi, T., Renfro, K.J., Lloyd, E., Wallen, K. Women's experiences of orgasm during intercourse: Question semantics affect women's reports and men's estimates of orgasm occurrence. *Arch Sex Behav* 2018; 47: 605–613.

Gleick, James. Faster: *The Acceleration of Just About Everything*. Vintage Books, New York. 1999.

Chapter 5: Pregnancy and Childbirth

ACOG committee opinion no. 742 postpartum pain management. *Obstet Gynecol* 2018; 132: e25–e42.

ACOG committee opinion no. 736 optimizing postpartum care. *Obstet Gynecol* 2018; 131: e140–e150.

Leeman, L.M., Rogers, R.G. Sex after childbirth: Postpartum sexual function. *Obstet Gynecol* 2012; 119: 647–655.

Jones, C., Chan, C., Farine, D. Sex in pregnancy. *CMAJ* 2011; 183: 815–818.

Chapter 6: Medical Maintenance

CDC cervical cancer screening guidelines. cdc.gov/cancer/cervical/pdf/guidelines.pdf, accessed 11 Nov 2018.

Guirguis-Blake, J.M., Henderson, J.T., Perdue, L.A. Periodic screening examination evidence report and systematic review for the US preventative services task force. *JAMA* 2017; 317: 954–966.

ACOG committee opinion no. 626 the transition from pediatric to adult health care: Preventive care for young women aged 18–26 years, 2015 (Reaffirmed 2017). *Obstet Gynecol* 2015; 125: 752–4.

Bates, C.K., Carroll, N., Potter, J. The challenging pelvic examination. *J Gen Intern Med* 2011; 26: 651–657.

Chapter 7: Food and Vaginal Health

Mirmonsef, P., Hotton, A.L., Gilbert, D., et al. Glycogen levels in undiluted genital fluid and their relationship to vaginal pH, estrogen, and progesterone. *PLOS ONE* 2016; 11; e0153553.

Jepson, R., Craig, J., Williams, G. Cranberry products and prevention of urinary tract infections *JAMA* 2013; 310: 1395–1396.

Holscher, H.D. Dietary fiber and prebiotics and the gastrointestinal microbiota. *Gut Microbes*. 2017 Mar 4; 8: 172–184.

Harlow, B.L., Abenhaim, H.A., Vitonis, A.F., Harnack, L. Influence of dietary oxalates on the risk of adult-onset vulvodynia. *J Reprod Med* 2008 Mar; 53: 171–8.

Chapter 8: The Bottom Line on Underwear

Runeman, B., Rybo, G., Forsgren-Brusk, U., Karkö, Larson, P., Faergemann, J. The vulvar skin microenvironment: Impact of tight underwear on microclimate, pH and microflora. *Acta Derm Venerol* 2005; 85: 118–122.

Mårdh, P.-A., Novikova, N., Stukalova, E. Colonisation of extragenital sites by Candida albicans with recurrent vulvovaginal candidiasis. *BJOG* 2003; 110: 934–937.

Mårdh, P.-A., Rodrigues, A., Genc, M., Novikova, N., Martinez-de-Oliviera, J., Guashino, S. Fact and myths on recurrent vulvovaginal candiosis—A review of epidemiology, pathogenesis, diagnosis and therapy. *Int J STD AIDS* 2002; 13: 522–539.

Alam, P.A., Burkett, L.A., Clark, B.A., Tefera, E.A., Richter, L.A. Randomized crossover comparison of Icon™ reusable underwear to disposable pads for management of mild to moderate urinary incontinence. *Female Pelvic Med Reconstr Surg* 2018; 24: 161–165.

Chapter 9: The Lowdown on Lubricant

Cunha, A.R., Machado, R.M., Palmeira-de-Oliveira, A., Martinez-de-Oliveira, J., das Neves, J., Palmeira-de-Oliveira, R. Characterization of commercially available vaginal lubricants: A safety perspective. *Pharmaceutics* 2014; 6: 530–542.

Use and procurement of additional lubricants for male and female condoms: WHO/UNFPA/FHI360 Advisory Note. World Health Organization 2012.

Steiner, A.Z., Long, D.L., Tanner, C., Herring, A.H. Effect of vaginal lubricants on natural fertility. *Obstet Gynecol* 2012; 120: 44–51.

Edwards, D., Panay, N. Treating vulvovaginal atrophy/genitourinary syndrome of menopause: How important is vaginal lubricant and moisturizer composition? *Climacteric* 2016; 19: 151–161.

Chapter 10: Kegel Exercises

Price, N., Dawood, R., Jackson, S.R. Pelvic floor exercises for urinary incontinence: A systematic literature review. *Maturitas* 2010; 67: 3019–315.

Bø, K., Sherburn, M. Evaluation of pelvic floor muscle function and strength. *Physical Therapy* 2005; 85: 269–282.

National Association for Continence; nafc.org/bladder-health-awareness-month-2018, accessed 10 Nov 2018.

Barnes, K.L., Dunivan, G., Jaramillo-Juff, A., Krantz, T., Thompson, J., Jeppson, P. Evaluation of smartphone pelvic floor exercise applications using standardized scoring system. *Female Pelvic Med Reconstr Surg* 2018.

Chapter 11: Vulvar Cleansing: Soaps, Cleansers, and Wipes

Farage, M., Maibach, H.I. The vulvar epithelium differs from the skin: Implications for cutaneous testing to address topical vulvar exposures. *Contact Dermatitis* 2014; 51; 201–209.

Schmid-Wendtner, M.H., Korting, H.C. The pH of the skin surface and its impact on the barrier function. *Skin Pharmacol Physiol* 2006; 19: 296–302.

Mendes, B.R., Shimabukuro, D.M., Uber, M., Abagge, K.T. Critical assessment of the pH of children's soap. *J Pediatr* 2016; 92: 290–295.

Aschenbeck, K.A., Warshaw, E.M. Allergenic ingredients in personal hygiene wet wipes. *Dermatitis* 2017.

Chapter 12: Vaginal Cleansing: Douches, Steams, Sprays, and Potpourri

Crann, S.E., Cunningham, S., Albert, A., Money, D.M., O'Doherty, K.C. Vaginal health and hygiene practices and product use in Canada: A national cross-sectional survey. *BioMed Central* 2018.

Grimley, D.M., Annang, L., Foushee, H.R., Bruce, F.C., Kendrick, J.S. Vaginal douches and other feminine hygiene products: Women's practices and perceptions of product safety. *Maternal and Child Health Journal* 2006; 10: 303–310.

Brown, J.M., Poirot, E., Hess, K.L., Brown, S., Vertucci, M., Hezareh, M. Motivations for intravaginal product use among a cohort of women in Los Angeles. *PLOS ONE* 2016; 11: e0151378.

Brown, J.M., Hess, K.L., Brown, S., Murphy, C., Waldman, A.L., Hezareh, M. Intravaginal practices and risk of bacterial vaginosis and candidiasis in a cohort of women in the United States. *Obstet Gynecol* 2013; 121: 773–780.

Chapter 13: Hair Removal and Grooming

Pauls, R., Cotsarelis, G. The biology of hair follicles. *NEJM.* 1999; 341: 491–497.

Schild-Suhren, M., Soliman, A.A., Malik, E. Pubic hair shaving is correlated with dysplasia and inflammation: A case-control study. *Infec DIs Obstet Gynecol* 2017.

Glass, A.S., Bagga, H.S., Tasian, G.E., et al. Pubic hair grooming injuries presenting to U.S. emergency departments. *Urology* 2012; 80: 1187–1191.

Butler, S.M., Smith, N.K., Collazo, E., Caltabiano, L., Herbenick, D. Pubic hair preferences, reasons for removal, and associated genital symptoms: Comparisons between men and women. *J Sex Med* 2014.

Chapter 14: Moisturizers, Barriers, and Bath Products

dermnetnz.org/topics/emollients-and-moisturisers, accessed 4 Nov 2018.

van Zuuren, E.J., Fedodorowicz, Z., Christensen, R., Lavrijsen, A.P.M., Arents, B.W.M. Emollients and moisturizers for eczema. *Chrane Database of Systemic Reviews* 2017.

Strunk, T., Pupala, S., Hibbert, J., Doherty, D., Patole, S. Topical coconut oil in very preterm infants: An open-label randomised controlled trial. *Neonatology* 2-18; 113: 146–151.

Lodén, M. Effect of moisturizers on epidermal barrier function. *Clinics in Dermatology* 2012; 30: 286–296.

Chapters 15–16: The Truth About Toxic Shock Syndrome and Are There Toxins in Tampons and Pads?

Faich, G., Pearson, K., Fleming, D., Sobel, S., Anello, C. Toxic shock syndrome and the vaginal contraceptive sponge. *JAMA* 1986; 255: 216–218.

DeVries, A.S., Lesher, L., Schlievert, P.M., et al. Staphylococcal toxic shock syndrome 2000–2006: epidemiology, clinical features, and molecular characteristics. *PLOS ONE* 6(8): e22997.

Centers for Disease Control and Prevention. Summary of notifiable infectious diseases and conditions—United States, 2015. *MMWR Morb Mortal Wkly Rep* 2015; 64 (No. 53).

Vostral, S.L. Rely and toxic shock syndrome: A technological health crisis. *Yale Journal of Biology and Medicine* 2011; 84: 447–459.

Nonfoux, L., Chiaruzzi, M., Badiou, C., et al. Impact of currently marketed tampons and menstrual cups on *Staphylococcus aureus* growth and TSST-1 production in vitro. *Appl Environ. Microbiol* May 2018; 84: e00351–18.

DeVito, M.J., Schecter, A. Exposure assessment to dioxins from the use of tampons and diapers. *Environ Health Perspect* 2002; 110: 23–28.

Hickey, R.J., Abdo, Z., Zhou, X., et al. Effects of tampons and menses of the composition and diversity of vaginal microbial communities over time. *BJOG* 2013; 120: 695–706.

Tierno, P.M., Hanna, B.A. Propensity of tampons and barrier contraceptives to amplify *Staphylococcus aureus* toxic shock syndrome toxin-1. *Infec Dis Obstet Gynecol* 1994; 2: 140–145.

Chapter 17: Menstrual Hygiene

Wyatt, K.M., Dimmock, P.W., Walker, T.J., O'Brian, P.M.S. Determination of total menstrual blood loss. *Fertil Steril* 2001; 76: 125–131.

Woeller, K.E., Hochwalt, A.E. Safety assessment of sanitary pads with a polymeric foam absorbent core. *Regulatory Toxicology and Pharmacology* 2015; 73: 419–424.

Beksinska, M.E., Smit, J., Greener, R. Acceptability and performance of the menstrual cup in South Africa: A randomized crossover trial comparing the menstrual cup to tampons or sanitary pads. *J Women's Health* 2015; 24: 151–158.

Tan, D.A., Haththotuwa, R., Fraser, I.S. Cultural aspects and mythologies surrounding menstruation and abnormal uterine bleeding. *Best Pract Res Clin Obstet Gynaecol* 2017; 40: 121–133.

Chapters 18 and 19: Menopause and Treating GSM

Hawkins, S.M., Matzuk, M.M. Menstrual cycle: Basic biology. *Ann N Y Acad Sci.* 2008; 1135: 10–18.

Suh, D.D., Yang, C.C., Cao, Y., Garland, P.A., Maravilla, K.R. Magnetic resonance imagine anatomy of the female genitalia in premenopausal and postmenopausal women. *The Journal of Urology* 2003; 170, 138–144.

Management of symptomatic vulvovaginal atrophy: 2013 position statement of the North American Menopause Society. *Menopause* 2013; 20: 888–902.

Lindau, S.T., Dude, A., Gavrilova, N., Hoffman, J.N., Schumm, L.P., McClintock, M.A. Prevalence and correlates of vaginal estrogenization in postmenopausal women in the United States. *Menopause* 2017 24; 5, 536–545.

Leiblum, S., Bachmann, G., Kemmann, E., Colburn, D., Swartzman, L. The importance of sexual activity and hormones. *JAMA* 1983; 249: 2195–2198

Rahn, D.D., Carberry, C., Sanses, T.V., et al. Vaginal estrogen for genitourinary syndrome of menopause. A systemic review. *Obstet Gynecol* 2014; 124; 5: 1147–1156.

Hickey, M., Szabo, R.A., Hunter, M.S. Non-hormonal treatments for menopausal symptoms. *BMJ* 2017; 359

ACOG. Committee opinion no. 659 The use of vaginal estrogen in women with a history of estrogen-dependent cancer, March 2016.

Chapter 20: Cannabis

Di Blasio, A.M., Vignali, M., Gentilini, D. The endocannabinoid pathway and the female reproductive organs. *J Molec Edocrinol* 2013; 50, R1–9.

Klein, K., Hill, M.N., Chang, S.C.H., Hillard, C.J., Gorzalka, B.B. Circulating endocannabinoid concentrations and sexual arousal in women. *J Sex Med* 2012; 9: 1588–1601.

Beigi, R.H., Meyn, L.A., Moore, D.M., Krohn, M.A., Hillier, S.L. Vaginal yeast colonization in nonpregnant women: A longitudinal study. *Obstet Gynecol* 2004; 104: 926–30.

Blumstein, G.W., Parsa, A., Park, A., et al. Effect of delta-9-tetrahydrocannabinol on mouse resistance to systemic candida albicans infection. *PLOS ONE* 9(7): e103288.

Chapter 21: Contraception

Hormonal contraceptive eligibility for women at high risk of HIV. Guidance statement. Department of Reproductive Health and Research, World Health Organization.

Chassot, F., Negri, M.F.N., Svidzinski, A.E., et al. Can intrauterine contraceptive devices be a *Candida albicans* reservoir? *Contraception* 2008; 77: 355–359.

Brooks, J.P., Edwards, D.J., Blithe, D.L., et al. Effects of combined oral contraceptives, depot medroxyprogesterone acetate, and the levonorgestrel-releasing intrauterine system on the vaginal microbiome. *Contraception* 2017; 95: 405–413.

Bahamondes, M.V., Castro, S., Marchi, N.M., et al. Human vaginal histology in long-term users of the injectable contraceptive depo-medroxyprogesterone acetate. *Contraception* 2014; 90: 117–122.

Chapter 22: Antibiotics and Probiotics

Morovic, W., Hibberd, A.A., Zabel, B., Barrangou, R., Stahl, B. Genotyping by PCR and high-throughput sequencing of commercial probiotic products reveals composition biases. *Front Microbiol* 7: 1747. *Genome Medicine* 2016; 8: 52: 1–11.

Kristensen, N.B., Bryrup, T., Allin, K.H., Nielsen, T., Hansen, T.H., Pedersen, O. Alterations on fecal microbiota composition by probiotic supplementation in healthy adults: A systematic review of randomized controlled trials.

De Seta, F., Schmidt, M., Vu, B., Essmann, M., Larsen, B. Antifungal mechanisms supporting boric acid therapy of Candida vaginitis. *J Antimicrob Chemother* 2009; 63: 325–36.

Senok, A.C., Verstraelen, H., Temmerman, M., Botta, G.A. Probiotics for the treatment of bacterial vaginosis. *Cochrane Database of Systematic Reviews* 2009, Issue 4.

Chapter 23: Cosmetic Procedures, Injections, and "Rejuvenation"

Yang, C.C., Cold, C.J., Yilmaz, U., Maravilla, K.R. Sexually responsive vascular tissue of the vulva. *BJU International* 2005; 97: 766–772.

ACOG. Committee opinion no. 686 Breast and labial surgery in adolescents. *Obstet Gynecol* 2017; 129: e17–19.

Crouch, N.S., Deans, R., Michala, L., Liao, L-M., Creighton, S.M. Clinical characteristics of well women seeking labial reduction surgery: A prospective study. *BJOG* 2011; 118: 1507–1510.

Fractional laser treatment of vulvovaginal atrophy and U.S. food and drug administration clearance. Position Statement. May 2016.

Chapter 24: General STI Information

2018 CDC STI Conference cdc.gov/nchhstp/newsroom/2018/2018–std-prevention-conference.html, accessed 10 Nov 2018.

Lewis, F.M., Bernstein, K.T., Aral, S.O. Vaginal microbiome and its relationship to behavior, sexual health, and sexually transmitted diseases. *Obstet Gynecol* 2017; 129: 643–654.

Gorgos, L.M., Marrazzo, J.M. Sexually transmitted infections among women who have sex with women. *CID* 2011; 53(Suppl 3): S84–S91.

Carey, K.B., Senn, T.E., Walsh, J.L., Scott-Sheldon, L.A., Carey, M.P. Alcohol use predicts number of sexual partners for female but not male STI clinic patients. *AIDS Behav* 2016; 20: 52–29.

Chapter 25: STI Prevention

ACOG. Committee opinion no. 595 Preexposure prophylaxis for the prevention of immunodeficiency virus. *Obstet Gynecol* 2014; 123: 1133–6.

AAP Committee on Infectious Diseases and AAP Committee on Fetus and Newborn. Elimination of perinatal hepatitis B: Providing the first vaccine dose within 24 hours of birth. *Pediatrics.* 2017; 140(3): e20171870

Holmes, K.K., Levine, R., Weaver, M. Effectiveness of condoms in preventing sexually transmitted infections. *Bulletin of World Health Organization* 2004; 82: 454–464.

ACOG. Committee opinion no. 704 Human papillomavirus vaccination. *Obstet Gynecol* 2017; 129: e173–8.

Chapter 26: The Human Papilloma Virus (HPV)

ICO. Human Papillomavirus and Related Diseases Report 2017.

Castellsagué, X. Natural history and epidemiology of HPV infection and cervical cancer. *Gynecol Oncol* 2008; 110(3 Suppl 2): S4–7.

Ho, G.Y., Bierman, R., Beardsley, L., Chang, C.J., Burk, R.D. Natural history of cervicovaginal papillomavirus infection in young women. *NEJM* 1998 Feb 12; 338: 423–8.

Park, I.U., Introcaso, C., Dunne, E.F. Human papillomavirus and genital warts: A review of the evidence for the 2015 Centers for Disease Control and Prevention sexually transmitted diseases treatment guidelines. *Clin Infect Dis.* 2015 Dec 15; 61 Suppl 8: S849–55.

Chapter 27: Herpes

Feltner, C., Grodensky, C., Ebel, C., et al. Serologic screening for genital herpes: An updated evidence report and systematic review for the US Preventative Services Task Force. *JAMA* 2016; 316: 2531–2543.

Langenberg, A.G.M., Corey, L., Ashley, R.L., Leong, W.P., Straus, S.E. A prospective study of new infections with herpes simplex virus type 1 and type 2. *NEJM* 1999; 341: 1432–1438.

Corey, L., Wald, A., Patel, R., et al. Once-daily valacyclovir to reduce the risk of transmission of genital herpes. *NEJM* 2004; 350: 11–20.

Johnston, C., Corey, L. Current concepts for genital herpes simplex virus infection diagnostics and pathogenesis of genital tract shedding. *Clin Microbiol Rev* 2016; 29: 149–161.

Chapter 28: Gonorrhea and Chlamydia

2015 CDC Guidelines.

Blank, S., Daskalakis, D. *Neisseria gonorrhoeae*—Rising infection rates, dwindling treatment options. *NEJM* 2018; 379: 1795–1797.

CDC gonorrhea fact sheet cdc.gov/std/gonorrhea/stdfact-gonorrhea-detailed.htm, accessed 10 Nov 2018.

Geisler, W.M. Duration of untreated, uncomplicated *Chlamydia trachomatis* genital infection and factors associated with chlamydia resolution: A review of human studies. *JID* 2010; 201(Suppl2): S104–S113.

Chapter 29: Trichomoniasis

Kissinger, P. Epidemiology and treatment of trichomonas. *Curr Infect Dis Rep.* 2015 June; 17(6): 484.

CDC 2015 STD Guidelines.

Bell, C., Hough, E., Smith, A., Greenie, L. Targeted screening for *Trichomonas vaginalis* in women, a pH-based approach. *International Journal of STD & AIDS* 2007; 18: 402–403.

Perieira-Neves, A., Benchimol, A. *Trichomonas vaginalis*: In vitro survival in swimming pool water samples. *Experimental Parasitology* 2008; 118: 438–441.

Chapter 28: Pubic Lice

CDC 2015 STD Guidelines.

Dholakia, S., Bucklet, J., Jeans, J.P., Pilai, A., Eagles, N., Dholakai, S. Pubic lice: An endangered species? *Sexually Transmitted Diseases* 2014 June; 41(6).

Izri, A., Chosidow, O. Efficacy of machine laundering to eradicate head lice: Recommendations to decontaminate washable clothes, linens, and fomites. *Clinical Infectious Diseases* 2006; 42: e9–10

Salavastru, C.M., Chosidow, O., Janier, M., Tiplica, G.S. European guideline for the management of pediculosis pubis. *JEADV* 2017; 31: 1425–1428.

Chapter 31: Yeast

Sobel, J. Vulvovaginal candidiasis. *Lancet* 2007; 369: 1961–1971.

Erdem, H. et al. Identification of yeasts in public hospital primary care patients with or without clinical vaginitis. *Aust N Z J Obstet Gynecol* 2003; 43: 312–316.

Ferris, D.G. et al. Over-the-counter antifungal drug misuse associated with patient-diagnosed candidiasis. *Obstet Gynecol* 2002; 99: 419–425

ACOG. Practice Bulletin, *Vaginitis Number* 72, May 2006.

Chapter 32: Bacterial Vaginosis

Kenyon, C.R., Osbak, K. Recent progress in understanding the epidemiology of bacterial vaginosis. *Curr Opin Obstet Gynecol* 2014; 26: 448–454.

Nassiodis, D., Linhares, I.M., Leger, W.J., Witki, S.S. Bacterial vaginosis: A critical analysis of current knowledge. *BJOG* 2017; 124: 61–69.

Bradshaw, C.S., Sobel, J.D. Current treatment of bacterial vaginosis-limitations and need for innovation. *J Infect Dis* 2016; 15; Suppl 1: S14–20.

Machado, A., Cerca, N. Influence of biofilm formation by *Gardnerella vaginalis* and other anaerobes on bacterial vaginosis. *J Infect Dis.* 2015; 15(212): 1856–61.

Chapter 33: Vulvodynia

Reed, B.D., Legocki, L.J., Plegue, M.A., et al. Factors associated with vulvodynia incidence. *Obstet Gynecol.* 2014 February; 123(201): 225–231.

Stockdale, C.K., Lawson, H.W. 2013 vulvodynia guideline update. *Low Genit Tract Dis* 2014 Apr; 18: 93–100.

Reed, B.D., Harlow, S.D., Legocki, L.J., Helmuth, M.E., et al. Oral contraceptive use and risk of vulvodynia: A population-based longitudinal study. *BJOG* 2013; 120: 1678–1684.

Andrews, J.C. Vulvodynia interventions—systematic review and evidence grading. *Obstet Gynecol Surv* 2011; 66: 299–315.

Chapter 34: Pelvic Floor Spasm and Vaginismus

Gyang, A., Hartman, M., Lamvu, G. Musculoskeletal causes of chronic pelvic pain: What a gynecologist should know. *Obstet Gynecol* 2013 Mar; 121(3): 645–50.

Crowley, T., Goldneier, D., Hiller, J. Diagnosing and managing vaginismus. *BMJ* 2009; 338: b2284.

Polackwich, A.S., Li, J., Shoskes, D.A. Patients with pelvic floor muscle spasm have a superior response to pelvic floor physical therapy at specialized centers. *J Urol* 2015 Oct; 194: 1002–6.

Holland, M.A., Joyce, J.S., Brennaman, L.M., Drobnis, E.Z., Starr, J.A., Foster, R.T. Intravaginal diazepam for the treatment of pelvic floor hypertonic disorder: A double-blind, randomized, placebo-controlled trial. *Female Pelvic Med Reconstr Surg* 2017.

Chapter 35 : Skin Conditions

Stockdale, C.K., Boardman, L. Diagnosis and treatment of vulvar dermatoses. *Obstet Gynecol* 2018; 131: 371–386.

Le Cleach, L., Chosidow, O. Lichen planus. *NEJM* 2012; 366: 723–732.

Vyas, A. Genital lichen sclerosus and its mimics. *Obstet Gynecol Clin N Am* 2017; 44: 389–406.

Ingram, J.R. Hidradenitis suppurative: Treatment. *UpToDate* 2018, accessed 16 Aug 2018.

Chapter 36: UTIs and Bladder Pain Syndrome

Chu, C.M., Lowder, J.L. Diagnosis and treatment of urinary tract infections across age groups. *Am J Obstet Gynecol* 2018.

Hooton, T.M. Uncomplicated urinary tract infection. *NEJM* 2012; 366: 1028–1037.

Nicolle, L.E. Uncomplicated urinary tract infection in adults including uncomplicated pyelonephritis. *Urol Clin N Am* 2008; 35: 1–12.

Little, P. Antibiotics or NSAIDs for uncomplicated urinary tract infections? *BMJ* 2017; 359: j5037.

Chapter 37: Pelvic Organ Prolapse

ACOG. Practice Bulletin no. 185 Pelvic Organ Prolapse November. *Obstet Gynecol*. 2017 June; 130: e234–e248.

Quality of life and sexual function 2 years after vaginal surgery for prolapse.

Pelvic organ prolapse and pessaries; acog.org/About-ACOG/ACOG-Departments/Patient-Safety-and-Quality-Improvement/How-I-Practice/Pelvic-Organ-Prolapse-and-Pessaries, accessed 28 Oct 2018.

Deng, M., Ding J., Ai, F., Zhu, L. Successful use of the Gellhorn pessary as a second-line pessary in women with advanced pelvic organ prolapse. *Menopause*. 2017 Nov; 24(11): 1277–1281.

Chapters 38–44: Symptoms Section

Cobos, G.A., Pomeranz, M.K. A general approach to the evaluation and the management of vulvar disorders. *Obstet Gynecol Clin N Am* 2017; 44: 321–327.

Clinical Practice Guideline. Vulvovaginitis: Screening for and management of trichomoniasis, vulvovaginal candidiasis, and bacterial vaginosis. *J Obstet Gynaecol Can* 2015; 37(3): 266–274.

Bohl, Y.G. Fissures, herpes simplex virus, and drug reactions. *Obstet Gynecol Clin N Am* 2017; 44: 431–443.

Allen-Davis et al. Assessment of vulvovaginal complaints: Accuracy of telephone triage and in-office diagnosis. *Obstet Gynecol* 2002; 99: 18–22.

Chibnall, R. Vulvar Pruritus and Lichen Simplex Chronicus. *Obstet Gynecol Clin North Am* 2017; 44: 379–388.

Subramanian, C., Nyirjesy, P., Sobel, J.D. Genital malodor in women: A modern reappraisal. *J Low Genit Tract Dis* 2012; 16: 49–55.

Alfhaily, F., Ewies, A.A. Managing women with post-coital bleeding: A prospective observational non-comparative study. *J Obstet Gynaecol* 2010; 30: 190–4.

Chapter 46: Internet Hygiene and Apps

Oliver, J.E., Wood, T. Medical conspiracy theories and health behaviors in the United States. *JAMA Internal Medicine* 201; 174: 817–818.

Marcon, A.R., Murdoch, B., Caulfield, T. Fake news portrayals of stem cells and stem cell research. *Regen Med* 2017; 12: 765–775.

Jolley, D., Douglas, K.M. The effects of anti-vaccine conspiracy theories on vaccination intentions. *PLOS ONE* 2–14; 9: e89177.

Pennycook, G., Cannon, T.D., Rand, D.G. Prior exposure increases perceived accuracy of fake news. *Journal of Experimental Psychology: General*: 2018.

Acknowledgments

THANK YOU TO Oliver and Victor, my amazing boys, who push me every day to be better. You bring me so much joy that I struggle to explain it. What amazing young men you have become. I know I was very busy writing this book, and you have been patient and kind and supportive. And tolerant of all the vagina and vulva pictures and articles lying around the house. But know that so many women and men are going to learn more because of you. After all, it was your health struggles that helped me see how hard it is for people to get quality medical information and how disempowering that can be. I vowed that when you were old enough and well enough, I would do my part to try to fix the information in my corner of the medical world.

To Cara Willems and Jennifer Schmitt—best friends are the family you choose. I love you both so much. You two have always believed in me. I have to stop there or I'll cry.

Tania Malik and Maya Creedman—you each read every word in this book several times, and I am eternally grateful. Your suggestions and questions were invaluable. You are amazing friends, gifted writers, and all-around fun people!

To Brian—I could not have started or finished this without your love and support. Although we are no longer together, I am a better person for having known you. I have never, ever had a lover and friend so firmly on Team Jen. I didn't know there were truly good men until I met you. You taught me that I should ask for no less than a partner who is tall enough to ride my ride. The world needs more Brians.

Jill Marr, my wonderful agent. Thank you for all your guidance and cheering! Lisa Clark, thank you for your amazing illustrations. They are breathtaking!

To all the amazing people at Kensington. Thank you. I know many of you worked so hard on this book. Special mention to Esi Sogah, thank you so much for sending me that letter that led to this book—snail mail for the win! You are a wonderful editor. You get me, and that means everything. I could not have birthed this beautiful book without you. You are my literary OB/GYN. Ann Pryor, thank you for keeping me on track! It's hard, but you are more than up to the task. And Kristine Mills—OMG, the cover! The cover!!! I love it so much. You are a genius.

Thank you to everyone who reads and shares my blog and columns, and to my extended social media family on Twitter, Facebook, and Instagram. Sharing my content means so much to me because *you* are helping me build a better medical internet. Many of you have made suggestions and also nudged me to be better in so many different ways and I really appreciate it.

And to every woman who has ever given me the privilege of being your doctor. Thank you.

Index